MEDICAL COSTS, MORAL CHOICES

Medical Costs, Moral Choices

A Philosophy of
Health Care Economics in
America

PAUL T. MENZEL

YALE UNIVERSITY PRESS
New Haven and London

Designed by James J. Johnson
and set in Zapf Book type by
P&M Typesetting, Inc., Waterbury, CT.
Printed in the United States of America by
Vail-Ballou Press, Binghamton, N.Y.

Library of Congress Cataloging in Publication Data

Menzel, Paul T., 1942–
  Medical costs, moral choices.

  Bibliography: p.
  Includes index.
  1. Medical care, Cost of—United States—Moral and
ethical aspects.   2. Medical care—United States—Cost
control.   I. Title.   [DNLM: 1. Ethics, Medical.   2. Cost
control. 3. Health policy—United States.   4. Health
services—Economics—United States. W 74 M551m]
RA410.53.M46   1983   338.4'33621'0973   83–3450
ISBN 0–300–02960–8

10 9 8 7 6 5 4 3 2 1

To my mother, Annemarie,
and in memory of my father, Theophil

Economists know the price of everything and the value of nothing.

—aphorism

[When countries are compared with one another,] the *share* of GNP ... devoted to medical care actually rises with income.... This is startling.... [It] is the pattern found for "luxury" goods such as foreign travel and fine wines, while exactly the opposite holds for "necessities" such as food.

—Joseph P. Newhouse, economist

Contents

Preface

At some point or other most of us have two very different reactions to contemporary health care. On the one hand we think that it is more important than anything else money can buy; we may even feel guilty or foolish if we find ourselves momentarily considering not using or providing it because of its price. On the other hand we are rankled by the incredible leverage over resources that the providers of medical care often appear to have. The doctor's income, the plush office, the elaborate hospital, the run-on list of astonishing cost items on a hospital bill can all cause us unease, even anger. When we don our societal hats and consider what we ought to do collectively to provide care for the poor, the same pair of reactions is present. It seems more urgent to make health care accessible to the poor than to provide perhaps anything other than food, but we wince at the irony of providing them their care in a typical, elaborate hospital, if perhaps they can't afford to fix the toilet when they get back home.

Until three years ago I had not realized what a host of fascinating moral issues amenable to careful, philosophical analysis were harbored in this pair of reactions. I had not thought of them, for example, as harboring a set of questions about social justice equally as important as the traditional debate about national health insurance and socialized medicine. I went to Washington, D.C., on sabbatical leave to size up the latter debate intellectually; however, my reading and discussion soon led me more and more into problems surrounding the issue of cost containment. The medical and health-policy journals were full of items ranging from passing comment on cost-effectiveness to sophisticated analysis of it. Little of that material, however, seemed to reflect any clear or justified methodology for thinking about the larger value judgment to which it all pointed: whether health care is *worth* the money it costs. I quickly became convinced that this was an area that could benefit from a philosopher's conceptual skills. The result is this book.

Being neither medically trained nor an economist, I need to be very clear about the limits of this study. I have had to work from an empirical background set by economists and medical and public-health scholars. I am not in a position to assess the competence of their writings in their own fields, though I hope I have gotten their claims straight and followed my nose sensibly in sniffing out their most significant materials. In relation to medicine, I hope I have never assumed that it is easy to assess the degree of a therapy's effectiveness. I assume only that sometimes it can be assessed; that even when we do not have the scientifically sound results of randomized clinical trials to work with, providers and scholars who are knowledgeable, critical, and experienced can often make educated guesses. The substance of few if any of my arguments is affected by this frequent lack of hard data. My significant conclusions do not have to do with whether this or that therapy finally is or is not costworthy; they are that we ought to follow certain conceptual paths and not others in trying to think our way through to a decision. In many cases the data necessary for a particular decision will have to be provided finally by someone else. I have tried to use statistics and empirical claims as examples to set a stage for discussion without resting my arguments on them or tying myself to dated information.

If the book is not scholarly social science or medical analysis, it also does not constitute careful, sustained work in philosophical ethics. Explicitly, it is applied normative ethics; I only hope that I have given intelligent consideration to the complex, general philosophical issues involved, which require more extended treatment elsewhere.

At many points it may seem that I naively adopt the narrowly individualistic notion of costworthiness espoused by the market economists—a notion so exclusively related to individuals' preferences about what to do with financial resources that it largely ignores broader notions of justice, social value, and intrinsic worth. Throughout the book, however, I try to connect that traditional notion of efficient use of one's money with those other values, which must be accounted for before we can conclude that some procedure is or is not costworthy in the largest sense. Thus I treat costworthiness as a much more elusive concept than many economists do. Sometimes, to be sure, I do not incorporate broader values into the final conclusion, but then it is generally with argument. And in any case, major parts of many chapters explicitly attempt to integrate the much less individual values of justice and fairness into the equation.

I present this book entirely in a spirit of exploration. At points I get quite daring in what I argue for—some will say foolish, or wrongheaded, or even dangerous. When I argue for such controversial claims it is because the more carefully I have tried to think out the arguments for and against them, the more I have become convinced of their merits despite my often contrary initial opinion. In any case, I put them forward in the hope that they will eventually propel us on to some productive and persuasive insights. Even when I seem to be defending a certain conclusion vigorously, I remain sensitive to my possible wrongheadedness.

Little of this book would have been feasible without the good graces of various institutions, colleagues, and friends. I can mention only some of them here. Very early on, Walter McClure opened my eyes to the problem of cost containment in medical care. Pacific Lutheran University granted me sabbatical leave for the 1979–80 academic year; I would like to thank the university for its unwavering support of research leaves despite these financially hard times. The Kennedy Institute of Ethics at Georgetown University generously provided me an office for an entire year; many of its faculty and staff, particularly LeRoy Walters and Robert Veatch, gave invaluable feedback and support. The Commonwealth Fund of New York City financially facilitated my subsequent writing back in Tacoma, as did Pacific Lutheran University through its Regency Advancement Award.

Parts of the draft manuscript were read and constructively criticized by various colleagues: Loren Lomasky in particular, as well as Baruch Brody, James Childress, Robert Coburn, Norman Dahl, John David Eatman, Benjamin Freedman, Gunnulf Myrbo, Norris Peterson, Jeffrey Reiman, Robert Veatch, and Albert Weale. I also benefited from making presentations of some of this material at the University of Washington, Reed College, and Pacific Lutheran University. A sharply abridged version of the first three chapters was published in *Hospital Progress* (January 1982); I learned much from the subsequent published exchange with Donald McCarthy and David Thomasma.

Dana Murphy extensively edited several early chapters, and Sally Serafim of Yale University Press was immensely helpful in editing the final manuscript. Marta Call was undaunted in typing various drafts of the manuscript; Debbie Florian in particular, as well as Kay Hirst, Ruth Jordan, Kathy Emge, Barbara Neeb, and Susan Trainer, provided much-needed help. Charles Bergman, Mary Bohn, and Susan Blank gave their own special moral support. At all stages of the review process Charles Grench of the Yale University Press accurately grasped what I was up to; no author could ask for a more understanding publisher.

CHAPTER ONE

Rising Costs: How Much Is Too Much?

1. THE ISSUE

At what point would a society be spending too much on health care? On care for whom, and on what kinds of care, might too much be spent? When are the benefits of additional care to patients, and to society, too few, or costs simply too great? Especially when we are dealing with "marginal" care—care with possible but statistically improbable benefits, and with still substantial costs—we look hard for a cut-off point. But how can anyone come to rational judgments on issues like these, and who should make them?

These questions underlie the current concern in many Western countries to halt the rise in health-care costs. In the United States, the containment of medical costs has virtually had to come into the public spotlight, given the facts. The costs of medical care have risen rapidly, not just in real dollar terms, but also as a proportion of gross national product—from less than 5 percent of GNP in 1950 to 10 percent at the present time. Put another way, per-capita annual expenditures on individual health care increased over ten times between 1950 and 1980. The cost of a day's stay in a hospital, which averaged $14 in 1950, had jumped to $133 in 1975, to over $200 in 1980, and to nearly $300 in 1982; in real dollar terms, it has more than doubled just since 1965.[1]

---

1. It is important to consider costs per unit of care, for example per hospital patient day, not just aggregate health-care expenditures. An increase in aggregate costs might be accounted for merely by population changes—for example, by the fact that the population is now older. In 1930 there were 12.1 workers for every retired person; today there are 6.1; in 2025 it is projected that there will only be 3.5. In 1970 5.4 percent of the population was over sixty-five; today 10.8 percent is. See Hellegers 1979.

In 1981 General Motors spent an average of $3,270 per employee on health insurance premiums (adding, incidentally, $370 to the cost of producing a car). Discounting for inflation, real per-capita expenditures on personal health care have more than quadrupled since 1950, and this general rise in costs has continued unabated through the 1982 recession. A substantial part of the growth in hospital costs has been an increase in the level and sophistication of care. It has included growth in "real inputs" such as staffing and technology. For example, the number of hospital employees per patient rose from 1.5 to 3.7 between 1960 and 1979.[2]

One final consequence is that today health care costs per capita in the U.S. are nearly three times those of Britain and over five times those of Japan.[3] Care is increasingly sophisticated, and it covers increasing numbers of detectable and treatable problems. We are getting further and further away from the day "when half...our ailments were cured by going to bed and the other half by getting up."[4]

We would undoubtedly be much less concerned by this rise in costs if we felt confident we were receiving as many benefits per real dollar now as we got thirty years ago. But in fact we are not confident. We wonder whether we are getting our *money's worth*—we wonder what proportion of present-day health care is still a "good buy."

Costs and Risks

Are the benefits, then, worth the costs we pay? This is the question at the heart of a comprehensive "cost-benefit analysis" of health care. Sometimes, however, the question highlighted by that term is not what the cost is in terms of money, a commodity which could be used just as easily for things other than health care, but rather the cost in terms of other health-related risks. This sort of calculation, more aptly termed "risk-benefit" analysis,[5] is importantly different from cost-benefit analysis in the full sense.

2. The figures cited in this paragraph are found in Greenburg 1979; Greenwald 1982; U.S. Health Care Financing Administration 1982; Hough and Misek 1980, pp. 162ff; and Russell 1979, pp. 1–2. Klarman (1979) estimates that of the 12.5 percent annual rise in hospital costs between 1966 and 1976, one-third was due to a higher level of care. Altman and Wallack (1979) claim that between 1967 and 1971 general inflation accounted for a 7.8 percent annual increase in hospital costs, and that better services and inefficiencies account for a 6.2 percent annual increase. Feldstein and Taylor (1977) claim that 75 percent of the increase in hospital costs between 1955 and 1975 was due to greater "real inputs." For an excellent general review of the extent that developments of new medical technology have driven up health-care costs, see Altman and Wallack 1979. For the viewpoint that many have actually saved money by alleviating the economic costs of sickness, see Mushkin 1979.

3. Godber 1976; Newhouse 1976a.

4. Irvine Page, in Bishop 1980.

5. Pauker and Kassirer 1975; Schwartz et al. 1973.

Suppose, for example, I have a sharp unexplained pain in the right lower quadrant of my abdomen. Suppose the diagnostic studies available imply that appendicitis is unlikely, but that still its probability is 10 percent. Should the doctor operate now, or wait and observe me? If I do have appendicitis, of course, it would be better to operate, but if I do not, the risks involved in any appendectomy mean it would be better not to. In this state of partial ignorance, we need to weigh the health-related risks of not operating against the benefits of not operating, and we need to compare that balance with the balance between the risk and benefits of operating. Then we would get a clearer idea of whether an appendectomy would be medically shrewd. (Some commentators, in fact, have concluded that the break-even point in this case—the point where the benefit-risk balance of operating is more favorable than it is for not operating—comes when there is only a 10 percent chance of my having appendicitis; with a greater than 10 percent chance I should have the appendectomy, with a less than 10 percent chance I should not.[6]) None of these considerations, however, focuses on the issue of *costworthiness:* Is the appendectomy worth the money it costs, even if it does have some health advantages over its alternative? Only this sort of issue is the concern of this book.

Efficiency, Medical Perfection, and Cost Containment

We wouldn't be much bothered philosophically if the failure to get our money's worth were simply an inefficiency—that is, if we could get more health or health care for the same money, or the same for less money. We might, of course, be angry. And economists, organizational analysts, and health-care providers might then spend some of their energies trying to offer equivalent health-care benefits at lower cost, or more benefits at the same cost. They might study, for example, whether hospitals could operate more efficiently with fewer beds.

The philosophically interesting problems occur when doubts about our money's worth arise not just about efficiency but about value: Is a particular instance of care, even when efficiently delivered, beneficial *enough* to warrant its cost?[7] This brings us to the crux of the philosophical problem of cost: What is cost*worthy* care? When life and health are at stake, how might we determine that a given sum of

6. Pauker and Kassirer 1975.

7. There are finer divisions than the three I have described (risk-benefit analysis, efficiency, and costworthiness). They include: (1) "Economic analysis" in the narrowest sense, that is, assessing whether a particular medical procedure results finally in fewer or more dollars being spent on health care. (2) "Efficiency" in the sense described in the text above, that is, "cost-effectiveness" in relation to a single set of health indicators. (3) "Risk-benefit analysis" in the sense described in the text above. (4) "Cost-effectiveness analysis," which considers varied and conflicting health indicators. For example, which

money spent on health care would give benefits of greater value were it used on things *other* than health care?

Obviously this is a question about value, and as such it raises the broader philosophical issues about how to go about assessing the value of anything. It also generates some rather unusual and intriguing philosophical puzzles of its own. But putting all that aside for the moment, we need to make completely clear that the focus of this book will be neither on the question of what health-care system is *medically the best* in terms of health produced, nor on the narrowly economic or strategically political question of *how to contain the costs* of health care. What one commentator says is sufficient to put aside the former question as less than ultimate: "Because of the law of diminishing marginal returns, the best conceivable medical care is a monster. It is no more desirable or affordable than the best conceivable defense system or . . . educational system."[8] What another says is sufficient to put aside the search for mere cost containment as shallow: "The statement that this nation cannot afford a particular program . . . reflects an implicit personal judgment of what is worth doing."[9] Quality health care and cost containment will at some points inevitably conflict, so cost containment per se is never an obviously justified goal.

The task of this book is, then, to explore the ideal of costworthy health care, not just the more limited goals of efficiency, cost containment, or quality health care, and to come to understand this ideal and its relationships to other moral ideals we have for our health-care system.

2. SOME CRITICAL VIEWPOINTS

If, at the outset, one looks for an explanation of the growth in medical costs, new technologies stand out as an obvious possibility. The

---

is more cost-effective, a $100 procedure that reduces the probability of the patient's being restricted to very light activities, or a $500 procedure for the same reduction in the probability of some pain and discomfort also? See Williams (1974) for one of the most detailed attempts to outline a model for such cost-effectiveness. (5) "Cost-benefit analysis" in the broadest sense, "efficiency" in the use of resources in the economist's broadest sense, or "costworthiness" judgments in my sense: Should the money spent on a given health-care service be spent on that or on something outside health care together? For major discussions of these distinctions see Cullis and West 1979, pp. 167–96; Klarman 1974; Roberts 1974; Stason and Weinstein 1977; and Cooper and Gaus 1979. For the most useful and comprehensive discussion of the ethical questions raised by cost-benefit analysis, see The Hastings Center 1980. For the most comprehensive discussion of cost-benefit and cost-effectiveness analysis in health care that I have seen, and for immensely helpful bibliographical information, see Warner and Luce 1982.

8. McClure 1978.

9. Klarman 1979. See also Pellegrino 1978; Joskow and Schwartz 1978.

much-talked-about CT scanner (computer tomography) might be an example. Yet many analysts think new technologies are only a symptom, not a cause. The real reason for the rising costs, they say, has more to do with the growth of health insurance, private and public. Hospital insurance, for example, has grown especially rapidly and, in one sense, has become surprisingly comprehensive. In 1950 annual hospital costs were $24 per U.S. resident, and $12 of that, or 49 percent, was reimbursed by insurance; in 1977 annual hospital costs were $297 per person, 94 percent of which was reimbursed by insurance. When we look at annual out-of-pocket hospital expenses, moreover, we see that they climbed from $12 per person in 1950 to only $17 per person in 1977. In real dollar terms, out-of-pocket hospital expenses have decreased significantly.[10]

Economist Louise Russell comments on this situation:

> Third party payment arises out of the philosophy that no one should have to forgo medical care that might save his life or preserve his health because he cannot afford to pay. As a means for putting this philosophy into practice, it has been thoroughly successful. . . .
>
> But the opposite side of the coin is that, because they pay little or nothing directly for hospital care, and because their own decisions about care have no perceptible effect on the insurance premiums and taxes they pay, people draw on resources as though they cost nothing. . . . When benefits do not have to be weighed against costs—when the only criterion is that there be *some* benefit—the number of good things that can be done in medical care is, for all practical purposes, unlimited.
>
> Freed of economic restraints . . . , the medical sector in general . . . has pulled in new resources almost as fast as it can separate them from other areas of the economy in order to provide all the care that might be of some benefit. The resulting flow of resources has been the primary component in rising expenditures.[11]

Russell thinks that her case studies—of intensive care units, intensive coronary care units, respiratory therapy, diagnostic radioisotopes, electroencephalographs, open-heart surgery, cobalt therapy, and renal dialysis—repeatedly demonstrate that "in the presence of extensive third party payment, investment in a technology will continue *until*

10. These figures were cited by former U.S. representative Al Ullman; see U.S. Senate, Committee on Finance 1979b, p. 322. This growth of insurance, of course, is only "comprehensive" or "complete" in one sense: in the relatively high proportion of aggregate hospital costs that insurance covers. It may still be the case that many individual people refrain from using beneficial hospital services for fear of incurring their costs because they have no or little insurance, and that some who are insured still face extremely burdensome expenditures for large hospital bills. Note that 4 percent of U.S. households pay over 25 percent of their income for health care; see McClure 1978.

11. Russell 1979, pp. 2–4.

the benefit from any further investment is zero" (emphasis added). As Cullis and West catchily put it, "the increasing role of third-party payments makes the additional treatment and care appear to be 'free lunch' for the patient, cooked by the physicians."[12]

If one doubts whether intensive care units, coronary bypass surgery, or renal dialysis can stand as examples of health services that are frequently used even when their benefits approach zero, another, more specific example illustrates Russell's general point more indisputably. To detect intestinal cancer, it has become common to perform a series of six inexpensive simple tests ("guaiacs") on a person's stool. The benefits of the first two tests are significant. However, when calculations are done for each of the last four tests to determine the costs of detecting a case of cancer (not even curing it), the costs are discovered to be $49,150, $469,534, $4,724,695, and $47,107,214 respectively. To some these calculations suggest that the routine should be reduced, say to a three-guaiac test.[13] In any case, surely the last two tests represent instances of procedures whose "benefits approach zero." A system accustomed to using third-party payment, however, will fail even to ask the question of whether those tests are worth the money they cost.

The Cycle of Costs and Insurance

No wonder, then, that health-care costs have escalated sharply. As costs rise, the need for additional financial protection grows; thus, people are exposed to greater financial risk from illness merely because of rising costs, even if they become no more, or no more frequently, ill. They then demand more insurance, and more actual insurance fuels further cost escalation. That, in turn, again raises people's financial risks from illness, and so forth. Cost escalation and insurance become natural allies. Any reduction in consumer demand for medical care that would be normally expected to occur as the price of care rises is offset by these forces. Since higher prices raise demands for more complete insurance, the cycle continues.

In fact, without external cost controls, the provision of insurance that is proportionally more complete may even end up being self-defeating. Since the cost of being treated for an illness has escalated, we may end up, despite our "better" insurance, having just as many out-of-pocket expenses for an illness. In fact, while the ratio of patient out-of-pocket expenses for hospital care to the total hospital bill

12. Cullis and West 1979, p. 254.
13. Neuhauser and Lewicki 1975.

dropped sharply in the 1960s, the ratio of total out-of-pocket expenses to total consumer income dropped only 0.01 percent.[14] These losses can wipe out the gains in financial protection that come from insurance *even when others provide us the insurance at their expense.* Witness, for example, the fact that the elderly today pay a higher percentage of their income for medical expenses than they did before Medicare.[15] In any case, even if the provision of more complete insurance is not in a strict sense self-defeating as protection from the out-of-pocket expenses of illness, it may still create an overall loss in welfare. One economist, Martin Feldstein, has estimated that lowering the average proportion of expenses borne by the patient from 50 percent to 33 percent actually lowers people's welfare.[16] The increased security and better care derived from the more comprehensive insurance coverage is more than offset by two sorts of losses that result from "better" insurance: Insurance that is more comprehensive naturally pushes prices up just by raising patient demand for services, and questionable, noncostworthy care is more frequently used—that, by definition, is a loss of welfare, for the money could be better spent elsewhere.

The pressure of insurance to draw more resources into health care beyond costworthy limits is even immune to most competition between insurers. Any increase in costworthy care must be absorbed by patients in the form of higher premiums. Suppose that patients are fully aware of this factor when they make decisions for care, and that they shop around for the most cost-constraining, "best-buy" insurers and the lowest premiums for a given level of benefits. *Individually, they will still gain nothing*—in fact they will usually lose something—*if they refrain from using this noncostworthy care, unless most others in their insurance pool also act in the same way.*[17] Unfortunately, it is very un-

---

14. Krizay and Wilson 1974, p. 95.

15. Senator Edward Kennedy cited this in congressional testimony. It is possible, of course, that the health care that the elderly are getting is sufficiently improved in quality and quantity to make their greater personal outlays a good buy for them. However, according to William R. Hutton, executive director of the National Council of Senior Citizens, the elderly today pay out of pocket twice as much of their income for medical care as they did before Medicare. Do they get twice the value from medical care now that they did in 1965? For Kennedy's and Hutton's testimony, see U.S. Senate, Committee on Finance 1979b, p. 505.

16. Feldstein, 1973.

17. Virtually the same point is made by Seidman (1979): "An appropriate analogy is restaurant bill splitting in a large group. All persons pay a share of an inflated total bill when everyone over-orders. Yet each person knows that if he orders less, but others continue to over-order, the total group bill ... will remain inflated. Thus everyone continues to order extravagantly."

likely that others will refrain from using such care; they, too, have little confidence that others will voluntarily refrain.

One Option: Compulsory Controls

By now we can see that this situation is most frustrating for those of us who both are concerned about costs and believe that some kind of more comprehensive insurance for presently un- or underinsured people is required. We see the tremendous value of protecting ourselves against the potentially devastating financial burdens of health care. But how, if then insured, can we correctly and accurately determine the real demand for—and value of—health care?

One option is to impose some kind of compulsory controls on the decisions of patients and providers. Here the classic "free-rider" argument for institutional control of individual choices applies. Consider another context. Residents who would benefit from street repair hold off contributing voluntarily to the repair, in the hope that others will get fed up first and carry it out without their assistance. Coercion of these would-be free-riders, i.e., a tax, is necessary to prevent them from unfairly gaining equal benefits without contributing an equal share.[18] Restraining noncostworthy health care is parallel. If everyone would forgo this kind of care they might be better off than they would if everyone used it. But, to prevent those who will not exercise restraint from taking a free ride on those who do, the restraint must be imposed. Mandatory denial of noncostworthy services is justified. The restrictions established by a prepaid practice, a health maintenance organization (HMO), or a sufficiently budget-strapped national health service may exemplify just such a justified denial of services. Though these institutions only rarely—and hesitantly—describe their practices in these terms,[19] the restrictions that they impose along these lines would seem to be as justified as the taxes that are imposed for roads or defense.[20]

18. For critical philosophical discussions of the principle of fairness that drives the free-rider argument for coercion, see Nozick 1974, pp. 90–95, and Simmons 1979.

19. Heysell (1979) writes: "I doubt seriously that the Kaiser people [Kaiser-Permanente, a West Coast health maintenance organization] think they are offering a product of lower quality!... In the Kaiser system, if a patient needs open-heart surgery or radiation therapy, expensive high technology care if you will, it is made available." I suspect, however, that prepaid plans do restrain somewhat the use of some less visible measures whose benefits are very small or speculative.

20. Here I slight a major problem, having to do with "coercive" denial of allegedly noncostworthy services, that arises in at least the national health service variety of such plans. It may be that some individuals have higher ceilings on noncostworthiness than those the plan operates with. They are willing to pay the insurance premiums for the additional care, but they cannot win the plan over to their standard and cannot afford the additional uninsured private care they might want.

How Much Should the Well Pay for the Ill?

But even after sorting through these considerations, and even after imposing some compulsory cost controls, the cost escalation problem isn't over. Suppose that individual patients (and their providers) are assured that others, too, will refrain from using noncostworthy care if they do. Patients will still have incentives to use such care. The total increased costs that result from this (and all other similar patients') use of care are spread among all the insured, both ill and well alike, not just among the ill. Suppose I am ill; suppose I can get all other patients to join me in refraining from the temptation to use marginally beneficial care, even though it does not cost me much at the time; and suppose I know right then how much extra I will have to pay in premiums because of any mutual lack on constraint among patients. I will still not have to pay more than a minor part of the costs of that care, for they are spread out among all the insured, not just among myself and other patients.[21] Thus, the ill have an incentive to take a partially free ride on the well, and costs continue to spiral upward.[22] Shouldn't the perspectives of *all those paying for the insurance*, not just *ill patients*, come into play in deciding what care it is costworthy to insure for, to encourage, and to use?

We have typically not taken this view. Instead, we have regarded assistance for the ill by the well as part of our obligation to help those struck by misfortune. Only the perspective of the patient, we have thought, needs to be considered, even if the costs generated by that patient are spread among the ill and well alike. But we have seen the odd and seemingly noncostworthy practices that are then generated. The people in a community that is arranging a health-care system for itself ought to be able to sign a mutual contract to minimize noncostworthy practices. As not-yet-ill people, *shouldn't they have the choice to sacrifice some of their future welfare as patients in order to stop the drain of resources into marginally beneficial health care?* Such a

21. The same point is made by Butler (1980): "The burden is spread over the population covered by the insurance...." Despite the increase in premiums, "the effect on the individual patient is negligible compared with the benefits he has received."

22. That incentive will evaporate well before the benefits of the care in question reach zero, for the well do not constitute a large enough proportion of the insurance pool to absorb most of the costs.

Some will take offense at my use of the term "free ride" here. I simply use the term descriptively, and I think accurately: The ill can choose to get the benefits of certain marginal or optional care without, even as a group, paying more than a fraction of its cost. Furthermore, before you think that the claim that the ill are taking a partial free ride on the well is unfair, remember another thing: Throughout this work the focus is on "marginal care" (with "marginal" benefits)—not on clearly lifesaving emergency care like, for example, surgery for a ruptured spleen.

choice will inject the perspective of the well, as well as that of the ill, into the heart of our determinations of when health care is worth the money it costs.

The Structural Incentives of the System

In the U.S. we have few mechanisms that impose any compulsory, mutual restraint on providers and the ill. We do not have a national health service with its budgetary ceiling, and HMOs and other prepaid group practices constitute only a small part of the delivery system.[23] Thus, built into our very delivery system are strong incentives for health-care providers to prescribe care and for patients to use it, even when its benefits approach zero. These incentives are not just occasional abberations, abuses, or accidents. Rarely are they counteracted by cost-containment forces. In the case of hospitals, the administrators' rewards lie not in being efficient or considerate of costworthiness issues; rather, growth of the hospital is related to its prestige in the eyes of area physicians who send it their patients. The practice of government and insurance companies of simply reimbursing hospitals at rates determined by their costs compounds the problem.[24] Physicians, too, are inclined by training to ignore the issue of whether care is costworthy. The advice of the American Medical Association to resident physicians in its guidebook on cost-effective care is "to learn to be efficient purchasing agents" in order to "assure affordable health care of the highest quality." Note that talking of "highest quality" care effectively avoids issues of costworthiness. A typical physicians' code of cost curtailment suggested by county medical societies mentions only considerations of efficiency: Avoiding unnecessary, or unnecessarily high-priced, care is emphasized, but any discussion of the conflict between cost and quality seems to be studiously avoided.[25] Indeed, if the interest of an individual insured patient lies in obtaining care whose benefits approach zero, the physicians' traditional professional ethic of loyalty to the patient seemingly obligates them *not* to consider costs when prescribing a particular service.[26] In fact, fewer than two-thirds

23. In the 1970s approximately 5 percent of the population used prepaid group plans or individual practice associations; see Krizay and Wilson 1974, p. 125, and Schwartz 1978. Even if these plans were to play a larger part, their internal limitations on costworthy care would probably still exceed those that their members would set by their values and preferences about the optimal health/non-health uses of money. For one thing, standards for the profession as a whole tend to be formed by the more prevalent, less cost-conscious practices of other non–prepaid-practice, fee-for-service physicians.

24. Pauly 1976; Enthoven 1979a.

25. Kridel and Winston 1978, pp. v and 35.

26. Butler 1980; Havighurst 1977.

of the house and attending physicians in one study had even a rough idea (within 20 percent) of the cost of a day in the cardiac care unit, and even fewer knew the approximate cost of other procedures.[27]

Furthermore, providers and patients are not the only groups motivated by the structure of the delivery system to use noncostworthy care. In addition, present tax policies furnish people with incentives to purchase noncostworthy insurance while they are still healthy. Employer-paid insurance premiums are entirely tax-free; they are not classified as income. Since most of these premiums represent forgone wages, the price to employees of additional health insurance is discounted by whatever tax on them they would have paid had they taken them as income. Individual purchases of insurance also provide personal tax deductions.[28]

Thus, significant use of noncostworthy care is built into the basic organization of our health-care delivery system. The main point here is that *we can predict, merely from noting the incentive structure of the system, that a significant amount of care whose benefits approach zero is being delivered.*

A Specific Estimate

Can we derive a more specific estimate of how much of our health care dollar is spent on such dubiously costworthy care? Arriving at a figure is very difficult. It first of all depends on empirical data about the statistical effectiveness of care, which is scarce. It also depends on a host of conceptual and moral complexities about how to put a monetary value on something that is related to an increased chance of living or maintaining health. It cannot, therefore, rest upon a simple, empirical judgment. To convince any skeptical readers who might suspect that the problem of costworthy care may be a philosophical chimera, however, we can attempt a quick estimate.

First we need to focus on the rather loose idea that "excess" health care is any service whose benefits "approach zero." We can begin with Russell's list of seven dubiously costworthy technologies. She gives a "conservative" estimate that intensive care units add 10 percent to a hospital's average cost per patient day. Suppose that half of this utilization of intensive care provides benefits that are only very marginal (she suspects that the situation is even worse). Then, on a total 1979 hospital bill of $80 billion, *$4.0 billion* a year can be consid-

---

27. This statistic is from Nagurney, Braham, and Reader 1979. It is corroborated by another study in which only one-third of medical students, medical faculty, and house staff were able to estimate charges for diagnostic tests within 25 percent of the actual fee; see Skipper et al. 1976.

28. Mitchell and Vogel 1975.

ered "excess."[29] Dubiously costworthy respiratory therapy, diagnostic radioisotopes, electroencephalography, and cobalt therapy involve excesses of *$995 million*. Open-heart surgeries for which benefits are dubious may absorb *$500 million*.[30] Renal dialysis absorbs *$450 million*, when we consider both the excessive use of dialysis centers, as compared with home care, and patients who gain very doubtful quality-of-life benefits.[31] Beyond Russell's seven technologies, we can add the CT scanner for another *$200 million*,[32] and unnecessary surgery for *$2.5 billion*.[33] The estimated savings in physician office-visit charges alone that would result from removing physician's financial incentives to use more and more technological procedures are *$6.5 billion;* savings from the elimination of excess clinical lab tests probably would amount to another *$4.0 billion*.[34] The total already comes to *$19.15 bil-*

29. Though I compute this figure from Russell's discussion, other sources can be cited. The study by Mather et al. (1976) about intensive coronary-care units is a classic. Griner (1972) adds support for the position that much of the use of intensive care is ineffective. For an excellent critical discussion of Mather, see Cochrane 1972, pp. 52–54.

30. These are estimated from Russell's discussion as follows: respiratory therapy, $325 million (half of a $650 million total); diagnostic radioisotopes, $500 million (half of a total in excess of $1 billion); electroencephalography, $70 million; cobalt therapy, $100 million. The $500 million in the case of open-heart surgery is one-quarter of a $2 billion total; see Randal 1982.

31. This is computed as follows: 10,000 of 50,000 patients who gain disputed benefits at $30,000 per year ($300 million), and 10,000 of the remaining 40,000 patients changed to home care at half the cost ($150 million). See Rettig (1979) and Rich (1980) for these figures, which are more precise than those that Russell provides.

32. This estimate comes not just from the cost of a scanner ($750,000) and estimates of how many duplicate, dispensable scanners there are in certain communities, but from the lower rates of scanner use in prepaid plans like Kaiser-Permanente in California. Willems et al. (1979) also consider the CT scanners' savings of things other than unneeded tests. I assume their estimate of a net annual 1976 cost for scanners of $300 million. If the number and use of scanners were cut in half, as the Kaiser-Permanente indicates it can be, the savings would be $150 million. Increase that to $200 million for 1979 dollars.

33. I am averaging two conservative estimates here. The much discussed estimate of the House Committee on Interstate and Foreign Commerce was $3.9 billion; see U.S. House of Representatives 1976, and Fineberg and Hiatt 1979. To be safe, I halve that figure, for $2 billion. Wennberg's noted study of different incidences of nine common surgical procedures in different areas of Vermont leads him to estimate a $3.8 billion saving nationwide resulting from the more conservative use of surgery whose benefits are dubious. See Wennberg 1977 and Gittelsohn and Wennberg 1977. Inflating Wennberg's estimate to $6.0 billion for 1979 dollars, and, to be conservative, taking half of that, yields $3.0 billion. I compromise, for present purposes, at $2.5 billion.

34. The former estimate is cited by Moloney and Rogers (1979) and Shroeder and Showstack (1979). The latter I compute from Fineberg's discussion (1979) of the 1977 total for clinical lab tests of $11 billion. One study he cites found that average lab test utilization of internists dropped 49 percent in a three-month period following a lab test audit in which they were simply informed how they compared with colleagues in the rate of lab tests per patient. Thirty percent of $11 billion is $3.3 billion, or, inflated to a 1979 value, $4.0 billion.

lion, over 10 percent of the 1979 medical-care budget in the U.S. This amount is clearly no pittance.[35]

Redistribution and Exploitation

We have not yet touched on one of the most interesting aspects of the growth of health-care costs: its redistributive character. Resources for non-health-care uses are drawn into health care, and "providers of medical care will be enriched at the expense of the rest of the population" as the medical-care sector expands its control over resources.[36] By itself, that development is perfectly unobjectionable—most transactions result in the same thing. But if noncostworthy choices are endemic to the basic organization of our health-care delivery system, then that organization *systematically* draws resources and dollars away from better uses. Most other uses are not provided with the same breaks, the same *structural* incentives. To set the limit of costworthy care very high is, of course, beneficial to health-care providers, and to all those who supply them necessary materials and services. This practice does not benefit most other people, however.

This redistributive aspect of the escalation of health-care costs suggests a possible exploitation of the poor. For one thing, claims that the society cannot afford to provide adequate insurance and care for the poor and near-poor because the total health-care burden assumed by the government is already excessive now begin to look like flimsy excuses. We should realize that, as one critic has put it, providing health care for those presently not covered "would look like a relatively cheap social program if it could be seen merely as taking medical care of small marginal utility from the more affluent and using the savings to give care of seemingly great marginal utility to the disadvantaged."[37]

For another thing, the dividing line between costworthy and non-

35. I have made this estimate without in any way depending on the claims of more radical critics about the pervasive impotence of medical care. Illich (1975) and Carlson (1975) are probably the most comprehensive and well-known of such critics. Their skepticism starts with the relatively undisputed contention that most of the improvement in health and the decline in death rates in Western Europe after 1800 was due to better nutrition and environmental sanitation, decrease in family size and birth rate, and specific preventive, rather than therapeutic, measures; see McKeown 1965, 1980. Studies of more recent expenditures for health care claim no evidence of greater aggregate health from increased spending. See Enthoven and Noll 1979; Fuchs 1979; Lembcke 1952; Wennberg 1977. Nagin (1978) notes that life insurance companies do not charge higher premiums for those who for religious reasons refuse all medical care. This then suggests that health insurance should more appropriately be called "sickness insurance"; see Somers and Somers 1977, p. 316.

36. Newhouse 1976b.

37. Havighurst 1977.

costworthy care, as that line influences the development of prevailing, available medical practice, is not likely to be drawn by the poor. If it were, they would probably set it at a relatively low point; many competing, nonmedical uses of dollars are just more urgent to the poor than they are to the better off. Now, if the earlier analysis is correct, the use of care that is noncostworthy to average middle-income Americans is not uncommon. But if such care is wasteful to middle-income people, as it is, it will be doubly wasteful to the poor. For the poor it will be "Cadillac care." Though Cadillacs may be better *cars*, the poor are very likely to find Chevies a better *buy*.

The poor are probably not sufficient in numbers or political power, either in government, insurance groups, or prepaid practices, to draw the line between costworthy and noncostworthy care where they would choose to set it by themselves. It is doubtful, for example, that in the entire U.S. there is a prepaid practice or HMO that reflects as low a ceiling on costworthiness, and therefore as low a premium, as the very poor would find to be a truly good buy. In Britain, the National Health Service limits its per-capita spending to only one-third the U.S. average.[38] To be sure, the quality of their care is undoubtedly lower than the average in the U.S., but it still seems respectable, certainly to most of the British. Would not Americans below the poverty line find a given $3 better spent by first spending $1 on that "British" level of health care and then $2 on non-health-care needs, instead of spending all of it on health care? They might even find it better than devoting $2 of the $3 to health care and $1 to other needs, which a restrained plan like Kaiser-Permanente probably represents.

Furthermore, suppose that some of this care becomes common practice—for example, perhaps, the use of hospital intensive care.[39] Suppose also that subsidizing *that* care for the poor is regarded by the society as meeting the poor's legitimate rights, and suppose that this view leads society to think it has thereby already accomplished a significant part of social justice. Then society may more easily ignore other allegedly just claims of the poor, such as for a general redistribution of income and wealth.

If all that is true, then surely the systematic, structural, and often noncostworthy attraction of excess resources into the health-care sector deserves some morally strong term of opprobrium. It constitutes a kind of "exploitation" in the name of the poor, or at least an ignoring of their overall, real needs. Remember, too, that this situation is made more suspect morally by the government's support of noncostworthy

38. Godber 1976; Newhouse 1976a.
39. Russell 1979, pp. 41–70.

insurance purchases through its provision of tax exemptions and deductions. The amount of that support which goes to middle- and upper-income citizens even exceeds the total of Medicaid funds for the poor.[40] Thus, in the final analysis, the organization of government support for health care seems hardly designed to serve the clientele for which it was originally established.

3. SOME CLAIMS TO EVALUATE

Admittedly this indictment of U.S. medicine may not represent the whole picture of how our health-care economy works. By arguing for it, however, we can examine which of its aspects hold up under scrutiny and which do not. It rests, to be sure, on a number of very disputable claims. This book's task will be to explore, and usually to defend, several of these moral and conceptual claims with much greater care.[41] They include the following.

The value of life, and the value of the kinds of health care that are sometimes necessary to preserve life, can be given a finite dollar price tag.

If, of course, the value of life cannot be given a dollar price tag, the value of health care and the lives it may save ought not to be compared with the value of other goods and services which the same money could buy. The notions of "costworthy" and "noncostworthy" care would then be meaningless in cases where care enhances longevity.

The monetary value of life, marginal care, and insurance for that care is lower for the poor than it is for the rich.

Admittedly, as an empirical matter, the poor do seem to draw a lower ceiling on the dollar value of life than do the rich. But does that mean that *in any morally relevant* sense the *value* of life, health care, or insurance is lower for them than it is for the rich? How can persons' wealth or income possibly affect the value of their very lives?

If insurance alters incentives so that a certain proportion of care is used by patients that otherwise, in the absence of this insurance, would not have been regarded by them as worth the money it costs, that care is not costworthy.

But insurance is designed precisely to make care affordable to people by spreading out its costs. Thus, the increased utilization of care stimulated by insurance may still be costworthy in the largest

40. Mitchell and Vogel 1975.
41. As a philosopher, I will seldom be drawn into debate about the empirical portion of these claims. I will, of course, have to cite certain empirical claims.

sense. Perhaps the value of the financial and medical security provided by insurance outweighs the waste it generates.

If a society subsidizes marginally effective care for the poor, the poor have a justifiable claim to get most of this subsidy in transferable form—cash—possibly to use for other things.

Without an extended defense of cash aid (income maintenance) over "in-kind" public assistance, however, this irritation of the poor has little moral weight. After all, others finance the care, and the poor may damage themselves with the freedom of cash. Then do the poor really have any complaint when others insure them for care which they, the poor, do not regard as costworthy?

An income tax deduction for health insurance indirectly benefits the rich more than the poor. It is therefore morally objectionable.

But if it is, are not *all* tax deductions and income exemptions other than those for business and occupational expenses—as distinct from tax credits—objectionable in a progressive income-tax system?

Continuing to expand rescue care without providing better prevention is yet another noncostworthy dimension of our health-care system. We can avoid more deaths and more suffering per dollar spent if we make use of currently neglected programs of preventive care than we can if we rely on our currently emphasized, more amply financed care for people who have already developed serious health impairments.

But doesn't rescue care still have a weightier moral claim on us than prevention does, despite its greater expense per benefit? The lives that medical care saves or improves are more easily identifiable, more concretely personal, and less a matter of statistics than those assisted by prevention.

The subsequent chapters will focus on these claims and the questions that revolve around them. Some other claims and questions that are less directly related to the critique presented in this chapter will also be discussed. In chapter 8, for example, we will look at questions of efficiency and justice that arise admist competing claims for scarce health-care resources by the young versus the old, the extremely ill versus the less sick, and the victims of rare versus more common diseases. In chapter 9 we will consider whether, morally, physicians' incomes are too high.

4. IDEALS FOR A HEALTH-CARE SYSTEM

In all this it will be important to discuss costworthy care within the total context of the other ideals we hold for an optimal health-care system. We do not want to disdain the important goal, for example, of adequate individual financial protection from the vagaries of accident and disease. Any respectable discussion of costworthy care must carefully take these other ideals into account. If care that is worth its cost in the broadest sense helps us meet these other goals, it may be much more expensive than care that is worth its cost only in a narrower sense. Our entire subsequent discussion will be infused with these other goals, though we will still focus most on the question of costworthiness.

Among the conditions we want in an ideal health-care system are the following. The difficulty arises when we try to meet all of them together.

The system would provide costworthy care, and costworthy care only. In its narrow sense, costworthy care can be formally defined without reference to the other ideals for health care: It is care which brings patients and other affected parties[42] benefits whose value[43] is at least as great as that which would be obtained by using the same money[44] to satisfy other needs and desires instead.

It would provide financial protection to individuals who need care. Choices about how comprehensive the financial protection should be will depend, finally, on a variety of other factors and value judgments, including those about what kinds of care are costworthy. Intuitively, however, it seems that what the very word "protection" calls most attention to are the largest, last-dollar, "catastrophic," albeit less frequent, expenses, not the more frequent, smaller, first-dollar ones. Protection, for example, from being thrown into bankruptcy or from

42. We should certainly include some other parties affected by the patient's care, e.g., family, dependents, or close friends, or in the case of immunization, e.g., others who avoid catching a disease because of the care I got. But I do not know exactly where or how to draw the line here. I certainly do not want to include *anyone* affected by the patient's care, for that would include, for example, health-care providers who might monetarily gain from a patient's otherwise noncostworthy care. See 2.6.

43. At this point in the discussion "value" is not restricted to what is measured ultimately by the patient's subjective preferences, even when they are corrected for inconsistency or ignorance. It includes as well the more externally derived and "objective" dimension that Scanlon (1975), e.g., terms "urgency" in contrast to mere subjective "preference." The term will be narrowed in chap. 4, where it will be argued that the morally relevant value to the patient should ultimately be determined by his or her individual, and possibly very idiosyncratic, preferences.

44. The full monetary price of the care. It includes not merely what the patient and the insurer together pay (that is, what the provider charges), but also any charitable or governmental subsidy of the provider (such as proceeds from hospital fund drives or the indirect subsidy that the government gives nonprofit hospitals when it allows them to raise capital by selling tax-free bonds).

spending more than 20 percent of one's income on necessary health care are thus among the plausible working standards for determining how well this condition has been met.[45] We are also inclined to include the degree of unpredictability rather than just the size of potential expenses in saying what "financial protection" connotes. It might be important to obtain protection against some smaller but unpredictable expenses first, before worrying about the more expensive but predictable ones.

It would make health care equitably accessible to all, assuring us that no one is denied timely access to costworthy and necessary health care because of any unwarranted geographical, social, financial, or other barrier.

It would equally distribute the costs of care between the ill and the well. The well would help pay a large portion of the costs of care of the ill, and those likely to remain well would share the actuarially higher insurance premiums of those more likely to become ill. Underlying this ideal is a more general principal of justice as equality: Any person's net welfare over a lifetime should be equal to any other individual's net lifetime welfare.[46] If, of course, a burdensome illness comes about through some equally beneficial or pleasurable but hazardous activity (e.g., smoking), then an ill person has not really been "disadvantaged" (that is, had his or her overall net welfare lowered). Thus such a person might not have a claim to assistance from the well.[47] More usually, however, illness seems to represent an act of fate which adds burdens that the well do not bear. Then the ill have a just

45. The U.S. has a long way to go to approach even such a moderate standard of financial protection as this. Four percent of U.S. households spend in excess of 25 percent of their income on health care and health insurance combined; see McClure 1978. Moreover, that figure does not include people who did not incur expenses for medical care that was in some sense needed but forgone because they decided they could not afford it.

46. This principle clearly demands not mere equality of benefits, health care, or income, but equality of *net* benefits. Thus if I accrue more burdens, say by hard work, it is not unjust or "unequal" that I receive more income. This principle also concerns total *results* over lifetimes; it is not fundamentally a matter of procedure, deontological rules, or rights. Such procedures, rules, and rights are not therefore less important; it is simply that they are derived from logically more fundamental principles of equality, autonomy, and welfare (utility) which I will subsequently expound (see 1.5). For detailed treatments of this sort of principle of equality, see Nagel 1979 and Ake 1975. For a slightly different conception of the relationship of rights to the three principles of welfare, autonomy, and equality, see Fried 1975.

47. For a detailed discussion of the claim that the well should not have to pay for the costs of illness contracted through a person's voluntary behavior, see Veatch 1980. See also Smurl 1980 and Macklin 1980.

claim against the well, at least to the extent of equally sharing the costs of illness.[48]

It would justly allocate the costs of care between the rich and the poor. Here again, the principle of justice as equality is the rationale.[49] If income and wealth are already justly distributed between the rich and the poor (for example, where greater income is a just reflection of greater burdens in one's work), both groups should equally bear the costs. If income and wealth are not already justly distributed, however, then the rich should pay whatever portion of the total costs will burden them no more than bearing the remainder of the costs will burden the poor.[50]

It would recognize and respect autonomy of patient choice. Informed consent to treatment would be required, and patients would be free to choose providers and types of insurance.

It would recognize and respect autonomy of provider choice. Pro-

---

48. Some doubt that fate ever creates such obligations. After all, if you are struck with illness through no act or oversight or inaction of mine, why should I be obligated to help you? Yet obligations of justice, as well as of benevolence, do get created in just that way. It begs the question against the principle of justice as equality to argue that *since* I have in no way created your misfortune, I am in no way obligated to help you.

49. It would be more defensible, but certainly more complex, if I stated this condition as the *fair* allocation of costs between rich and poor. That statement reflects the same principle of justice as equality, but outcomes are modified by the autonomous choices of actual disadvantaged persons. They may even choose to accept unjust inequalities for themselves if so doing raises their benefits or lowers their burdens. When I am on the short end of an inequality, and when I freely choose to accept it because I would even be worse off in a society without it, then the resulting inequality is *fair.* I, after all, would knowingly bargain for it. Fairness is the principle of justice as equality, as departed from by only the autonomous choices of actual worse-off persons. It is equality compromised by autonomy. See Appendix.

This concept is different from Rawls's notion of *justice* as fairness. My use reserves the term "justice" for a more exclusively egalitarian principle. Also, my modification of equality by autonomy to get "fairness" is not equivalent to Rawls's second principle of justice, which is generated by his hypothetical contractors. The main reasons for my dissatisfaction with Rawls's second principle are largely taken from Ake 1975. They also derive from the fact that in Rawls's model only hypothetical contractors, not actual persons, can choose to depart from a strictly egalitarian distribution. See the Appendix.

50. This position reflects the same ideal as the attempt to graduate income taxes so that tax losses to individuals with different incomes constitute equal burdens. I might have made a more radical statement of the ideal for the distribution of health-care costs between rich and poor: The rich should pay however high a portion of costs that still leaves their overall net benefits in life no greater than those of the poor. That ideal would often imply that all health-care costs for the poor should be borne by the rich. Instead, I choose the less radical version of the ideal because I am unsure that *health care* is the proper vehicle to bring about as much of a general justice of income and wealth as the more radical version seeks to do.

viders would not be forced to become providers, or to deliver care against their moral or medical judgment.

In such an ideal health-care system, cost containment would simply never be perceived as a problem. Even if aggregate costs were high, people would still be getting their money's worth. People would be insured for the care that was costworthy, and thus financially protected. They would have equitable access to health-care providers, and thus they could equally make use of the financial protection provided by insurance. The well and the ill, and the "likely well" and the "likely ill," would equally share tax expenses for health care, premiums for insurance, and the costs of actual care. Rich and poor would equitably share these costs also. Patients would have autonomy of choice about what care, providers, and insurance to use. Providers would never be forced to give care that contradicted their moral or medical judgment, or to become or remain providers when they did not want to.

Achieving all these conditions at once, of course, is a utopian ideal. In discussions of cost containment and the costworthiness of health care, however, we must not lose sight of this entire list of ideal conditions. If we compromise, it should be *between* these goals; we should not simply discard or disregard any of them. Costworthiness itself, in the largest sense, needs to take account of them all.

Readers may have noted the conspicuous absence in this list of any statement about a separate principle of the right to health care. That omission is fully deliberate. The notion of a right to health care is notoriously unclear. The first question we ask about it is, a right to *how much* health care?[51] It would seem preferable to generate whatever rights to health care people should be said to have out of the other ideals previously described. Conclusions about the justifications and scope of the right to health care will be made only in the course of relating these other ideals to the problem of costworthy care.

5. AN ETHICAL FRAMEWORK

Infused throughout this statement of ideal conditions for a health-care system is a philosophical view in ethics. While the present work is not a study in the theory of normative ethics, I still need to reveal

51. See especially Fried 1976, and also Bell 1979; Childress 1979; Daniels 1979; Veatch 1979b; and Lomasky 1981. Bell argues that "a right to health care can only be understood within the context of a ... program of funding ... whose limits are already circumscribed by ... scarcity." Veatch and Daniels, on the other hand, argue that part of what a right to health care means is that a society of a certain level of economic well-being is morally obligated to spend a certain amount on care for those who need it.

my philosophical colors. While it may often seem that I use no unified, coherent theory of ethics to drive the analysis and augmentation herein, no useful and coherent work of the scope of the present one can escape presupposing a philosophical position.

I have not worked out this philosophical position in ethics with any genuine rigor. Nevertheless, certain principles used throughout this work can be identified as a "position." It is first of all pluralistic: Not all principles emerge from one way of reasoning, and there is no *one* fundamental principle. Instead, three principles are assumed to be fundamental and independent: maximum human welfare, justice as distributional equality, and individual autonomy or consent.

Human "welfare" covers the same ground as "well-being," "utility," or "satisfaction." Welfare as a moral principle is teleological, aggregative, and maximizing: Other things being equal, we should try to do what results in the maximum aggregate welfare of all people affected by our action. People's welfare, in turn, is ultimately defined by their own individual preferences. Of course they can choose things that do not ultimately give them satisfaction, but, somewhere down the line, what ultimately constitutes that satisfaction is determined simply by what their words or behavior reveal to be their preferences.[52]

The principle of distributional equality has already been explicitly stated in the previous section: the equal lifetime net welfare of all individuals. It is also results-oriented, but, unlike the principle of welfare, it concerns relations between individuals. It matters not simply how much welfare is created, but to whom it accrues. The difference between any person's benefits and burdens in a lifetime should be equal to the difference between the benefits and burdens of other individual persons in theirs. All people should have equal lifetime net welfare. Yet, different as it is from the principle of welfare, the principle of equality is thoroughly and equally teleological: An action is favored if it is likely to *result* in less inequality of net welfare than the other available alternatives are.

Individual autonomy or consent is the one principle of the three that is not results-oriented. Prima facie, we ought to respect a person's freedom even when the exercise of freedom results in lower total welfare or unequal net benefits. This principle is also the more rigidly procedural and deontological of the three. It grounds many of our i

52. I am tempted to say "their *knowledgeable* preferences," for we wonder whe' even intrinsic preferences ultimately count if they are formed and expressed in i rance. But this is a complicated and two-sided issue. See chap. 2, n. 11 and ch; n. 17.

dividual rights and protects them even in instances when infringe-
ment upon one individual's rights would reduce the ultimate infringe-
ments upon others' similar rights.[53]

My supposition for this book is that no one of these three principles can be derived from the others. It is relatively easy to defend the
independence of the equality principle from the principle of welfare.
It may be more difficult to defend the independence of consent from
equality or welfare, although perhaps that can be done persuasively,
too. I also suppose that there is no further, more sophisticated, com-
bining principle that could effectively adjudicate the real conflicts
among these three, ground all of them, or somehow assume the role
of a more coherent and fundamental level of reasoning in ethics. It
would certainly be nice if there were—we would not be left with the
kinds of irresolvable conflicts that we may face in the present arrangement. John Rawls's theory of justice can be viewed as just this kind of
complex, superseding principle.[54] As dominant as his view has been
in discussions during the last decade, its role will nonetheless be rejected here (see Appendix).

Of course this kind of pluralism will seem philosophically unsatis-
fying. For one thing it means that at points in the arguments that en-
sue, fundamental moral conflicts will be noted, without any apology.
It is perfectly possible that these fundamental clashes of principle simply cannot be resolved. Even if they can be, an adequate framework to
resolve them has not yet appeared. Moreover, it is pleasantly surprising to see how many issues can be resolved by even this pluralistic
methodology.

6. PROSPECTUS

While this work is exploratory and its importance more the process of
discussion than its particular conclusions, it may be helpful to see
ahead to the package of claims to be defended. I will argue the
following:

Life does have a morally relevant monetary value, which is determined by properly understood "willingness to pay." This value varies
with the income or resources at a person's disposal; that variation represents the greater competing, non-health-care needs of the poor.

53. I have not analyzed or explained what "freedom," "consent," or "autonomy"
are. There are plenty of ambiguities. For one thing, we would want to know whether a
person is free if left to do what he or she wants, but wants completely ignorantly. See
the analogous problem for utility and welfare mentioned in n. 52.

54. Rawls 1971.

With the exception of maternal-child and possibly some emergency care, cash aid for the poor is preferable to in-kind health-care programs. Yet while for the poor less health care is costworthy than for the comparatively wealthy, it is even more important for the poor to be insured for whatever care *is* costworthy.

The present system of tax deduction and income exclusion for health-care expenses unjustly favors the rich, though this question is much more complicated than at first meets the eye. Plans that feature cost-containing, competitive vouchers face an almost impossible dilemma if they appeal both to diverse values about health care and to the ideal of equitable distribution and care between rich and poor, ill and well. A national health service, unlike competing prepaid plans, impinges on the autonomy of its clients.

In general, prevention is not as morally important as crisis treatment, but prevention of congenital defects is. The young ought to have some limited, highly qualified priority over the old in any competition for scarce health-care resources. The most ill patients ought not to be given automatic priority over any less but still seriously ill competitors. Those with rare diseases ought not to take second place to those with more common but equally severe diseases, just because the expense of their individual treatment is greater.

Finally, I will claim that while on average doctors' earnings are not as objectionably large as the public commonly perceives them to be, they are still unjustly high. Recognizing that life and lifesaving health care has a limited monetary value will help solidify a society's determination to keep those incomes in line.

CHAPTER TWO

Pricing Life

1. WILLINGNESS TO PAY

Does human life have a dollar value? Can full, real human *life*, not just some of its products, be given a monetary price? Is it morally obnoxious to think it can be? What amount, roughly, might such a value be? Is the amount the same for everyone? Ought we use these amounts to determine when a procedure that is possibly lifesaving is worth its cost, and when it is not?

In the last two decades, the two methods most frequently used by policy analysts to put a price on life have been "human capital" (or "livelihood saving") and "willingness-to-pay." With the human-capital method the value of life is assessed to be the amount of earnings and contributions that would be eliminated by a person's early death.[1] To most of us, that method seems obviously inadequate and crassly "materialistic." Isn't it clear that we do not view ourselves, or others, as mere receptacles of capital investment for future earnings? What does it matter to the real value of our lives if my future earnings add up to $500,000 and my sixty-four-year-old colleague's to only $30,000? People attach a monetary value to life out of considerations that are far more complex than simply assessing the value of their future earnings. To be sure, the human-capital method has a proper role, but what it assesses is limited to much less than any general monetary valuation of life. It may provide us with a floor for estimates of the monetary value of life, if empirical data for other models are difficult to obtain or interpret. Or, if we are calculating the contribution of

1. Cooper and Rice 1967, 1976.

health care to the growth of economic resources, or trying to compensate fairly the next of kin for the loss of earnings from a death, assessments of future earnings will be relevant.[2] But in other instances, human-capital assessments seem fundamentally, theoretically wrong as a method for pricing human life.[3]

The second method, willingness-to-pay, is much more promising. It simply focuses on the willingness of affected parties to pay to reduce the risk of death. For example, suppose ten of us are each willing—barely willing—to pay $10,000 to eliminate our individual one-in-ten risks of death. Suppose that the lifesaving program which we thus support is likely to save one of our lives. Each of us will then have placed an identical price of $100,000 on our individual lives. Note that this approach can equally well be called "willingness-to-sell": If for $10,000 more in salary, for example, I would be willing to take a job with a one-in-ten annual risk of death, then I am willing to sell my safety for $10,000; my valuation of my life would be $100,000.

This method seems to offer some immediate advantages that are germane to health-care settings. Since it respects the autonomy of the person who pays (or sells), it seems eminently consistent with the requirement that the informed consent of individual patients be obtained before they are treated. That requirement may even seem to demand the willingness-to-pay approach. For on the one hand, if people are willing to pay something to increase their chances of survival, shouldn't they be allowed to pay and reap the possible benefits of life? And on the other hand, if they are not willing, who would think of forcing them to undergo a treatment which, for them, has too steep a price?[4] Even if others are paying for their care, why should they be required to take that assistance in the form of health care when they would rather use the resources for their other needs?

2. Conley 1976; Conley, Cook, and Jones-Lee 1978; Cullis and West 1979, pp. 209–10.

3. My quick dismissal of the human-capital approach should not lead readers to think it has not been taken seriously in health policy. Since Schelling's (1968) and Mishan's (1971) definitive arguments against it, one gets the feeling it has been almost laughed at in most academic circles. It seems still to be taken seriously in some quarters, however. One cannot help but be struck, for example, by the detailed disease-by-disease empirical estimates in Cooper and Rice's 1976 update of the approach; their detail gets us far closer to specific policy implications than any willingness-to-pay estimates have yet done. Mushkin has also used the method and called it the "traditional" approach (1979, p. 160).

4. This is roughly Zeckhauser's articulation of Schelling's willingness-to-pay position, couched by Zeckhauser in a way that makes Schelling's point seem unobjectionable. See Zeckhauser 1975, and Schelling 1968.

Yet its initial attractiveness by itself hardly means that willingness-to-pay is any more correct or complete an approach than that of
human capital. It, too, suffers from significant possible flaws. Among
them are: (1) It dubiously transforms a willingness to pay to reduce a
risk to life into a valuation of *life*. (2) It transforms willingness to pay
money into a measure of the *value* of life. If money has no value without life, how can money be used to establish a limit to the value of
life? Let us put first things first, it will be said. (3) It generates value
out of people's irrational and inconsistent preferences, and it plays
largely on choices they would make in ignorance. (4) It apparently
generates different pricings of life for richer and poorer persons, yet
after all, when we are talking about life itself, how can any method
which generates such differentiations be morally justified?

    In the next two chapters I will try to show that willingness-to-pay
can be persuasively defended against these criticisms. The fourth criticism above is sufficiently crucial, and the response to it is sufficiently
involved, that I will devote the entire third chapter to it. Overall, my
defense of willingness-to-pay will end up addressing first the *conceptual* appropriateness of the model (what are the reasons for calling
what willingness-to-pay measures the "monetary value of life"—is
either "value" or "life" a correct description of what it measures?). Second, it will address the model's *moral* justification (does it give us information which morally we ought to use in deciding whether a procedure that is possibly lifesaving is worth its cost?).

2. FINITE MONETARY VALUE

It is first necessary to clarify how we derive distinctly finite monetary
values of life from willingness-to-pay. Such values are crucial to seeing
how willingness-to-pay is helpful in putting a costworthy cap on
health care costs.

    Initially it isn't obvious that the method generates finite monetary
values. What, for instance, would we be collectively willing to pay to
avoid the otherwise certain, entire extinction of the whole human
race? Wouldn't it be everything that could be paid, without limit? Suppose we saved something. *Save it for what?* Unless the situation were
one of extortion, in which some kind of moral honor demanded that
we pay less than everything we could, merely posing the question
seems to turn any species of financial conservatism into folly. Isn't the
proper conclusion, then, that human life has neither an estimable dollar "price" nor even a rough approximation of it? And, since life is a
prerequisite to the value of money, and since without life we can't buy

anything with money, we wouldn't exchange life for any amount of money. Thus life has no finite monetary value. What good does it do me if I save a million dollars but die in the process because I was miserly on health care?

But even in contexts of certain and immediate death these questions can be approached differently. We can get some finite prices for answers. Suppose, for example, that I know that unless I pay $1 million for lifesaving care, my death will be certain and almost immediate. If I pay, however, I will probably live another healthy year. And suppose that I have just about that kind of money available to spend. I, for one, would still almost certainly choose to die; for one thing, I would rather have something to leave my heirs. There is another, more direct and startling, way for me to express this preference, and, if I do not have $1 million to spend, it is a much more appropriate way: I would *sell* my last year of life, and a good one at that, for something less than $1 million.[5] At least for most people, the selling price would be finite.[6]

Reducing Risk

But suppose that many people are not willing to sell the last year of their lives for *any* amount of money. And in any case, the figures for those who are willing to sell are very high. At that point the willingness-to-pay model makes a crucial move. Even for these people, the model states, there are respects in which life still has a finite monetary price. The more common, realistic context in which we assess the value of life is deciding to pay in order to reduce the risk of death, not in order to assuredly avoid its certainty. But in this context we can see that the amount we would be willing to pay is very limited indeed. For example, one widely cited study of this kind of situation in the early 1970s found that on the average people were willing to pay only

5. Bayles (1978) raises the question in this form about selling. Here I assume that the selling form of the question is equivalent to the more standard form, what I will pay to buy myself out from under the threat of death. The two may not, however, be strictly equivalent. To some, selling a last year of life may seem to be very different than not spending to save or preserve it. 'Selling' may connote the fact that I am *unwilling to take what comes* (life's continuance); instead I am looking for an offer for my life. Not paying to save my life, by contrast, seems to be in this respect precisely the opposite—a matter of *being willing to take what comes*. If I see acceptance of a 'natural' course of events which leads to death (letting die, refusing to pay, taking what comes) as morally more acceptable than actively creating the course of events which leads to my death (killing, selling, not taking what comes), then I may be unwilling to sell for the amount I clearly say I am unwilling to pay. For analyses of the distinction between letting die (not saving) and killing, see Menzel 1979 and the essays in Steinbock 1979.

6. Weinstein, Shepard, and Pliskin 1976.

$56 each to reduce a 1-in-500 risk of death to zero.[7] The consequent price that each person was thereby putting on his or her own life was $28,000—that is, $56 × 500, the total amount in dollars that they were willing to pay reinflated by the inverse of that low probability of death that presumably deflated their actual response.

Now another question intrudes. What are we really measuring when we use this computation on an individual's "$56" response? Was the "$56" a deflation of that person's *full valuation of life* by the 1-in-500 improbability of death? Might the $56 response, instead, be simply and only a valuation of eliminating the 1-in-500 *risk* of death, rather than some fractional valuation of *life*?[8] The correctness of the $28,000 price-of-life computation becomes apparent *only* if we regard it as derived from the sum that a large group of people *together*, say one thousand, would be willing to pay to avoid two deaths among their number.[9] This group would be able to collect $56,000 to implement safety measures to save two lives, that is, $28,000 per life saved. Looking at the matter in this way slightly shifts our view of what it is strictly that we are computing. In a sense it is not the value of an individual's life to him or her at all; it is *the aggregate of all the community members individual valuations of their separate reductions in risk of death, averaged out to an only theoretically individual life value.* We come face to face with one of our gravest doubts: Is what we are computing in this model still a value of *life*, or does willingness to pay now express only a valuation of reducing the *risk* of death? This is crucial, for after all, what bothers us so much in most health care contexts is that we vividly see the life that might be lost, not just the risks that are taken, if we forgo a procedure.

To be sure the matter is tricky, but I still think it is life whose value is being measured. After all, two real lives are saved in the example cited above, and *that* is what the people are paying for. To be sure, they achieve this end indirectly, by paying a certain amount of money to reduce the risk of death. But the reason they are willing to pay anything at all is the risk of losing *life*. Consider a parallel case. Since I care about my house, I install smoke alarms and fireproof insulation to keep it from going up in flames if it should catch fire. Presumably, I am not merely placing value on a reduction in the risk of my house burning down; I am also demonstrating the value I place on the house itself. The latter is simply part and parcel of the former. Likewise, valuing reductions in risks to life cannot be separated from

7. Acton 1973.
8. Williams et al. 1976.
9. Rhoads 1978.

valuing life. If there is a difference in the computed dollar values of life in situations in which death is nearly certain, as distinct from those of low risk, it does not arise because one figure represents a monetary value of life while the other represents an appraisal of something else. Both are monetary valuations of life, although they are made from different perspectives.

Anxiety and Gambling

Two further doubts about the validity of transforming a willingness to pay to reduce risk into a valuation of life must be considered. One concerns anxiety, which undoubtedly inflates the prices of life obtained by willingness-to-pay. Maybe part of what we are willing to pay for is a reduction in our *anxiety* about death rather than the avoidance of death itself.[10] What then are we measuring with the willingness-to-pay approach—the value people place on life or the value they place on life absent so much anxiety about death? Our desire to reduce anxiety inflates what we would otherwise be willing to pay.[11]

Another factor, however, probably works in the opposite direction, deflating the valuations of life we may derive from willingness-to-pay responses: For most of us a degree of gambling "instinct" lowers our willingness to pay. Wouldn't we be willing to pay more to secure our lives were it not for our love of gambling? The real value we put on life, then, is higher than what our willingness to pay would indicate. The best evidence for this interpretation is simply that after any gamble they take, those for whom gambling is significantly attractive express just as much relief that they are still alive as others do.[12] They

10. We still must preserve a distinction between "valuing" and "liking." For example, if one morning I say I like orange juice and the next morning, in the very same situation, I say of qualitatively identical orange juice that I dislike it, I am expressing only likes or desires, not values. Values require a further element of consistency; see Hare 1952, 1963. But this type of consistency does characterize our monetary valuation of life—in *all similar* (similar-risk) situations, I may express roughly the same monetary value of life.

11. Schelling 1968. He illustrates his belief that this anxiety has a definite disvalue with an interesting example: "Let me conjecture that if one among forty men had been mistakenly injected with a substance that would kill him at the end of five years, and the forty were known to the doctor who did not know which among them had the fatal injection, and if the men did not know it yet, the doctor would do more harm by telling them what he had done. . . ." Schelling may be mistaken to imply the rightness of what seems to be paternalistic action here, but he is undoubtedly right about the disvalue of the anxiety.

12. Maybe we should not even try to filter anxiety of death out from death itself. We are as interested in the disvalue of the dying process for patients as we are in what is actually only one part of that process, the final absence of life. The same might be said for the gambling factor, though not filtering this out seems to me more questionable than not filtering out anxiety about death.

evidence as much gratitude for life as more risk-averse people do. The enjoyment that they take in a risky activity does not seem to reflect any deflation of the value of their own lives. It is merely enjoyment of the suspense of gambling or whatever activity they are engaged in. They want to gamble, yet even then they would prefer not to risk their lives if somehow they could get the same enjoyment without the risk. They may want, say, simply to climb mountains; they would prefer to do that without risking their lives if they could. They do not want to die, nor do they want to live any less than nongamblers.

Perhaps it is then reasonable to view this deflation effect of gambling and the inflation effect of anxiety about death as canceling each other out. At any rate, it seems reasonable to view the finite monetary values that willingness-to-pay generates in low-risk situations as in great part genuine pricings of life.

3. ARE OUR PREFERENCES IRRATIONAL?

In this way we have solved one problem: The relatively modest dollar prices generated by the willingness-to-pay approach are monetary values of life, not merely values of avoiding risk. But we have thereby created another problem—possible inconsistency and irrationality among those values. If people do price life lower in situations of mere risk than they do when faced with certain death which they can assuredly avoid, but if in either case they are valuing the same thing, *life*, then aren't they simply being inconsistent? Furthermore, it will be said, the responses that in low-risk situations generate modest prices of life are made out of psychological ignorance, when harms seem remote or unreal. Thus, either the entire model denigrates human dignity because it is built on irrationality and ignorance, or, if we should discard low-risk responses and consider only those responses made in cases of near certainty of death, we end up back with the very high, perhaps infinite, prices of life that argue for placing virtually no cost ceiling on lifesaving health care at all. We can't have it both ways.

This line of attack is wrong. Before I proceed with the argument to that effect, however, it is best if we have our facts straight. How much of an actual difference is there in values of life computed from low- and high-risk perspectives? While Mishan first emphasized the importance of this variation in 1971, empirical data are still sparse. Acton's responses indicated that, as risks get higher and more concretely and immediately related to the individual, willingness to pay for an assured reduction of a given risk rises; later, Jones-Lee got similar ɒ-

sults.[13] Both investigators utilized questionnaires, with all their attendant problems of sample size, interpretation, and the potential for self-
delusion among respondents.

Fortunately these same results can be verified intuitively.[14] Suppose that I am willing to pay roughly $50,000 to reduce to zero a 1-in-
2 chance of losing my last year of relatively healthy life, or, alternately,
that I would be unwilling to sell my last year of relatively healthy life
for less than $100,000. Considering these high-risk perspectives, the
monetary value of a relatively healthy year of my life exceeds $100,000.
But if this were all true, what would I be willing to pay per year for
fifteen or twenty years to reduce to zero a 1-in-5 chance of dying five
years earlier than otherwise I would? Very likely it would not be
$5,000, or anything close to it. Yet, that is what I would have to be will-
ing to pay to generate the same $100,000 value for a year of life. To get
that same value, it would also be necessary for me to pay $2,000 to
eliminate a 1-in-1,000 chance of dying twenty years prematurely. I am
surely not likely to be willing to pay that, either. Thus, my actual responses in the lower-risk situations generate valuations of a year of
my life that are considerably less than $100,000.[15] In fact, eventually
the risks would become sufficiently low that I would probably be willing to pay nothing to eliminate them. The computed value of life,
amazingly, would plummet to zero.

These intuitive conjectures are bolstered by other theoretical explanation. When my life is relatively unthreatened my assets are more
valuable to me than when I am near death. That is, I will not be willing to pay as many of those assets for a given reduction in risk.[16] (This
reveals, incidentally, that it is not necessarily the nonmonetary value
of life which drops as risks diminish; it is only the *monetary* value
which drops. That is, I am willing to pay fewer *dollars* for a given reduction in a risk to a thing which I nevertheless value just as much.)

13. Fromm 1968, pp. 172–74.

14. Jones-Lee 1974; 1976, pp. 93–99.

15. Throughout I am assuming that the valuation of a year of life is "quality-
adjusted." See Zeckhauser and Shepard (1976) for the notion of a "quality-adjusted life
year." Suppose an operation has probability $1 - x$ of being fatal. What value of x would
leave me indifferent between having and not having the operation? That is the quality-
adjusted-life-year level (from 0 to 1) for my particular impairment. In other words, when
I am indifferent about an operation with a one-third chance of restoring full function
and a two-thirds probability of killing me, a year of my present life is discounted to one-
third the quality of a fully functioning year.

16. Fuchs (1979) works from a similar observation: "A person facing almost certain
death would usually be willing to pay a great deal for even a small increase in the
chance of survival; that same person, facing a low probability of death, would not pay
nearly so much for the same increase.... This behavior is not necessarily irrational."

Thus, despite the shortage of empirical data, we are on perfectly safe ground in assuming that the prices of life computed from willingness-to-pay rise with the level of risk.[17]

Inconsistency

Yet I am claiming that these varying dollar figures are valuations of the same thing, life. How can we be consistent and yet value the same thing so differently?

Any inconsistency is merely apparent. If the value of life were something "objective," something "there" in life itself rather than something "subjective" reflecting ourselves as evaluators, we would have an inconsistency. But the value of life needn't be something objective, in that sense. At least its monetary value need not be, and that is all we need to see to get out of the problem. There is nothing at all contradictory in saying that the value of something evaluated by a subject in one situation differs from the value of the very same thing when it is evaluated by that same subject in another situation.[18] We are only saying that the value rests on something within the subject, rather than on something intrinsic to the thing itself. The fact that willingness-to-pay yields different monetary values for the same life in different situations thus indicates only that these pricings of life are subjective.

17. This point is made by Weinstein, Shepard, and Pliskin 1976. Viscusi (1978), how-ever, gives two theoretical arguments for precisely the opposite conclusion. (1) As the size of the risk to be reduced increases, people have already paid more to try to reduce part of that risk. Thus their extra payment for some additional reduction in the risk is made as much poorer persons. (2) Reducing, say, a 50 percent risk to a 40 percent one is less attractive than reducing a 20 percent risk to a 10 percent one. The assets with which the person pays have a higher value at 20 percent risk than at 50 percent. Thus the per-son is really richer at 20 percent risk and will be willing to pay more.

The first argument, while possibly correct, could merely lean away from an initially greater willingness to pay for a given reduction in high-risk situations. Though the ar-gument would be correct about marginal additional reductions in risk, there could still be more than proportionately greater total willingness to pay for safety as situations get riskier.

The second argument is simply mistaken. To be sure, the assets with which a per-son in the low-risk situation pays are worth more, but instead of just making that person wealthier, this means that a given dollar unit of assets is worth more and therefore harder to part with. In any case Viscusi's citation of Weinstein, Shepard, and Pliskin (1976) as supporting his view is mistaken; they seem to come to precisely the opposite conclusion.

To be sure, this entire issue is complex, a mixture of scanty and somewhat ambig-uous empirical data, of clear intuitions (but still intuitions), and of theoretical arguments that are not entirely clear. Nevertheless, I think it not too treacherous to assume that monetary valuations of life which are computed on the basis of willingness-to-pay rise as the level of risk increases. At least the majority of commentators think they do.

18. See n. 10.

Now in fact, who would ever have thought otherwise? The subjectivity of the monetary value of life is precisely one of the cornerstones of the willingness-to-pay approach. It cannot simply be argued that this point is exactly what reveals the wrongheadedness of the approach, for to say that would beg part of the question. Why should we have ever thought that the dollar value of life could be an "objective" value in the first place? If the bottom-line criticism that can be leveled against willingness-to-pay is that it fails to measure some "objective" value of life itself, the case against willingness-to-pay is weak indeed. The disparity between the values of life computed for situations where a person is subjected to risk, as opposed to those values computed for situations in which a person is faced with certainty of death, is no indication of inconsistency.

Ignorance

A vigorous criticism will still be made: Pricing life with the relatively low figure that we would be willing to pay in a low-risk situation simply stems from our ignorance. People come to a full realization of exactly what the life which they might lose is *really* worth only when death, as we say, stares them in the face:

> If a definite number of people are going to die, can it really make such a vast difference whether or not it is known who they are? . . . Their interest is to refuse every offer of compensation [for the imposition of a risk], but they do not know this. . . . If there is to be a death, we know at once that the cost, defined as the compensation required for the loss, is infinite [or very, very large]. Any other conclusion is a deliberate and unfair use of people's ignorance.[19]

Furthermore, specific contradictions seem to emerge from any premise that the price of life varies according to the degree of risk. For example, when tomorrow we will know just who in particular will be likely to die, but today we do not know that, why should life's real value be higher then than it is now?

This objection to placing limits on the worth of lifesaving programs by working from low-risk responses is echoed in concrete situations. If park commissioners refuse to take down diving boards even when each summer one child dies from using them, but they would agree to take them down if several died, haven't they so distanced themselves from human feeling that they should no longer be given our public trust?[20] Furthermore, if some business or government pro-

19. Broome 1978.
20. Hapgood 1980.

gram distributes the risk it imposes among a large enough group of people, the risk to each individual may become extremely low, so low that people will not be willing to pay *anything* to remove the small risk that remains, and then the lives lost as a result of the program will apparently have a monetary value of *zero*.[21] This might well happen in some cases of pollution. But surely any life actually lost must have some monetary value.

The willingness-to-pay model for valuing lives should simply bite the bullet here. *If it will be known tomorrow—but not today—exactly who will likely die, and if there is no way to know today what we will know tomorrow, and if there is still a need to make some decision to-day on reducing risk, then there really is a difference between the value of life assessed today and the value of life assessed tomorrow.* And this is not at all an unfair way to think about the effects of people's igno-rance. If we adopt a policy that imposes risks on people before they know about them, *and* if we create that situation by withholding infor-mation, then it certainly is unfair to say that the risks are justified be-cause people are not willing to pay what is necessary to reduce them. But this is hardly the typical situation in health-care settings. Further-more, park commissioners may indeed *be* justified in taking down the diving boards when several deaths are predictable, but not when only one is. It might be that the positive value of diving boards, as ex-pressed by people's knowledgeable willingness to pay to install them, is higher than the monetary value of one life computed in a low-risk situation, but lower than the monetary value of several lives.

Nonrational Preferences

Some critics will still dig in their heels and continue to charge irra-tionality. They might bring up the disturbing experiments by Milgram about psychic distance.[22] In these studies the suffering that one per-son was willing to inflict on another varied according to how imme-diately and vividly the person inflicting the harm was able to see or hear the victim suffer. To be sure, *this* variation in response is irra-tional. But why? Precisely because *the victim* does not evidence the same response variation. If the persons inflicting the harm had also been the victims, they presumably would not have shown the dis-tancing effect that Milgram documents. Thus, Milgram's respondents are irrational. At least they are *morally* irrational: They are not willing

21. Adams 1980.
22. Milgram 1973.

to impose their own behavior upon themselves. In precisely this respect, however, the variations in the value of life with level of risk that
are implied by willingness-to-pay are not at all irrational. They are expressed by people *for themselves,* imposed by people on themselves.

Saying any of this is not to deny that being unwilling to pay proportionately as much in low-risk situations is *non*rational. Any portion
of the variations in the pricings of life with the degree of risk that represent a failure to imagine the less likely sufferings and deaths in low-
risk contexts indeed is irrational. But clear this factor aside and we
still have a residuum of willingness to spend proportionately more per
life saved in high-risk situations. That this variation may be utterly
without a rational basis is no defect: What *ultimate* preferences are *not*
nonrational? We can hardly eliminate nonrational preferences from
moral relevance any more than we can do away with subjective
values.

We can say all this in favor of the willingness-to-pay model without saying that preferences have equal moral weight regardless of the
ignorance or irrationality behind them. Some economists, to be sure,
may make that further claim. They may argue at length that we should
never discount the moral relevance of preferences simply because
they are based on ignorance or irrationality.[23] They argue largely out
of respect for the autonomy of the person who expresses the particular preferences, as if autonomous choice always had the same moral
force regardless of the knowledgeability or rationality behind it. Indeed this is an arguable position.[24] But all that the willingness-to-pay
approach needs to maintain at this point is that the ignorance about
individual deaths which is entailed in low-risk situations is not a *re-
movable* ignorance, and that therefore preferences about using resources to reduce those risks are only *non*rational.

Even if there is no rational basis for variations in willingness to
pay according to perceived levels of risk, they are not irrational. They
do not present an undignifying picture of humankind. There is no reason to deny that they generate morally relevant differences in pricings
of life.

23. Mishan 1971.
24. This is a very basic issue in moral theory. It has not been adequately explored
in the philosophical literature. What are the subjective preferences that define morally
relevant "welfare" in a utilitarian framework? How rational or knowledgeable do autonomous choices have to be in order to count as autonomous, or how knowledgeable does
an autonomous choice have to be in order to be morally relevant? It is not clear to me
why we shouldn't somewhat discount a certain preference when it is formed in greater
ignorance than another, though perhaps we should not discard it.

4. MORAL FOUNDATIONS

So far I have argued two things: (1) The monetary value of life can be measured by the amount one is willing to pay to reduce the mere risk of death. (2) Nonrational variations in that value that have to do with the level of risk and the amount of its reduction do not undermine the moral significance of measuring it that way. But the underlying moral thrust behind willingness-to-pay pricings of life still needs to be developed. Why should we use such monetary values at all in deciding what kinds of care to develop, to provide, or to insure ourselves for? Even if the benefits of a certain kind of care statistically approach zero, maybe we should still insure ourselves for it.

Two Basic Reasons

Willingness-to-pay limits on care seem most relevant when the same person is not only the payer but also the person at risk, the care's predominant beneficiary, and the one using willingness-to-pay pricings to make decisions about it. The situation is then analogous to a market in which only seller and consumer are affected by a purchase. When that is the case, a strong argument can be made for allowing individuals to choose for themselves. The same reasons underlie the moral relevance of the entire willingness-to-pay approach to valuing lives. Basically, they are two: maximizing overall welfare and respecting individual autonomy.

People's knowledgeable preferences comprise the ultimate standard for determining what constitutes their welfare. Of course people can make choices which defeat their own interests. But assuming that they are knowledgeable about available alternatives, there is no *ultimate* test for what constitutes their welfare other than the preferences that at some point they actually voice or reveal by their behavior. If, for instance, people insist that eating at the local ice cream parlor creates greater well-being for them than spending the same $5 on nourishing ingredients to eat at home, and if they have tried eating both sorts of things and know their respective long-range effects, then eating at the parlor just does result in their greater welfare.[25] Analogously, the worth or "welfare" of life must ultimately be measured by human preferences. Willingness-to-pay works up from the same ground.

Willingness-to-pay also respects the autonomy of consumers. If one state of affairs is freely and knowledgeably chosen over another, that constitutes a moral reason of some significance for allowing it

25. For more detailed discussion of this matter, see 4.3.

rather than its competitors to obtain. Other things being equal, individual preferences ought to count. In our approach to pricing life, this principle is followed; people price their own lives.

With this underlying moral footing for the willingness-to-pay approach, no one has committed any "naturalistic fallacy." The model does not *sneak* from an empirical willingness to spend only so much to a moral conclusion that no more ought to be spent. Principles of maximizing welfare and respecting people's autonomy, openly acknowledged, are the moral underpinnings of the model.

Intrinsic Worth and Monetary Value

To be sure, it will be conceded, willingness-to-pay pricings of life then have *some* moral weight. But is there any connection between monetary values determined this way and what is allegedly more important, life's "intrinsic worth"?[26] How can willingness-to-pay pricings possibly get at the intrinsic worth of life? Perhaps this more elusive value underlies the belief that society should not give up on a person's life in order to save money, even a great deal of it. Why shouldn't that value dominate any monetary value which life may have? Doesn't this consideration then render our defense of a finite price of life largely impotent for a genuinely sophisticated, humanistic health policy?

To be sure, the intrinsic worth of life—of anything—cannot be represented by its monetary value. There is more than a grain of truth in the quip about economists: They "know the price of everything and the value of nothing."[27] Isn't this the reason to have policies that do not use pricings of life to limit what the society will pay to save lives? Those policies are adopted precisely to express the conviction—we are prone to say the "fact"—that not much of the worth and value of life can be expressed monetarily.

Defenders of pricing life on the basis of willingness to pay should simply grant that there is a distinction between monetary valuation and some other more elusive "intrinsic" worth. But even granting that, a health-care system that, in deciding what care to develop, provide, and cover, regards life as literally priceless still flouts the autonomy of patients and diminishes their welfare. I find it hard to conceive of what the argument would be for letting any nonmonetary, intrinsic worth of life trump this autonomy and well-being. The principles of freedom and welfare demand that we relate the use of medical resources to the rest of the economy.

26. Zeckhauser 1975.
27. Newhouse 1976a.

This is especially true when we are considering whether to cover one or another marginally beneficial kind of care in our health-care plans, rather than making life-and-death choices for identifiable people who already are in a hospital. Should people be prevented from binding themselves to a more restrained manner of care? In a hospital setting, of course, such cheaper models of care may not seem available. But that is because we are letting our sights be limited by the setting of that hospital and our society's accustomed level of care. Why shouldn't people band together to procure an admittedly medically less perfect health-care system for less money, if for some reason they think the savings are worth it? Health care is often a life-sustaining service, to be sure, but *why should it not be a service under our control?* Lacking a conception of pricing life to rein in health care before its benefit-to-cost ratio approaches Louise Russell's prophetic zero, we are simply rolling over in the face of a medical imperialism that has caused our thinking to become pervaded with the pernicious idea that we have no choice.

Of course, in some sense it still is crassly materialistic to give a monetary value to life. But it may also be materialistic to give one to friendship, love, ecstasy, or whatever else is not strictly or easily replaceable. Yet people surely do trade life, love, friendship, or ecstasy for other things that may be on or off that list. Consider the essence of monetary value, which lies in its convertibility (it signifies that a given amount of one thing can be freely traded for one, and not another, amount of another thing).[28] Doesn't life, too, have some usable, finite, monetary value? This conclusion follows conceptually from money's essence (convertibility), empirically from the fact that people do make trade-offs, and morally from the prima facie weight of the principles of autonomy and preference-based welfare that drive the use of willingness-to-pay.

Of course, even by using willingness-to-pay, a rough dollar figure for the monetary value of life is difficult to determine. It is difficult for us to discern what responses other people would make to willingness-to-pay dilemmas. It is even difficult for us to decide in our own cases what we are willing to pay. Moreover, we are not entirely clear, even theoretically, from what perspectives the appropriate expressions of such willingness are to be generated. To try to estimate the price of life may then appear to be a mess, both theoretically and practically. Thus, many will be tempted to discard the model. The complexity of the problem does indeed make it perfectly easy to understand why

28. Walzer 1973.

deliberate decisions to limit health-care expenditures within some ceiling for costworthy care come so reticently, so hard, and so seldom. The attractions of more complete insurance coverage are not the only roots of escalating expenditures. In the absence of any easily estimable dollar ceiling on the value of life, providers have understandably felt free to act as if there were hardly any ceiling at all. Into this vacuum the providers of expensive medical procedures whose benefits approach zero have moved, swiftly and effectively. But no matter how difficult it is to decide just where to draw the line on costworthiness, they should not be allowed to continue to hold center stage. Nothing short of people's autonomy and welfare are at stake.

Some Misleading Cases

Certain prominent cases in the public consciousness may have blinded us to this justified pricing even of individual lives. Despite the fact that Karen Quinlan, for example, was permanently comatose, questions about the cost of preserving her life did not seem to arise in the debate about whether to remove her respirator.[29] If her *comatose* life seemed priceless, how can conscious lives have any price? Perhaps, however, the absence of cost considerations in her case does not indicate that life has no price. This absence may stem from wariness about the dangerous precedent of starting to assign monetary values to *others'* lives in cases *where they cannot express their own preferences*. Furthermore, even an extremely conservative policy of rarely, if ever, acceding to competent patients' own refusals of lifesaving treatment can be justified by the need for extreme caution about the dangers that such an accession could create—subtle, unwitting coercion, and improper enticement of people to decide to end their lives. A conservative policy in this regard, however, need not rest on the belief that life has no monetary price. It can rest instead on a cautionary bias in favor of life when people cannot express their preferences, or on an awareness of the danger of coercing the preferences they do express. Both of these reasons are eminently consistent with

29. Blumstein (1976) has noted this absence. For those readers not familiar with the case, in 1975 at the age of ten Karen Ann Quinlan of Morris County, N.J., lapsed into what was believed by medical observers to be an irreversible coma. For many months thereafter she was aided by a respirator, thought to be essential to preserving her life. She was not brain dead—not quite. Her parents wanted to have the respirator removed, and nearly two years later the New Jersey Supreme Court upheld their right to do so. The respirator was then removed. Although undoubtedly she would have died had that been done much earlier, and although there is not the slightest evidence to reject the original and continuing judgment that her comatose state is irreversible, she is still alive at this writing. See Branson et al. 1976.

the freedom of choice which underlies the moral attractiveness of willingness-to-pay.

Another example in which we have experienced great discomfort
in attaching any finite monetary valuation to people's lives has been
renal dialysis. The government's assumption of the costs of dialysis is
usually thought to represent the belief that society should not give up
on lives just because it is very expensive to preserve them. But even
for such a policy, realism about how best to spend scarce resources
can be a determining factor. Rettig argues that in the debate about
funding dialysis "the reluctance to sacrifice even identifiable lives to
dollars was articulated not as an absolute value, but as one that bore
some relation to national wealth or affluence."[30] The impassioned 1972
speech of Senator Lawton Chiles of Florida in support of federally
funding dialysis can be cited as evidence: "In this country with so
much affluence, to think that there are people who will die this year
merely because we do not have enough of these machines and . . .
dollars . . . , while we are working out other improvements and everything else necessary."[31]

In the case of dialysis we are dealing with identifiable lives that
will certainly be lost without the procedure and will almost certainly
be extended with it. Probably the cost of dialysis in such situations of
high risk is not too high. We are likely to consider the monetary value
of life to be much more limited when risks are lower and benefits are
more marginal and less clear. Then pricing life comes more easily.
Take, for example, the American Cancer Society's recision of its recommendation for annual health examinations. The cost per case of
cancer thus detected was roughly $100,000, and in only one out of five
cases did the marginally earlier detection that resulted from yearly
check-ups enhance the effectiveness of treatment.[32] The consequent
$500,000 price tag for each life saved was simply too high. Economics
won.

But moral values did, too. Such a decision reflects no depravity or
callousness, but instead a deep respect for both the welfare and freedom of patients and consumers.

5. OTHERS' WILLINGNESS TO PAY

In a sense this concludes the main argument of the chapter: Life has
a morally relevant and finite price, determined roughly by willingness-

30. Rettig 1976.
31. Quoted by Rettig 1976.
32. Greenberg 1980b.

to-pay. Several important details, however, have yet to be discussed; they will occupy us in the next three sections.

If considerations of autonomy and welfare provide the moral foundation for using willingness-to-pay valuations of life, shouldn't we take into account not only the person's own willingness to pay, but also others'? My life may affect yours, and drastic damage to your welfare can result from my death. Isn't your freedom to spend resources to save my life also morally important? If my willingness to pay were the only consideration to be used in pricing my life, we would be left with the impression that no one else cared about my life, or that if someone else did, that that concern or lack of concern didn't matter. But some people do care, and that they do matters a great deal. If we fail to take others into account here, we are making the mistake of viewing individual lives as atomistically isolated. Society is morally obligated to avoid that error in constructing a model for pricing lives.

Yet the decision to count others' willingness to pay confronts us with distinct, new problems in obtaining and interpreting data. What *are* others willing to pay? It is even harder to find the data to answer this question than it was to get information on individuals' willingness to pay in their own cases. Theoretically, it seems clear that in both situations there is some willingness. People are willing to pay to reduce their own risks, and they are often prepared to increase their own risks to help reduce those of others. We must then interpret them as willing to pay to reduce others' risks.[33] Suppose, for example, that we know what risks people are willing to undergo in donating a kidney for transplant to save another person. Then, since we also know something about their willingness to pay to reduce their own risks, we can estimate their monetary valuation of another person's life. One analyst has thus estimated that the pricings of a person's life by his or her relatives add, on the average, nearly 50 percent to the original valuation; another estimates nearly a 90 percent addition.[34]

It is not *measurement* that raises the most serious problem with this component. Even if we can measure a certain dollar amount, should we *use* it in computing the monetary value of life? If we include the preferences of others in the computation, we are led to give more weight to someone who is loved and desired by others than to a person who is less loved or more reclusive. That weighting makes the procedure clearly disputable. Even worse, we would also have to consider the preferences of those who would feel *worse* if the person were saved. To say at this point that malevolent preferences should

33. Needleman 1976.
34. Jones-Lee 1976, p. 142.

simply be denied public recognition is merely an ad hoc reason for not counting them.[35] If, in order to arrive at a price of a life, we have to filter people's preferences through some sort of moral screen ("malevolence") to see whether people ought or ought not to have them, we will have lost the empirical footing of the willingness-to-pay approach. It is not only the distinctly negative preferences about a person's life that will be discarded; the role of others' positive preferences about a life will also be thrown into doubt—we could always wonder whether people should care *more*. Perhaps we would even have to consider using a moral screen on a person's own preferences; we would wonder whether people *should* be willing to pay more to secure their own lives than they are.

Furthermore, the issue discussed in the next chapter becomes far more problematic if we must consider the preferences of others, rather than just people's own preferences about themselves. That issue is how, after all, it can possibly be morally proper to count willingness to pay if it varies so much with income and wealth. In the next chapter I will argue that variations in willingness to pay that stem from income in people's preferences about themselves are a morally acceptable component in pricing their lives. But I will also argue that these variations are acceptable only if the poor can use the "savings" that accrue from their lower investment in risk reduction to meet their other needs. If we need to say the same thing about our preferences concerning other people's lives, to whom do the savings accrue? We sit here stumped—perhaps theoretically, and certainly practically.[36]

Apparently, then, we should not include others' willingness to pay as a factor in calculating the monetary value of a person's life. Or at least if we do, we should use some standard increment index instead of the particular preferences that vary with a person's popularity, interdependence, and the income of others.

6. IMPOSED RISKS

The welfare and autonomy of people in assuming risks about their lives are the moral grounds for using willingness to pay as a criterion for pricing life. But do those two principles still apply when the people whose lives are at stake haven't themselves chosen savings over safety? Voters' or representatives' decisions about funding coverage for

35. Rhoads (1978), however, claims this.

36. There is, by contrast, a practical solution for this point when we are dealing with preferences of persons about themselves: Give aid in the form of cash, not in-kind assistance. See chaps. 3 and 4.

other people come to mind. And we think particularly of defective newborns: May we put the same monetary limits on their care as the limits we derive from adults' willingness to pay only so much for a given reduction in risk? Shouldn't we use higher monetary values of life, or none at all, in delivering care for people who have *never* bargained for its restraint, and *never would*? This is one of the nastiest problems in seeing how usable the notion of pricing life can be.

Hypothetical Consent

We might argue that prices of life that have been gathered from our own choices to reduce risks to ourselves are much too low to be used in deciding what should be spent to reduce risks that we have imposed on others. For one thing, isn't our autonomy diminished when risks are imposed by others? At this point the standard reply of advocates of willingness-to-pay is to take note of what a person *would* spend to reduce risks *were he or she in control* and then transfer that over to the current imposed-risk situation. Yet in at least one respect, it is claimed, doing that does not meet the argument; a decision by *others* to let risks stand still does not constitute *that* person's autonomous choice. The *hypothetical* consent of actual persons to their own risks is morally insufficient; only real consent in real markets will do.[37]

But now the argument is losing ground. *Why* would I *not* want others to use what *I* would consent to as a basis for their decisions about my care? If they, not I, are the ones to keep the savings, then of course I would not want them to use the price to which I would choose to limit myself if I were the one to get the savings. But that is not the entire issue of whether we can use prices of life in deciding whether to leave others exposed to risk; it is the different and only occasionally associated issue of whether we can impose risks on others who will not share (or have not had a chance to share) in the benefits. Assume, however, that I *have* a chance of benefiting from letting risks stand. Why should I not want others to use, as a basis for their decisions, the prices that I would generate? *Won't they be respecting my free choices a lot more if they do use them? Won't they be ignoring my will if they don't?*

There are, nevertheless, some plausible reasons why I might not want them to. Though these reasons do not imply any generally higher spending to avoid imposed risks, and while in fact they leave the willingness-to-pay model entirely intact, they are important qualifications: If I don't actually do the consenting to let the risks stand in

37. Sagoff 1981.

order to save resources, I will lose out on the subjective satisfaction of incurring the risks myself. I may also fear that others will overestimate the risks I would consent to let stand. Both of these concerns, however, are limited. Surely the first is a marginal factor, and the appropriate response to the second is not to dispense with the model but simply to focus as accurately as possible on the prices that the people for whom we are making decisions actually do put on their lives in voluntary risk-reduction cases. If after that I am still suspicious that others will underestimate my price of my own life, why should we make more than a marginal adjustment in my voluntary pricing when we shift from voluntary to imposed risks? Our thinking fits squarely into willingness-to-pay pricing of life. Just as we will take account of higher pricings in high- as imposed to low-risk situations, so also we will have to take account of somewhat higher pricings in choices to reduce imposed as compared to voluntary risks.[38]

There is thus a legitimate difference between imposed and voluntary risks, but we can still use the willingness-to-pay model to deal with both. When others *would* consent to higher risks because of the cost of reducing them, the risks to them can be left standing as long as several conditions are met: *(a) if there is no way in which we can presently discern their actual consent; (b) if they share in the benefits of not spending more; (c) if we are already spending what they would knowledgeably consent to spend; and (d) if we have inflated that figure both for any real losses in satisfaction from not making the decision themselves and for the real danger of underestimates.*

Is this highly qualified conclusion still useful in actual health-care policy? Indeed it is—we can use willingness-to-pay pricings of life in setting limits on costworthy care even when people have not actually

38. How much higher? I am strongly inclined to refer only to specific factors—to the two factors mentioned earlier in this paragraph and any other specific ones we may come to perceive. We could, of course, grant that these factors are relevant but then use *whatever* higher pricings of their lives people espouse when they know that others will be using the prices to make decisions for them later. Why not proceed that way? Have I not already set a precedent for doing that by accepting at face value the actual differences in people's pricings of life in low- and high-risk circumstances? I do not think so. I suspect that some of the resentment people feel about others making decisions for them, and consequently some of their higher pricings of life for later imposed risk contexts, is not only non- but irrational. The argument for using whatever actual low-/high-risk pricing differences they happen to espouse was that nonrational preferences were completely unobjectionable as a base for judgments of welfare and expressions of autonomy. If, of course, people's voluntary/imposed risk pricing differences are likewise only nonrational, then we should gladly accept them and run our willingness-to-pay model from there. But if they are somewhat irrational, then to be consistent we can still discount them. In any case, in the attempt to limit what we spend to reduce risk we need not jump to some very different sort of consideration from willingness-to-pay. We are merely making adjustments within the model.

consented to them. If they, too, stand to benefit from having such limits, and if there is no feasible way to elicit their actual consent, and if we account for our possible underestimation of their own pricings of life, why shouldn't we set limits generated by their willingness to pay? Under these conditions many hospitals, research institutions, government programs, and insurance and private health plans may set limits.

People Who Never Benefit

We run into much nastier moral problems, however, in situations where patients have never *had* a chance of benefiting from the savings. We get back to the literally awful cases of some defective newborns, among others. The bothersome aspect of such cases is not so much that these people have not expressed their preferences, or currently cannot express them. Suppose they have not, and cannot; if we could judge what their preferences *would* be were they only able to form and express them, or if we could extrapolate hypothetical preferences from some predictable, later interest of theirs, we would have some reason for their sake to impose a definitely limited price of life on their care.

But in these cases we may not be able to do either of those things. An infant with multiple congenital problems already has serious limitations placed on its later life prospects; its welfare is hardly likely to be increased by saving resources for other things later in life. If, of course, its welfare were to be increased sufficiently through those savings, we should restrain care now in order to use the savings later. But seriously defective infants often seem to stand no chance of gaining from putting a ceiling on what is spent for care. When that is the case, there seems to be no sense in which their implied consent or welfare can ground pricing their lives. Don't we just have to admit that in such cases we can put no monetary price on life at all—that, for example, pricing of life cannot act as a moral anchor for cost limits in the design and operation of intensive-care units for newborns? Instead, the only possible legitimate ceilings would have to emerge from considerations that the individual infant itself would actually be better off not receiving additional treatment.

Our argument in these cases needs to proceed carefully, however. The case against pricing-life limits on the cost of care for newborns is not that closed. For one thing, our opinions here may be bent by essentially different cases of actively imposing risk on unconsenting people who don't sufficiently share in the benefits. If, for example, a small number of lung-cancer deaths are likely to result from coal generation of electric power, if the monetary value of these lives assessed by the willingness of exposed people to pay is outweighed by the aggregate economic value of more abundant electricity, and if the people exposed thereby to the risk—those downwind, say, from the air pollution—will never share in the benefits of the more abundant power, then, to be sure, these people will seem to have been unfairly used as means to the economic gain of others.[39] Why should I be free to pursue for my benefit a project which imposes risk of serious harm on you, who stand little chance of gaining anything from the project?

It may be that here it is only because the risk is imposed by action that we are as cautious as we are in limiting the right to expose others. Why, after all, should I have the right to adopt projects which *disrupt* your life like that? Note that our caution may properly diminish when we shift to a different case, my *not reducing* your risk because I have chosen *not to help* you. It is this latter sort of case that is represented by defective newborns. To place a ceiling on what we should spend for their care, we needn't defend a right to expose others actively to risks from which they will not gain. We need only to delimit the extent of our obligation to come to their aid.[40]

Articulating the limits of that obligation may take us far afield from the narrower domain of willingness-to-pay pricing of life. For defective newborns, then, that kind of life pricing may directly generate few important conclusions. Though we want to know in these cases, too, what legitimate ceiling we can place on the cost of care, it is not simply willingness-to-pay from which such moral limits seem to emerge. We could then still call whatever limit finally did emerge a "monetary value of life" if we wished, but it would be a very different sort of measure than the values that emerge from willingness-to-pay. In a sense, the term "monetary value of life" would not fit it well at all: We aren't making a valuation of others' *lives* when we recognize such a ceiling, only assessing the extent of our obligation to them. A *moral relationship*, not their lives, is being examined. Cost ceilings can still be set, perhaps, but not out of any willingness-to-pay pricings per se, nor out of any limits on the obligation not actively to endanger others; they will have to be set out of our obligation to *help* others in need, which is, significantly, more limited.

39. Von Magnus 1980.

40. Whether the obligation not to "impose" risks by failing to aid is weaker than the obligation not to impose risks by action will finally depend on whether the action/ omission distinction is morally relevant. I am inclined to argue that it is, though not nearly as straightforwardly as many of its defenders do. See Menzel 1979 and many essays in Steinbock 1979.

Suppose we do get to that issue explicitly. If we were in their shoes, what would we consent to? If we couldn't benefit from the savings, would we set limits? What limits would we set? Would we want to tie down our community with very, very large bills for our care? *If* I understood the problem, and *if* I knew what others could do with the savings, I am sure that at some point I would say "no" to more and more sophisticated care. Indeed, we are on much murkier ground here than we are in situations that are more amenable to willingness-to-pay assessment. Certainly we will have higher cost ceilings here. Yet that must not blind us to what limits there still may be.

Furthermore, it should not blind us to some very substantial but hidden benefits that may possibly come to patients from the savings. A risk may be imposed on people who would consent to a *general policy* of permission to impose that sort of risk on others. We prize our freedom to pursue individual projects enough that we will readily consent to a general policy that allows people to impose on others very small risks of serious harm and larger risks of nearly trivial harm.[41] That same reasoning may extend to even greater risks. In any case, we need to see the general point: People do not have to consent to or benefit from imposing the *particular* risk in question.

What can we see out of all this? For people who are dependent on us and on whom we are imposing some decision, I suspect we should insist that what we pay to reduce their risks ought not to be lower than *their* pricing of their own lives. But also, why should we ever pay *more* than the price that they themselves would put on their own lives if they had access to our resources? We still get back to willingness to pay.

7. PATIENT, OR BUYER OF INSURANCE?

There is another question outstanding. Suppose we are using willingness-to-pay to establish some kind of cost ceiling for proper care. We saw in 2.2 and 2.3 that the computed prices of life vary with the level

41. Within the framework of a Rawlsian hypothetical contract conclusions of this sort are developed by Coburn 1981. An elaborate theory of legitimate imposition of risks on others is also provided by Nozick 1974, chaps. 4 and 5. Nozick's theory revolves around concern for efficiency: The harm that might come about must be compensable, the person exposed to it must not fear the joint event of exposure and later compensation, the persons imposing the risk must gain enough so that they would be willing either to buy from the potential victim his or her right not to be exposed or to fund the later compensation, actual sale by the victims of their right not to be exposed must for some reason be impractical, etc. As Von Magnus points out (1982), the problem with this theory is that it rests on a presumption in favor of action, the active projects of the people imposing the risks.

of risk and the amount of risk we are paying to reduce. Given these variations, we will wonder: When we make decisions to cap the costs of health care, from what perspective should we assess the monetary value of life? Should we use a low-risk or a high-risk perspective? The answer could make a significant difference; a high-risk perspective may generate almost no cap at all, while a low-risk vantage point will impose sharp limits.

Two answers represent opposite extremes. The first focuses on whatever level of risk constitutes the immediate context in which the care is given. This answer can be called the simple patient's perspective: The costworthiness ceiling for different kinds of care should simply depend on whether the care is administered in high- or low-risk situations. Preventive care, for example, is usually given to its recipients in low-risk situations, whereas the context for hospital intensive care is more often high risk. The context for kidney dialysis is very high risk; not only are people who need it certain to die rather soon without it (assuming that a transplant is not available), but with it they are nearly certain to live.[42] Perhaps, then, it is quite correct for a society to spend much more per life saved on kidney dialysis than on preventive care. (This will be discussed in much greater detail in chapter 7.)

The other answer is what we can call the simple insurance-buyer's perspective. Low- and high-risk perspectives correspond, respectively, to the viewpoints of buyers of insurance or voters on a national health plan on the one hand and ill patients on the other.[43] To patients whom illness has already transported to a high-risk situation, low-risk pricings appear to be no longer relevant, but they will be relevant to buyers of insurance or to voters. If the latter groups are asked now to give prior consent to cost limitations, it would seem that they would choose a plan whose operating limits are based on their current, low-risk situation, not on the much higher-risk perspective of the patient.[44] This is an important practical matter. The care that we can

42. Weinstein, Shepard, and Pliskin 1976.

43. Henceforth I will usually speak only of buyers of insurance, but I do so merely for the sake of convenience. Most of the discussion will also apply to voters and legislators when they consider what to cover in a government health plan.

44. Weinstein, Shepard, and Pliskin (1976) say that for decisions of insurance coverage the lower-risk valuations "may well be" the correct ones; I do not know the source of their hesitation. In a paper that came to my attention shortly before my last revisions, I see that Gibbard (1982) argues for what I would take to be the low-risk perspective in this discussion. In any case, he develops a philosophically systematic defense of limits on very expensive or marginally beneficial care on the basis of the "ex ante Pareto principle." The principle is similar to what I more loosely call "prior consent." The gist of much of what I argue in this and the next chapter is very close to what he argues. He is not be saddled, of course, with the details, mistakes, and weaknesses of my own argument. See also Gauthier 1982.

actually use when we do become ill is greatly influenced both by how comprehensively we are insured and by whether we pick a cost-conscious insurer who readily draws lines of costworthiness beyond mere efficiency. How thrifty a health plan should we purchase (or vote for)? Though we are insuring ourselves for possible high-risk situations, our current vantage point as insurance buyers or voters is one of low risk; people usually don't know whether the health care they will need in the future will be extensive or limited. Autonomous voters or insurance buyers will thus be more willing to forgo expensive, marginally beneficial care than patients will.

This difference in perspective between patient and purchaser of insurance may partially explain why physicians and economists so often are at odds on the matter of cost containment. When doctors consider the monetary value of life, they usually adopt the perspective of the patient. It has been thought that they should, out of loyalty to the individual patient.[45] Their perceived ceiling on costworthy care will understandably exceed the ceilings proposed by economists, policy-makers, and other nonmedical observers, who usually speak more from the lower-risk viewpoint of buyers of insurance.

In general, a strong case can be made for using the insurance buyer's lower-risk perspective. Shouldn't people be thought of as banding together to procure a health-care plan that is admittedly medically less perfect for less money, if the savings are worth it? If it is objected that people themselves seldom explicitly do that and that any decision to limit health care will be a matter of other people imposing risks on them, can't pricings of life with the qualifications we have stipulated in the previous section still be used? Apparently, then, prior consent from the insurance buyer's perspective should generate most of our decisions on cost containment.

What Do We Insure For?

The matter, however, is not that simple. Some complications begin to tilt this very argument from prior consent back toward the patient.

45. The dilemma in which physicians' loyalty to insured patients obligates them to prescribe seemingly noncostworthy care is most effectively posed by Havighurst 1977. He concludes that the individual physician should not be removed from this obligation; other points of institutional decision-making need to be devised to handle the problem. If the physician still has that obligation, most of the argument by Eisenberg and Rosoff (1978) that physicians should be held liable for part of the cost of any unnecessary services that they prescribe loses its practical import. "Unnecessary" care may really be care that is somewhat beneficial though noncostworthy, so significant physician liability is generated by their argument only if the physician is not obligated to prescribe the large segment of noncostworthy care that is still in the insured patient's interest.

What are the eventualities that we insure ourselves for when we buy insurance? For getting ill and needing care, of course—for being a patient. Thus Michael Bayles argues that in deciding how much care to cover in an insurance plan, the crucial consideration is what reasonable persons who are insuring would choose "for themselves were they in similar situations as patients, taking into consideration the proportional increase in the cost of insurance.... The question is not whether most reasonable people *now* want the services, but whether they *would* want them if they were afflicted by the conditions in the specified circumstances."[46] Thus healthy insurers have to decide how much care they would regard as worth its cost if they were ill, whether they expect to be or not. Bayles can admit that the insurance-buyer's perspective may be the correct one, but what precisely is that perspective? Since putting ourselves prospectively into the patient's situation is the very point of insurance in the first place, the buyer's perspective on the value of life really is the patient's perspective as well. A buyer's perspective that appears to yield a lower ceiling is simply deceptive.

To be sure, right at the time when you are buying insurance, deciding on a plan which excludes certain care is a relatively low-risk decision. So how can it be rational for you *at that time* to transport yourself into the patient's perspective? In this objection, however, we are ignoring what we should always be doing when we vote for a policy. We should realize that in the future we may value a policy's results differently—for example, when we are ill. We know *at the time* that we will, in higher-risk situations later on, price life higher. We look not only into future *events* but into ourselves as future *reactors* to events. Thus prior consent—the insurance-buyer's perspective itself—generates higher cost limits on health care than we at first expected.

The matter, however, is far from that simple. For purposes of discussion let us admit Bayles's point: Insurance buyers have to decide what they *would* regard as costworthy care if they *were* ill. As he says, they must still consider the proportional increase in the cost of insurance that would result. And if they take into consideration the fact that the insurance powerfully fuels the escalation of health-care costs, they might be led to lower even more their reflective costworthiness ceiling. Furthermore, even if we do admit that insurance buyers are to imagine themselves as patients, there are two other important questions about what they should consider.

46. Bayles 1977.

Patients, or Highly Insured Patients?

Premiums will increase for another reason besides the coverage of some disputably costworthy care that is justified by insurance-buyers' acknowledgment that they would regard it as costworthy were they ill. As actual patients, they will come to use services which they will judge costworthy because, *once they are insured,* the out-of-pocket cost of these services to them will be low. We begin to get skeptical again: Are buyers of insurance supposed to transpose themselves imaginatively first into ill people, but then also into *highly insured* ill people? Must they *only then* ask themselves what care is costworthy? Note carefully what they would really be asking themselves: "If we become ill, would we want (a) to get all that care nearly free and (b) to spread the resultant increase in premiums among the larger number of people insured rather than merely among ourselves (that is, among other ill people)?" If they were ill, of course they would want both those things! Already, in the process of deciding what insurance to purchase, they would be choosing as if they were both ill *and* highly insured.

This way of selecting among our options as insurance buyers would reflect an overly exclusive identification with the ill. It would *automatically* make costworthy those elements of care whose benefits approach zero, destroying, right from the start, the attempt to achieve any control of the costs aggravated by insurance. It would require us to give up entirely our search for costworthy limits to the resources that health care absorbs in a highly insured economy. The proper conclusion is this: Whereas in choosing plans that cover this and not that degree of care insurance buyers should consider that they will be patients, they must not slip into simply envisioning what as patients they would want when completely insured. This is not to say anything against having insurance; it is only to warn against a slippery manner of thinking that may be involved in deciding what is the costworthy care for which we want to insure.

Should the Ill Have to Imagine Being Well?

A further question arises about Bayles's suggested solution. Rarely are the ill in a position to realize the full value of the benefits from more restrained, less costly coverage. Suppose that premiums are $500 for a more restrained policy and $750 for the less restrained.[47] Why

47. That is the ratio of Blue Cross to Kaiser-Permanente premiums in the San Francisco area. See testimony by Alain C. Enthoven, U.S. Senate, Committee on Finance, 1979b p. 252.

shouldn't not only the healthy imagine how they would want the available funds to be spent if they were ill, but *the ill* also try to imagine what it would be like if all *the well* were able to use the $250 savings on other things?[48] Making a fair assessment of the worth of the $250 gained by choosing the more restrained plan is not the same as adopting the high-risk perspective of the already ill. The issue is this: Isn't it perfectly legitimate for real people—*"total"* people, people who are sometimes healthy, sometimes ill—to opt for the $250 they could save, even though they know, to be sure, that the skinnier plan will leave them more restricted if they do get ill? If we are to have any respect at all for actual, real people's autonomy, the answer, I think, must generally be yes.

The congenitally and chronically ill, of course, pose a problem of fairness here. Their point of view is not the insurance-buyer's low-risk perspective, in which it would be in their self-interest to consent to sharp limits on costworthy care. Still, wouldn't even they probably opt for some savings? When they buy insurance, why should they choose a plan for future care in which they prospectively consider themselves as highly insured, not merely ill? Won't even they offer some resistance to the drift toward care whose benefits approach zero?

A Final Assessment

What is the outcome of this complex of considerations? Perhaps the insurer/low-risk and patient/high-risk perspectives will merge to generate one potential ceiling for costworthy care. Yet even if the two perspectives merge, the patient's perspective does not just displace the view of buyers of insurance. While the proper price of life may well be closer to the estimation by a hypothetical patient than to that by a purchaser of insurance, the proper value still falls somewhere between the two.

This, of course, is precisely the problem that confronts us in our health-care system. Most people are highly insured—or at least most of those whom health-care providers are used to dealing with are. In defining standard care, the perspective of the high-risk, uninsured, ill patient has—operationally—nearly dropped out of sight. But the finite prices of life that emerge from willingness-to-pay responses in hypo-

48. It seems less fair to ask this of the chronically ill, especially the congenitally chronically ill, than it seems it is to ask it of others. For the congenitally ill, to adopt partially the perspective of well buyers of insurance is to move outside their own lives entirely. Asking the temporarily ill to do that seems fairer; they themselves (as future well people) either have benefited, or might benefit, from a more restrained policy. However, see the subsequent comment about the chronically ill in the next paragraph.

thetical *uninsured* contexts—albeit contexts of illness—should provide the relevant limits on costworthy care. *In our medical economy this perspective will not be gained by soliciting opinions from actual patients or providers. The proper limits on costworthy care will have to be imposed somehow from "outside" the provider-patient relationship,* either by insurance buyers or by some other party who is trying to ascertain dispassionately what prices people place on life.

A further observation is equally important. The high-risk dimension of the patient's perspective has often been exaggerated. To be sure, a seriously ill patient often faces a high risk of death, but the available care may reduce those risks only very marginally. Note this combination, for example, in Russell's quarrel with the widespread use of hospital intensive-care units.[49] By my willingness-to-pay responses I may imply that I place a lower price on life when responding to the prospect of a very slight reduction in a large risk than when responding to a potentially large reduction in the same risk.[50] Even the knowledgeable *patient's* perspective on valuing lives will thus rarely yield the same high ceiling on costworthy care that admittedly is appropriate for procedures like kidney dialysis.

8. AN AFTERWORD: EMPIRICAL DATA

I have focused on the theoretical structure of pricing life and the moral justification of its use. There is another, related, empirical inquiry: What are people actually willing to pay to secure their lives? This author is not competent to pursue this inquiry, but a few impressions on the matter can be relayed from the literature. Consider this section, then, a sort of long footnote to the main line of theoretical inquiry in these chapters.

Acton's study of responses to the threat of heart-attack fatalities has already been mentioned.[51] His responses generate a price of life of $28,000 in a situation where the chance of death is 1 in 500; adjusting his 1971 data upward to current dollars would put this value at something over $60,000. Viscusi notes problems in Acton's data: People had no particular incentive to give thoughtful responses to his questionnaire, the sample was small, and the hypothetical program asked

49. Russell 1979.

50. Fuchs (1979), to the contrary, apparently thinks that there is no significant variation in the valuations of life by amount of risk reduction. He thinks the variation occurs only according to whether the situation itself is high- or low-risk. See n. 16 of this chapter.

51. Acton 1973.

about saved post-heart-attack lives that were probably therefore less highly valued.[52]

Most other extrapolations arrive at considerably higher prices than Acton's. One of the most interesting of these is Thaler and Rosen's interpretation of the higher wages that are paid in certain relatively high-risk occupations.[53] Thaler and Rosen conclude that life is in fact valued somewhere between $154,000 and $286,000 (1969 dollars). Viscusi points out that an aspect of this estimate is misleading, too: Individuals vary in their valuations of life, and those who are least averse to risk are likely to take the risky jobs; most people would demand greater compensation.[54] Thus, Bailey adjusts Thaler and Rosen's range to $170,000–$584,000 in 1978 dollars, or a single estimate of $303,000.[55] Bailey himself arrives at a range of $170,000–$715,000, or a single figure of $356,000. Zeckhauser and Shepard use a range of $140,000–$900,000, and translate that into a per-year-of-life range of $10,000–$65,000.[56] We can use roughly the same translation ratio of 1:15 on the other figures. Then Bailey's price, for example, comes out $12,000–$50,000 per year of life saved.

It is interesting to compare these estimates with some actual policy decisions. Ford Motor Company passed over an improvement of $11 per car on Pinto gas tanks. That translates to a price of life exceeding $200,000.[57] Since forgoing the improvement is statistically a very low-risk decision for car buyers, the $200,000 price that Ford could use to defend its decision appears plausible, if borderline (note that the lower limit of Bailey's range is $170,000).

In this light, the decision on cancer detection previously mentioned also appears plausible; it stated that $500,000 per life was too high a price. Philip Cole based a suggestion to perform routine hysterectomies on consenting women over thirty-five years of age on a price of life of $15,000 per year of life.[58] The use of the third stool guaiac to detect intestinal cancer (see 1.2) prices life at over $12,288 per year; a decision *not* to use the fourth guaiac would price it under $117,384

52. Viscusi 1978.

53. Thaler and Rosen 1976.

54. Viscusi 1978. Almost any group of voluntary risk takers, in fact, will provide misleading data on the price of life used to set spending ceilings on reducing *imposed* risks. That is one reason why the Occupational Safety and Health Administration (OSHA) should probably use higher figures in determining when to require safety improvements in jobs for which workers have not in any sense knowingly and voluntarily assumed risk.

55. Bailey 1980.

56. Zeckhauser and Shepard 1976.

57. Greenberg 1980a.

58. Neuhauser and Lewicki 1976.

per year. Both of these decisions appear plausible. Many critics contend that OSHA's standards for coke oven emissions and occupational exposure to acrylonitrile price life too high—at least $1,963,000 and $4,500,000 per life, or $120,000 and $300,000 per year of life respectively. Undoubtedly they do, even if we decide to consider that the workers in these jobs did not voluntarily assume the risks involved.

One final example. Cost-benefit analysis of cholecystectomies for silent gallstones on forty- and fifty-year-olds has indicated a requisite price of $80,000–$150,000 per year of life saved.[59] Doing the analysis should lead us to reject routine performance of this test; its price is undoubtedly higher than we should pay, given the empirical data about our underlying preferences. Such a decision increases the overall welfare of our lives, and it protects our autonomy from a medical imperialism that is as threatening to society as any allegedly safety-mad OSHA. Medicine has no more right to adopt the routine practice of performing this test than OSHA has to impose its particular standard for coke oven emissions regardless of costs. Our autonomy and our welfare are at stake.

59. Fitzpatrick, Neutra, and Gilbert 1977.

CHAPTER THREE

Pricing Life: Rich and Poor

1. THE ISSUE

The claim that the monetary value of life and health is generally lower for the poor than for the rich is the basis for the hardest hitting critique of rising health-care costs. When expensive or marginally beneficial care is not costworthy for the middle class, it is then even less so for the poor.

That claim must now be defended. Its importance in the larger moral argument for pricing life by willingness-to-pay cannot be overestimated. The gravest objection to the willingness-to-pay method is that it rests the value of life on inequitable and unjustly distributed abilities to pay.[1] If income and wealth were distributed justly, even the critics of willingness-to-pay grant that the approach might not be objectionable. But income and wealth are not distributed justly, and even if they might be, would we ever want to rest the life-and-death matters of health policy on the extremely disputable premise that they are? One critic has expressed this objection by characterizing willingness-to-pay as the "lobster-tank" theory for pricing lives. Just as each lobster in its restaurant tank gets a tag for weight that then determines its price, so willingness-to-pay tags the value of people's lives with their "weight" or standing in the community as indicated by their income.[2]

Let us agree with this much of the objection: Income and wealth are unjustly distributed. Still, I will argue, when properly understood,

1. Bayles 1978; Veatch 1979a.
2. Thomasma 1982.

willingness-to-pay's income-related variations in the monetary value of life do not have the morally objectionable features that critics allege. I will take the offensive in this respect: Willingness-to-pay's implication of different pricings of life for rich and poor is morally a positive factor in its favor. Unlike the admittedly obnoxious pricing of the life of one person by another according to status, like lobsters in a tank, these differences represent people's autonomous pricings of their own lives.

Two initial clarifications of the question at issue are needed to eliminate unnecessary confusion. First, people put somewhat different prices on their lives simply by virtue of different desires and values, regardless of any differences in income.[3] A wealthy individual who is rationally suicidal may be willing to pay nothing to preserve life, while an indigent person, addicted to life, may not be willing to part with a last year of it for millions. Different pricings of life might thus be only associated and statistically correlated with differences in income, not a direct result of them. Imagine, for example, that an increased incidence of preference for suicide is statistically correlated with poverty. The poor would then be placing, on the average, a lower valuation on their own lives than would the rich. Yet such a difference should not be taken as evidence that, in the sense of the current question, their monetary valuations of life differ. Here we will disregard differences in their other desires and values and simply focus on whether the mere financial situation of the poor and the rich leads them to different pricings of their lives.[4]

We should also not be misled by the term "willingness-to-pay" into thinking that the poor ought to pay for their health care themselves. The term does *not* connote that one's health care is finally a commodity *for which one oneself must pay*. It only claims that in establishing what risk-reducing care is worth, we should ask what people would be willing to pay for its benefits. Then, once we have determined that certain care is costworthy, it is a far different matter to go on to claim that we should not assist the poor to get the care that they themselves have determined to be really worth the money it costs.

3. Bayles 1978.
4. I am not sure that we should finally draw this distinction at all. Why shouldn't the same respect that we show for the poor's preference to spend less than others do on health care so they can attend to greater, competing needs be extended to the poor's other preferences? For purposes of discussion, however, I want to avoid considering a context in which the substantive desires about life and health of poor people are different from those of the rich. I want to assume equivalent desires of rich and poor, say, for life and health itself, and then work only from the differences in their competing needs that are directly signified by "rich" and "poor."

While the model makes us very skeptical about paying for any care of the poor above *their* lower ceiling of costworthiness, it needn't lead us to throw the poor to the winds of neglect. The question in this chapter is whether that ceiling is lower for the poor than for others, not whether we should assist the poor in getting costworthy care.

2. WHAT IT IS THAT VARIES

Economist Thomas Schelling has been the most ardent defender of wealth-related differences in the value of life. "...Is it worth more to save the rich than the poor?" His answer is yes, "if the question means is it worth more *to the rich* ... than it is *to the poor*.... [Thus] an expensive athletic club can afford [and should buy] better safety equipment than a cheap gymnasium ... and a rich country can [and should] spend more to save lives than a poor one."[5] We should add: The answer is yes *only* if that is the meaning of the question. And more: only if "worth more" means worth more *dollars*, not necessarily worth a greater fraction of income or greater other value.

We need to proceed with extreme care about this. Suppose we ask the rich and poor how much they will pay for lifesaving care. Are we to conclude from the $100,000 answer of a rich person and the $10,000 answer of a poor person that life is worth those respective sums to the two different persons? Aren't both the question and the conclusion we draw from the answers unfair? For one thing, poor people may have access to no more than $10,000 and have no collateral for credit; they may not even have the opportunity to choose to spend more. The question should be changed. It is fairer to ask the rich and the poor what the minimal amount of money would be that they would require, several years in advance, in order to give up their last year of life.[6] Relatively poor people would then ask a lower price than the relatively rich would. Suppose that for two particular individuals those prices were $10,000 and $100,000, respectively. The price of a year of life to the poorer person is then a lower number of the *poor person's* dollars than the price to the rich person is in the *rich person's* dollars.

5. Schelling 1968, emphasis added. See also Schelling 1976, 1979, and 1981.

6. Lead time needs to be inserted into the bargaining situation so that people have some interval of life left in which to use the money. The money is then more valuable to them than if their only use of it were to pass it on to inheritors. Now they have the opportunity to spend it also on themselves.

No Aggregation

But now we come to the likeliest confusion of all: We could conclude—entirely wrongly—that the poor person's life is worth ten
times less to him than the rich person's life is worth to her, or that
the difference between the two pricings is $90,000. Consider for a mo-
ment the latter suggestion: 90,000 of *whose* dollars? To subtract
$10,000 from $100,000 does not give a meaningful figure, for the dollar
units in the two amounts are not the same in value. They are both
dollars, but we are interested in dollars as a medium of exchange
which has value to the people who use it. Since poor people generally
get more value out of an average one of their dollars than richer persons get out of an average one of theirs, subtracting the one pricing
from the other simply leaves us in confusion about what the $90,000
result really means in terms of value. For the same reason it would be
a mistake to conclude that the value of the life of someone who would
sell a last year of life for $10,000 was one-tenth the value of the life of
another who would sell that year for $100,000. One-tenth the value of
whose dollars?

The same point is made when we consider variations in willingness to pay within one's own lifetime. I may be willing to pay five
times as much for a given reduction of risk now as I was when I was
a relatively poor student. It is "implausible and morally outrageous
that anyone should [therefore] consider that my life is five times more
valuable now ... simply because my income has increased during the
natural course of my career."[7] One of my earlier dollars was worth
more to me then than one of my present ones is to me now.

All this has an extremely important implication: Since the value of
dollars varies, *we cannot aggregate any of these pricing-life dollars and
get an entity that is of meaningful value to people*. If we use the willingness to pay of actual individuals to determine the value of one use of
resources as compared to another, we cannot merely aggregate those
dollar figures to determine which use produces the greatest total
value.[8] Not only is there no necessary reason within the willingness-
to-pay model to aggregate different individuals' willingness to pay, but
such adding up, if it is judged from within the perspective of the
model itself, is an outright misconception.

7. Veatch 1979a.

8. Robert Veatch, himself a critic, makes this point about willingness-to-pay:
"... There is no necessary reason within the [willingness-to-pay] approach why a poor
person's willingness to pay should be averaged with the rich person's." See Veatch
1979a.

To be sure, some will want to talk about a totally impersonal dollar value of life—the price that is abstracted from any particular individual's value of the dollar and signifies a society-wide market value. Then there indeed might be some sense in aggregating across individuals, and thus to the "one-tenth" and "$90,000 difference" comparisons. That may be how we use prices for most items in our economy; as "monetary value," one dollar is just one dollar, regardless of the different satisfaction values various individuals put on it.

But while this sense of dollar values is very useful when we are exchanging a commodity between individuals, in the case of the price of life the responses which generate our estimates do not emerge from trading lives *between* people. That is impossible—I simply cannot trade my life to you. The responses emerge instead from a person's trading *within* his or her own life. Willingness-to-pay is a morally attractive approach to pricing life primarily because it offers a way of estimating how people value their own lives. Talk of the "monetary value" of life would seem to make life into a commodity, if we were not interested in the dollar figures as reflecting value *for the person willing to pay*. Economists and makers of health-policy decisions may indeed often want to use "the dollar value of life" in the more impersonal sense. If so, it is no wonder that the notion of "costworthy care" founded on their conception of monetary value strikes others— health-care providers, patients, and most of the rest of us—as crass. It is.

Greater Competing Needs and Desires

Yet we shouldn't swing to the tempting, opposite view that the $10,000 price in the poorer person's dollars and the $100,000 price in the richer person's simply represent the same value of life. To be sure, rich and poor ultimately *care* equally about continuing to live. Surely—it is even offensive to note so obvious a point—it is just as personally difficult for the poor as it is for the rich to part with life, leave loved ones behind, and so forth. Heaven forbid that economists or smart policy analysts should ignore that. But "equal caring" about continuing to live doesn't lead to the conclusion that the *monetary* values of lives are equal. "Monetary valuation" has some greater connection with persons' own *dollar* pricings than that.

Now it is a plain fact that the poor have more unmet, non-health-care, non-lifesaving-related needs than do the rich. *Relative to their other needs and desires, which money can often be of great and even indispensable help in meeting,* of course marginal reduction of the risk of death has less value to the poor than it does to the rich. The qualification that I have emphasized is absolutely crucial. *Relative* to their *own* respective needs for *other* things, a poor person's need for health care of a particular expense is lower than a rich person's need. Even that sharply qualified, this value of life still deserves the term "monetary." Money is essentially something that can be used by a person to meet other needs. Therefore, the monetary value of life—not just the numerical dollar figures people are willing to pay—can properly be said to be lower for the poor. The *overall* value isn't lower; the *monetary* value is.

Admittedly we will still be tempted to ask: lower by how much? We have already dismissed as answers both the $90,000 difference and the factor of ten. At this point no further constructive suggestions are apparent. Rather, we should simply make no attempt at all to determine a proportional relation or dollar difference. All we need do is clarify what we mean when we say, "The poor place a lower monetary value on their lives"—that to the poor the use of money to meet other needs is more valuable than it is to the rich. It means nothing more, and nothing less. We need no *dollar* difference.

Some critics, however, think that willingness-to-pay has been predominantly used and defended in the literature without being qualified in these respects. To them, the direct implication of the whole approach seems to be that decreasing the chances of a particular death for a wealthy person is *more valued* than the same decrease in risk for a poor one.[9] That may be correct in terms of what the proponents of willingness-to-pay have often thought they were about. In any case, we shouldn't come close to defending such a confused version of the model. Three crucial clarifications have to be made. (1) It is only the *monetary* value—the "price", not the overall value—of poorer persons' lives that is lower than the monetary value of richer persons' lives. (2) The price of poor persons' lives is only lower *for the poor persons* than the monetary value of rich persons' lives is *for the rich*. It is not "lower, period" (whatever that might mean), or "lower for society." (3) The price is lower, to the poor, *only relative to their other unmet needs*.

3. THE RELEVANCE FOR HEALTH CARE

Despite all these qualifications, variations in the pricing of life are still relevant for estimating the monetary value of health care. They are es-

9. Veatch 1979a, emphasis added.

pecially relevant for marginal care that reduces risks of death or morbidity only slightly. Relatively poor people might choose to use only $20 of an additional $100 monthly income to upgrade a high-deductible, "major medical" insurance policy to a comprehensive, low cost-sharing, very cost-conscious, prepaid plan; they might reserve the remaining $80 for use on other things. Richer people might choose to use half of the $100 to upgrade the same initial policy to equally comprehensive third-party insurance with no restriction on choice of providers, insurance that presumably is more willing to cover services whose benefits approach zero. Given the very meaning of the notion "lower monetary value," this variety of preferences would constitute direct evidence that poor people place a lower monetary value on the most expensive policy than wealthier people do. It would tell us something very important, and it would do it without our having to aggregate the valuations of separate individuals or mention any dollar differences: We will be meeting weightier needs in the eyes of the poor people if we provide $20 of additional health-care coverage and $80 for other needs than if we provide an additional $50 for health insurance.

Furthermore, these differences in the monetary value of most health care may even be greater than the usually conceived differences in the monetary valuation of life. Much health care deals with low risks, or the purchase of it results in only slight reductions in risk. As we slide from high-risk to low-risk (or slight-reduction-in-risk) cases, the poor may become even more willing to gamble with risks of death than the rich. When the gamble only slightly risks your life, when it immediately saves you money, and when you are poor, it may be both attractive and actually a good bargain; it will probably be neither if you are rich. Even if the monetary values of the lives of rich and poor were equal, the monetary value of most health care would still be lower for the poor.[10]

10. At the same time, relatively cheap preventive care may in one sense be a better buy for the poor than it is for the rich. *Compared* to expensive, large reductions in large risks, poor persons will probably value inexpensive reductions in smaller risks more highly than richer people will; of course they will still monetarily value those inexpensive reductions by themselves less than the rich do. The explanation is this: "When an individual is put in a position where he must purchase a bigger (and more expensive) reduction, he is in effect poorer"—while a poor person may willingly sacrifice what amounts to 10 percent of his income to avoid a 1 percent chance of death, he could hardly sacrifice twenty times that much to avoid a 20 percent probability of death. See Zeckhauser 1975. Inexpensive preventive care, as opposed to expensive curative care, is likely to be more valuable to the poor than it is to the more well-to-do. That is, while some expensive emergency care for high-risk situations may be a good buy to the rich but not to the poor, inexpensive preventive care may remain a good buy to both.

Precisely at stake here, of course, are the two fundamental moral reasons behind the entire willingness-to-pay model for pricing life: maximizing human welfare from our resources, and, in particular, respecting the autonomy of free agents. We are different from lobsters, who just lie there in the tank and get tagged by us. If people put prices on *their own* lives and health care, and if we pay attention to their prices even when different than those we put on our own lives, we are acknowledging their *equal worth as free agents*. We are doing that despite the ironically unequal monetary pricings which we thus respect.

At precisely this point it will be objected that we have sunk to merely fanciful theory: In health care there is no realistic outlet for this autonomous choice. Your life is on the line, and there are no cheaper brands of care to pick from. And when you're ill, the contrast with health is so profound that you're not willing to settle for second-best care even if there are cheaper brands from which to choose.[11]

But follow out that logic to its conclusion. Honestly faced, the conclusion is simply Louise Russell's observation quoted earlier: "Investment in a technology will continue until the benefit from any further investment is zero."[12] Think of what we would then be spending, and developing to spend on. To be sure, people aren't realistically going to get hold of this escalation of costs by very often saying, when sick, "Well, that costs too much; don't use it." But they may very well choose to bind themselves ahead of time by buying into a cheaper plan with tighter cost controls. Should we ban people from binding themselves to a more restrained manner of care? Autonomous choice is still at stake after all. In the midst of a modern hospital it may not seem that there are cheaper models of care to choose from. But that's because we are letting ourselves be trapped by the whole setting of that hospital's and our society's accustomed level of care. Why shouldn't lower-income people band together, for example, to have an

---

There is a major problem with Zeckhauser's illustration, however. It seems unfair, since poor persons hardly have the choice to spend what amounts to 200 percent of their income. The unfairness can be removed by the same substitution we used earlier: Shift the question to whether people would be willing to incur a 20 percent risk of death in return for compensation equal to twice their current income. It is possible, of course, that poor people would be willing to take this bargain, and that their preference here would be consistent with their willingness to pay 10 percent of income to eliminate a 1 percent risk. Seeing the matter this way makes Zeckhauser's claims dubious. Maybe, relative to the desire to use available money to avoid large risks (or take money to incur them), the poor are not more willing to use money to avoid small risks than the rich are.

11. Thomasma 1982.
12. Russell 1979, p. 4. See 1.2.

admittedly less perfect health-care system for a third of the money? (In fact, that's roughly the amount of money with which the British run their system.) *Really*, why shouldn't they, if it would enable them to pocket the savings? Health care is admittedly often a life-sustaining service for us, not just another commodity, but *why shouldn't it be a service under our control?* Simply to say that in a hospital there are no cheaper brands of care to choose from and let the matter rest is to flee from the real freedom that groups of like-minded people have.

The real autonomy of the poor will increase, of course, only if more restrained, cheaper health-care options emerge. And it will be difficult to translate into reality this autonomy that morally fuels the willingness-to-pay conception of pricing life. But without some such conception to control health care before its benefit-to-cost ratio approaches Russell's prophetic zero, the poor (and all of us) are simply rolling over (like lobsters?) in the face of some medical culture that has crept into our heads with the pernicious idea that we don't really have any choice.

4. MISUSES IN POLICY

Misunderstanding what precisely is meant by saying that pricings of life and health care vary with income can lead to gross misuses of the concept of willingness-to-pay in public policy. These misuses must be carefully guarded against.

Schelling follows one of his most vigorous arguments for the variation with this insistence: "...A hospital that can save either of two lives but not both, has no reason to save the richer ... on these grounds...."[13] It is absolutely crucial to understand this point. If for the poorer person the value of this care relative to his other unmet needs is lower, why shouldn't the hospital save the richer one?[14] The key is found directly in the earlier discussion. The value of life to the poor person is lower *only* relative to her other needs, and therefore in willingness-to-pay terms; it is not lower in any other, more absolute

13. Schelling 1968.

14. Some have interpreted Richard Posner's well-known economic analysis of law to imply similar things generally about the use of resources; see Posner 1972. One critic wonders "who is the 'party whose use is more valuable'? The most 'obvious answer,' and the only answer consistent with Posner's definition of value, is the party who ... is willing (and able) to pay the most for the right...." See Baker 1975. That answer may in fact be what Posner has committed himself to, but in any case, willingness-to-pay models for valuing lives need not draw for themselves any such implications of Posner's analysis of law.

sense. It would be clearly fallacious—indeed outrageous—for the hospital to claim that it could maximize welfare or meet more unmet needs by giving the care to the rich. It would be confusing higher monetary value with higher value.

We might imagine the hospital making a further case to the poor for its proposal: "By your own admitted preferences you have told us that your need for this care *compared* to your other unmet needs is lower than a richer person's comparative need. So we think the rich have a slightly greater claim on this care than you do, as long as your medical need for it is no greater than theirs. We are, of course, only in the business of providing health care, not meeting other needs. If we were meeting other ones, you would often have a greater claim on those scarce resources than the rich would. We hope the many institutions whose job it is to meet those other needs will follow the same policy in principle as we do, and thus, that they will give *you* preference for *their* services. The *general* principle we are following is not unfair to you at all, but highly advantageous. It is just that we are merely a health-care institution."

This argument fails, too. Other institutions seldom follow the principle cited. Services for most of the poor's other unmet needs do not even have "institutions" to mete them out, but are distributed through the market. And even if an "institution" exists, the market clearly does not follow the policy described by the hospital above. In fact, since the rich also have more money with which to bid for those other services, they usually end up getting more of them, too, regardless of the poor's greater relative need for them. The hospital could meet these objections if, every time it gave health care to the rich, it gave cash or other services to the poor in lieu of the marginal health care that they value less. Obviously it does not do that. It will then have to fall back on the fallacious claim that it will maximize welfare by giving the care to the rich rather than the poor. That claim involves precisely the same mistaken interpretations of income-related differences in the value of life and health care that were noted earlier.

This same mistake can be made on a more society-wide level. Suppose that the costworthiness of developing and providing a medical advance were determined this way:

> Each person is asked how much he would be willing to pay for a technology which would have a [certain] probability ... of saving his life or ... [a given] number of lives. One then totals the amounts individuals are willing to pay. If the total amount people are willing to pay exceeds

the cost of the technology, then it is worthwhile.... If the total amount people are willing to pay is less than the cost of the technology, then it is not worthwhile.[15]

This method could make one technology costworthy and another one with equal health benefits and costs not, *merely* because the former benefited a wealthier population than the latter.[16] But then the method would seem to entail that the National Institutes of Health, for example, should research and fund the former technology but not the latter.[17] That seems intolerable, and clear grounds for rejecting willingness-to-pay.

Sensing these objections, Bayles proposes a modification: A particular medical advance is worth the money it costs if that amount is no more than the sum created by whatever *equal percentage* increase in each person's *already justly graduated income tax* everyone would willingly contribute to make this care available.[18] In this formulation willingness to pay would supposedly reflect the equally strong desires of everyone for the care, abstracted from their varying abilities to pay (an already justly graduated tax would presumably place burdens on everyone strictly according to ability to pay). That may or may not be the appropriate modification.[19] In any case, to conclude that because rich and poor are willing to pay different amounts, *society* should not develop care that the poor especially need but should develop analogous, equally expensive care for a problem more common among the rich commits the same fallacy as the previous hospital argument did.

15. Bayles 1978.

16. Bayles 1978; Veatch 1979a.

17. Jones-Lee, for example, admits that conventional cost-benefit analysis tends "to recommend the utilization of scarce safety-improvement resources in relative high-income areas." See Jones-Lee 1976, p. 103. He then tries to cushion himself from the unwanted final policy conclusion: Fully responsible decision making, he says, considers not only the results of cost-benefit analysis, but also the distributional effects. In what follows I claim that the results of cost-benefit analysis itself, correctly understood, do not tend to recommend any such utilization of scarce, *public* resources in relatively high-income areas.

18. This is probably what Bayles calls his more "complex method," designed to correct the previous and objectionable "simple" one. See Bayles 1978. Actually Bayles does not quite commit himself to what I here take him to mean—the lowest equal percentage increase in justly graduated income tax which everyone would willingly contribute.

19. Why and whether it is *in principle* the correct modification is unclear. What it should be designed to do is confusing. (1) Should it make the method simply reflect equally strong desires for *the care itself,* abstracting from desires for other needs to be met? (2) Should it yield an amount equal to the sum of what each person would actually be willing to pay if *all* (hypothetically) put themselves in the position of being *as likely to benefit* from the care as the target population? With the latter, while the willingness-

The lower monetary value put on care by the poor is not an overall valuation of the care itself; it is lower than the value which the rich person puts on the care only relative to competing, unmet needs.

Nevertheless, despite their misuse, under certain limited conditions willingness-to-pay determined variations in the price of life are related to what society ought to pay. It is relevant, for example, that low-income sufferers from sickle-cell disease would generally pay less to remove a death risk than wealthier sufferers of ulcers would pay.[20] The savings from not developing a treatment for sickle-cell disease[21] could be given to the poor who have the disease, and they might well knowingly choose to use it on other things. Or the rich might contribute their own money to find a treatment for ulcers. In either of these circumstances—but *only* in something like them—there would be nothing wrong with trying to find a treatment for ulcers but not for sickle-cell disease.

It is to the positive credit of the willingness-to-pay approach that it maintains the variation of the monetary value of life with income. Properly understood, the approach forces us to notice how important it is that the health-care system not use its pull to distract us from the poor's other unmet needs. As Schelling notes, providing the poor "the same level of medical services as the rest of the population wants to provide itself" is "an evasion of the fact that they are poor and have urgent unattended other needs, too." It is, in fact, a misapplication of the principle of equality. Equality concerns much more than health-care needs.[22] Amidst the admitted urgency of much of its work, the health-care system can easily forget the fact that poor patients are

---

to-pay inputs vary with income, no disease gets more or less money than another, all persons regardless of income each (hypothetically) voluntarily "contribute" to every disease's fund. Though Bayles's modification and the first principle just suggested avoid objectionable funding of research on the diseases of the rich before those of the poor, they remain open to other criticisms of unfairness. They would, for example, generate low priority for attention to rare diseases, while the second suggested principle would not. Whether or not that is fair to the victims of rare diseases is the vexing problem—should the mere numbers of afflicted or benefited persons count in our moral calculus? For more on that problem, see 8.3.

20. Here I am in direct contention with Veatch 1979a. The example is his, though I make the opposite claim of relevance about it.

21. There might, of course, be no overall savings once we consider all the real costs of the disease itself, not just the monetary ones. But then the poor might well be more willing to pay to find a treatment than the rich, who can bear at least the monetary costs of such a disease more easily. This is especially likely if the poor could in fact do what they usually can't, spread out their payments into the future time when they would reap the savings from the treatment.

22. See 1.4, 1.5, and chap. 1, n. 46.

poor, not just ill. A similar point can be made in relation to the previous chapter's discussion of the different perspectives of insurance buyer and patient on costworthy care: Medical providers tend to forget that patients are also buyers of insurance. These mistakes are readily understandable, but not therefore justified. They fail to respect people's equal moral worth as free agents.

5. UNJUST INCOME DISTRIBUTION

One objection still remains to even such a qualified defense and interpretation of variations in the price of life with income.[23] *Willingness* to pay, it will be said, harbors a further ideological bias. A choice to pay a certain, limited amount for lifesaving care is voluntary only *given* a certain income to divide between various things. But the poor do not choose that key background condition itself. The poor have not chosen to be poor, and they have often remained poor while struggling to improve their economic lot against far greater odds than most of the relatively rich have ever had to face. To be sure, in some individual cases people become relatively rich by their own free choices, determination, and shrewd decisions. Nevertheless, poverty is usually a condition for which a poor person is not responsible. Thus the poor have not chosen the situation in which they can meet fewer of their non-health-care needs than the rich can. Their "willingness" to pay less for care is therefore a mere superficial willingness. Since the predictable result of society giving to the poor less money with which to meet their other needs is that the poor will price reductions in risk at a lower level than the rich will, it is ultimately society, in fact, not the poor, which places a lower monetary value on their lives. Responsibility lies with society for the background conditions behind variations in the monetary value of life; it ought to be shared by the health-care system, since the same overall social/economic/political system that makes non-health-care needs a greater burden for the poor than for the rich is also the one that provides health care. How, finally, can the foundation for a morally relevant and voluntary variation in the monetary value of lifesaving health care be an immoral and involuntary distribution of income?

This critique raises the most fundamental questions about the structure of a just society, the reality of individual freedom of choice,

---

23. There are surely other objections. This is just the one which seems most troublesome, given the way the previous arguments have developed. It has been privately pressed against my position by Jeffrey Reiman of American University.

and the scope of individual responsibility—questions that can hardly be pursued carefully here.[24] But we can make a separate response here in defense of willingness-to-pay. Assume that the present distribution of income and wealth is indeed as unjust as this critique alleges.[25] To be sure, we must then face the correct and sobering point: The poor's other, greater unmet needs, to which the lower monetary valuation of their lives is inherently relative, are unmet largely because of society's unjust arrangements. We could simply add this point to our list of qualifications on the interpretation of "lower valuations of life by the poor" summarized at the end of 3.1. But it does not destroy the moral relevance of income-related differences in pricing life. That relevance is simply that there is at least a prima facie case for giving as much priority to meeting poorer persons' *other* unmet needs as poorer persons themselves give to meeting them. We should not give the poor assistance restricted to health care at any level beyond the contours of costworthiness shaped by their actual income, unless we give aid for all their other needs at levels just as far beyond their income.

Whether the current critique of the moral relevance of varying monetary values of life is persuasive may be partly determined by the political context in which those values are being discussed. Suppose we are considering a full-scale revamping of the social system to make it much more just. Then, yes, the immoral distribution of income that generates the present lower pricings of life may become the *exclusive* focus of our attention. So firmly will our sights be set on a more egalitarian distribution that we will not entertain the relevance of pricings of life that emerge from present inequalities. Even then, however, the precise moral relevance of variations in the monetary value of life which is emphasized at the end of the last paragraph does not distract our attention from these revolutionary goals. At least it does not say anything inconsistent with them.

24. A very useful volume of contemporary philosophical writings on economic justice is Arthur and Shaw 1978. The wider literature, of course, is huge.

25. At this juncture a different, but I think much less important, defense of willingness-to-pay could be made. A just distribution of income for many committed egalitarians will still contain inequalities of income and wealth. On Ake's principle of justice as equality, for example, some people in a just economy will take part of their "income" as leisure or more enjoyable work and thus have lower monetary incomes. See chap. 1, n. 46, and Ake 1975. The same question of whether the monetary valuations of life vary with income will still arise in that society. Admittedly, that point can hardly be used as a defense of willingness-to-pay as appropriate for use in actual American society; current inequalities in income and wealth here may not correlate well with different tastes for leisure or work. Nevertheless, this is a valid theoretical point.

Let us consider, alternately, a less "revolutionary" context: We are discussing what assistance the present government ought to give to individuals; we have put the longer-term, fuller, more revolutionary ideal on the back shelf for the moment. We have granted the current critique its claim that income-related variations in pricing of life depend on immoral inequities. Don't the poor still have to be dealt with as living, real persons in their present world? In this context *isn't it an insult to the poor to treat them only as lenses through which some future, less unjustly treated, not so poor people are envisioned?* Poor persons' present choices should be taken more seriously; certainly they should if the poor weren't tricked into expressing lower pricings of life by advantaged exploiters.

Variations in the monetary value of life and health care need not distract us from any revolutionary reconstruction of the society that we may be intent on encouraging. It is not merely that the dangerous ways of thinking to which those variations may give rise are avoidable. The variations can be seen to have a positive role as well. They make it less likely that we will ignore the broader conditions of the present poor. They are morally relevant, even if present differences in income and wealth are grossly unjust.

6. CONCLUSION

Willingness-to-pay should be used regardless of the frequent differences that result from it in the monetary value of the lives of rich and poor. In fact, when properly qualified and understood, these differences are a positive moral factor in support of the model. Critics of willingness-to-pay correctly argue that there is no necessary connection between what particular persons would pay for a program to add years to life and what society ought to pay for it.[26] For example, in the willingness-to-pay approach there is no implication whatsoever that governments ought to pay more for care to save the life of a wealthier person than they pay for a poorer one, or that scarce resources ought to be given to the wealthy before the poor when there are not enough for both. In part the lack of such a close connection between the monetary value of my life and what society ought to pay to save it is due to the fact that the different pricings of different people's lives cannot be aggregated or numerically compared. In part it is also due to the realistic political context: Any allocation by society of extra, marginal, scarce health-care resources to the relatively rich would not be paired

26. See, for example, Veatch 1979a.

with an allocation of monetarily equal, non-health-care-restricted benefits to the poor.

In other words, because they constitute a prima facie moral case for giving aid to the poor for things they would prefer over health care, income differences in the monetary value of life are morally relevant to decisions about what health care society ought to provide them. Then it becomes clear that the whole business of using prices of life and health care derived from willingness-to-pay pushes strongly toward either of two policies: Provide public assistance to the poor in transferable cash, not in-kind aid restricted to health care; or, in the very same spirit, meet the non-health-care needs of the poor through programs that are equally well-funded and are, in the eyes of the poor, equally beneficial. The moral thrust behind the willingness-to-pay approach to the monetary valuation of life is the same thrust that pushes the case for cash aid. There is no adequate justification of the willingness-to-pay approach to valuing life that is not also a prima facie justification of cash aid. The driving question behind both is, why give the poor aid in one form when *they* prefer it in another? There are, of course, many complications to the cash/in-kind issue. Those will be considered in the next chapter.

The debate between cash assistance and in-kind aid is a basic issue in political philosophy. The fact that these two chapters on the monetary valuation of life end by referring to this debate reveals that no discussion of the valuation of life and health care can be independent of underlying political philosophy.[27]

27. Mooney 1977, p. 72.

CHAPTER FOUR

Cash or In-Kind Aid?

1. THE ISSUE

Most of us believe that, for those who remain in greatest need, the results of birth, social status, and market choices need to be supplemented by government assistance. We believe this for a variety of reasons—expediency, general welfare, justice, individual rights. Short of wholesale changes in the way people get their shares of the economic pie to begin with, we then have two major options: Either make provision for the poor "in kind"—providing particular kinds of aid such as legal services, public housing or rent subsidies, food stamps, education, job training—or more directly redistribute income in the form of "cash"—that is, providing income maintenance. In between lie two variations: cash with required advice about how to use it, or vouchers that let a recipient choose whichever public or private provider to use for a designated service.[1]

The last chapter unfolded a connection between the problem of costworthy health care and this choice between cash and in-kind aid. Putting a limit on what care is costworthy involves assigning a finite price to life. The most plausible way of doing that uses willingness-to-pay, which generates lower prices of life for the poor than for the rich. The lower ceiling for the poor on what health care is costworthy that results is morally relevant in *only* one respect: The poor often have other needs which they prefer to meet before spending on health care. This very fact constitutes a prima facie case for cash as opposed

1. Thurow 1976. As I use the terms, cash with advice is included under "cash" and vouchers under "in-kind" assistance.

to in-kind aid for health care—after all, with cash the poor can choose to meet those other needs. If, after more thorough consideration, we were to decide not to give the poor that choice, an important part of the relevance of the willingness-to-pay model would be lost. To see whether we can preserve one of the most important implications of using willingness-to-pay to put limits on costworthy care, we need to take up the arguments for and against cash aid.

There is another, more practical side to the cash/in-kind aid debate. Giving poorer people cash rather than restricting assistance to services like health care will undoubtedly lead to the use of less care. One observer estimates that a 33 percent cash increase in the income of a poor family will result in only an 11 percent increase in health-care demand.[2] This means that if the $2,000 Medicaid expense for a family of four were all changed to cash, a relatively small portion of it would be used for medical care.[3] Policy makers and health-care providers who deplore the present low level of health care for the poor will understandably think automatically of specific health-care programs, not income maintenance.

The Initial Case for Cash
Economists have traditionally defended cash.[4] Foremost among their defenses of it is a general respect for consumer autonomy. If the market is unacceptable because of unjust distributions of resources, shouldn't it be corrected by redistributing the resources rather than by removing consumer choice? Individuals differ in their pricings of life, in their risk aversions, and in the elasticity/inelasticity of their demand for medical care.[5] Not only does the principle of autonomy favor cash; that of maximizing welfare does also. In relation to risk aversion, for example, "the economist is no more inclined to look behind [dispute] the taste for risk than he is the taste for pickled herring."[6] The

2. Acton 1975. Other kinds of evidence are relevant to the empirical question of how much health care the poor would buy with cash. That they would buy distinctly less than higher-income people is suggested by Mosteller's figures (1978): While demand by the poor in 1970 for the "necessary" surgeries for appendicitis, cataracts, hernia repair, and prostate problems was approximately the same as by the population as a whole, their demand for "less necessary" operations of tonsillectomy, hysterectomy, and lumbar laminectomy was roughly half of the general population's. Grossman and Colle (1978) document income variations in demand for pediatric care.

3. Allen cites an average 1978 Medicaid expense of $1850 for a family of four. See Allen 1981, p. 97.

4. Rhoads 1978.

5. Elasticity of demand is the degree to which a lower out-of-pocket price for medical care will increase the use of care.

6. Posner 1972, p. 127.

point can be extended to health in general. People not only have different aversions to risk but also diverse opinions about the degree to which health care increases health and the relative importance of health itself. One can "imagine a whole community rejecting most personal health care and pursuing, instead, say, the free provision of wine, good art and formal gardens, with only an investment in preventative medicine and minimal acute care."[7] Given who they are, that might maximize their welfare.

Cash aid also provides a solution to the terribly difficult problem of where to draw the limits on health-care coverage for the poor.[8] Do we cover expensive totally implantable artificial hearts, if and when safe versions of them have been devised?[9] Do we cover abortions that are not strictly medically necessary? Wigs for elderly women (or men) with thinning hair? Psychotherapy? These are not fanciful issues. The British National Health Service recently spent one million pounds on wigs for elderly women.[10] The traditional opposition of blue-collar labor unions to covering psychotherapy is well known, and the inclusion of psychotherapy in public insurance coverage has been regarded by some as urgent and necessary and by others as a spillover from upper-middle-class indulgence.[11] The point is that if redistribution or assistance to the poor is provided in cash, no *societal* decisions need to be made on *any* of these questions. A diversity of coverages could flower.

An economist like Schelling finds this case for cash so convincing that he attributes our reluctance to adopt it to our self-serving middle-class sensitivities and the defensiveness of medicine:

> If novocaine in the mouth costs $30 a shot and the well-to-do usually paid it, there would be many among the poor to whom 30 minutes of pain for half a day's wages would be a bargain.... But it may offend us to let the poor suffer pain because they'd rather have the money.... And it may be good for the morale and pockets of the medical industry not to let the poor trade their medical privileges for cash.[12]

To all this, one objection is immediate. *Equal* health care is a right, it will be said, so the economist's traditional arguments for cash

7. Englehardt 1980a.
8. Throughout, my use of the term "coverage for the poor" includes the possibility that this is part of universal coverage for everyone. It need not be a separate plan for the poor. In either case it does cover the poor.
9. See National Heart and Lung Institute 1976; Havighurst 1976; and Jonsen 1975.
10. Bayles 1977.
11. Cummings 1977 and Albee 1977.
12. Schelling 1979.

fail in the case of health care. But should we *start out* this discussion by assuming that *equal* health care is a right? To do so would beg the very question at issue. The case for cash is precisely a case for what will certainly turn out to be unequal health care. While recipients may well have a right to *something* equal, that something need not be health care. Though some principle of justice as equality may drive the acknowledgment of whatever the poor have a right to, it need not yield a right to equal health care.

We have seen briefly the attractiveness of cash aid. We now need to scrutinize the arguments against it. Because in-kind aid restricts freedom of choice, there is a prima facie case for cash. Therefore I will take up various arguments for in-kind aid one by one—as if they carried the burden of proof.

2. PUBLIC GOODS AND EXTERNALITIES

The market is usually thought to do its best job in distributing goods which are "rival" and "excludable." If you consume such a good, I too cannot consume it. We compete for it, and if you win, you can exclude me from it.[13] These are "private goods": Whether provided publicly or privately, they are distributed to and enjoyed by separate individuals.

By contrast, consider a lighthouse or a system of national defense, both pure "public goods." Their consumption is not rival, exclusion is impossible (you *can*not keep me from sharing in the benefits of the lighthouse), and roughly identical amounts of the good get consumed by everyone.[14] Leaving their distribution up to individual, private market choice will either decrease welfare or be unfair: Either the lighthouse will never get built though everyone would find its per-capita cost a good buy or "free-riders" will hold out for others to build it and then unfairly enjoy its benefits. Such goods ought to be publicly funded.

Certain public-health measures seem to be public goods—clean air and water, or certain immunization programs, for instance. The argument for in-kind government provision of these kinds of health care is overwhelming. But notice that this is the case whether anyone is poor or not. Moreover, medical care and individual preventive care seldom qualify as such public goods.

A more plausible argument for in-kind aid focuses on "externalities," a looser notion than "public goods." Though my *own* welfare

13. Cullis and West 1979, pp. 36–37.
14. Thurow 1976.

may be maximized by spending only $10 of $100 of public assistance on health care, for example, my spending more on health care may have greater benefits to others. As I do not take those benefits into account when spending cash, in-kind aid is needed as a corrective. The benefits to others are of two kinds: They are able to satisfy preferences that they have about their own lives, or preferences that they have about my life. An example of the former is the interest which "those who want to be safely promiscuous have ... in paying for a service to prevent and cure venereal disease in others."[15] An example of the latter would be the greater satisfaction that people get if a welfare recipient spends more on health care and less on alcohol, even when neither kind of spending in any way affects their desires about their own lives.[16]

Once we recognize the external benefits of in-kind aid, we can create a so-called Pareto-optimality argument for it: No one will lose, and someone will gain.[17] Imagine whatever level of *cash* aid people are willing to be taxed for, or that recipients have a moral right to. Taxpayers may find that it increases their own welfare to pay for more amply funded in-kind programs. If the recipients also gain more from that financially enlarged in-kind program than they gain from the cash aid it replaces, they and taxpayers alike will gain by shifting to more expensive in-kind aid.[18] Compared to cash, restricted aid raises everyone's welfare.

Weaknesses

The externalities argument, however, is simply not a general argument for in-kind assistance.[19] As a Pareto-optimality argument it works only if recipients gain at least as much from the enlarged health-care assistance which the taxpayers find it in their interest to provide as they do from the lesser cash aid which it replaces; taxpayers must gain enough from restricting the form of the aid that they will willingly pay for increases in aid large enough for recipients to gain from the change. Suppose, instead, that there are real welfare losses to recipients when we shift from fewer dollars of cash assistance to more amply funded health care. Suppose, furthermore, that there is still an ag-

15. Abel-Smith 1976, p. 33.

16. Thurow has some convenient terminology here: The former kind of externality is based on what he terms "private-personal preferences," and the latter on "individual societal preferences." See Thurow 1976.

17. Blumstein and Zubkoff 1973.

18. This Pareto-optimality argument for in-kind aid is described by Thurow 1976.

19. Cullis and West 1979, p. 59.

gregate gain: These losses are smaller than the gains to the taxpayers. Then the argument can be saved by only two moves. Both are dubious. (1) We could emphasize that aggregate welfare, both parties combined, is still increased. Then the argument becomes baldly utilitarian. It will be vulnerable to any nonutilitarian rights or principles of justice which may have been the initial moral force behind the assistance program. (2) We could resort to "prerogatives of taxpayers": The price taxpayers exact for funding the program is that the aid be used in the form they stipulate, despite its lower value to the recipients. One proponent puts the argument this way, giving away its true nature: ". . . The price exacted by these *voluntary* donors is control of the way redistributed funds are spent."[20] *Aid has become charity,* a privilege given to the poor by those who pay for it. It has ceased to be a *right* of the poor.

Some, of course, will not be upset by this, but *it surely reveals how far away from a right to health care the case against cash has drifted.* For those whose original rationale for supporting aid at all was some claim of justice for the poor, not the interests or largesse of others, this move in the argument will be hard to swallow. Thus, ironically, precisely those people who most vigorously defend in-kind health-care aid as necessary to avoid a second-class system of care that would violate the *rights* of the poor cannot resort to either of these turns in the argument. The fate of the whole argument should be placed back in the hands of the recipients: If in fact the recipients ultimately prefer the smaller amount of cash over the more amply funded health care, the externalities argument for in-kind assistance is dead.

Suppose, however, that the poor do gain by switching from the smaller amount of cash to the larger dollar amount of in-kind aid which taxpayers are willing to provide. Wouldn't their consent then justify in-kind aid? Serious questions would still arise. *Why would a society be willing to provide aid in kind that is more expensive than aid in cash?* We are driven back to problematic arguments based on paternalism, taxpayers' prerogatives, or Schelling's suspicion that society wishes to propagate its middle-class values or serve the interests of professional providers. We should not for a minute, of course, criticize *the poor* for deciding to take the greater in-kind aid. But that does not justify *the society* in paying less for cash and creating the very political reality under which the poor consent to in-kind assistance as the best they can get.

20. Blumstein and Zubkoff 1973, emphasis added.

But the externalities argument is even weaker yet. It is more likely that taxpayers' preferences about the lives of recipients, not about their own lives, are at stake. Of course, if the poor affect the state of others' lives by their choices, then taxpayers' preferences may count for something in restricting the poor's behavior. But if the poor disappoint others' preferences when those preferences are merely about the poor, the poor's choices hardly seem to be these other people's business.[21] If the poor's lower priority on health care does not affect others' interests in their *own* lives, why should any effect it does have matter?[22]

The argument from general externalities is self-contradictory at worst, and at best inconclusive.

Children

There remains one externality which survives these criticisms. If the poor choose to spend little of their cash aid on health insurance or health care, one effect of such choices seems unfair: Their children will also get little health care.[23] How in good conscience can we put the health and lives of innocent children at risk just to preserve a relatively small area of freedom for their parents? If in fact health care made little difference to the outcome of health, the problem would hardly be bothersome. But in the arena of prenatal and pediatric care in particular, some relatively modestly priced health care does appear to have considerable health payoffs.

Still, the reasonable implication to draw is merely that *maternal and child health care, not health care in general, should be provided for the poor in kind.* While the present system of prenatal/well-baby clin-

21. The philosophical literature on this issue is longstanding and extensive. J. S. Mill's *On Liberty* (1859/1947) with its "right to private action" is the classic. For contemporary reactions see Wasserstrom 1971. A distinction between "external" (other-regarding) and "personal" (self-regarding) preferences is delineated by Dworkin 1977, pp. 231–38. He argues that the former should not be counted in public policy calculations.

22. We can now see that one of the arguments for in-kind aid that Lester Thurow (1976) articulates is fundamentally mistaken: "The *reasons* for the preferences" that a neighbor has about me "are basically irrelevant. The only relevant fact is whether such preferences do or do not exist. If they do exist, there is an ... argument for restricted transfers aimed at particular goods" (emphasis added). *The only way this argument can work is by making others' preferences, not the poor's, the very ground for transfer of resources to the poor.* As explained above, any defense of a *right* of the poor to in-kind health-care aid which takes this direction is likely to be self-contradictory.

23. Twenty-seven percent of low-income families (under $7,000 income) in 1976 were without insurance coverage for their children. Four percent of families above $15,000 were without child coverage. See Rice 1979.

ics and childhood immunizations could serve as elementary parts of such a strategy, there is neither an a priori nor a definitive practical reason why such a very narrowly delineated in-kind program should spill over into providing all health-care aid in kind. And while health care for parents can admittedly—and drastically—affect the welfare of their children, the argument for government restrictions on aid is still very tough to make. We do not intervene with parental decisions to drink, to fail to work, or to do a thousand other things which indirectly but seriously affect a child's welfare. How, then, can the indirect effect of a parent's health on a child justify our restricting aid for health care to in-kind aid?

We need to ask a further question before we finally settle on this limited conclusion for in-kind maternal/child care. While we do require a child to undergo blood transfusions in special life-or-death situations in which its Jehovah's Witness parents refuse to give consent, we do not, for example, require Christian Science parents to use general medical care for their children. If we do not give the poor the freedom to spend less on child health care, why do we so easily give Christian Science parents that freedom? That religious freedom is at stake in the one case does not solve the essential problem. Nonpoor parents are at liberty to forgo health insurance or health care for their children for entirely *nonreligious* reasons. If transfer payments to the poor are a matter of justice or rights, not a privilege bestowed at the largesse of the more well-to-do, why should poor parents be required to do more than these other parents are?[24]

Perhaps there just is an inconsistency. Perhaps nonpoor as well as poor parents should be restricted in their choices, or neither should. Nevertheless, as bothersome as these points are for our society's particular legal arrangements, on balance the argument that part of any public assistance should be restricted to minimal maternal and child preventive and emergency health care still seems persuasive. The costs to innocent third-party children would otherwise seem simply too unfair to them.[25] Other externalities mount a much less effective argument for providing general health-care aid in kind.

24. It seems especially disturbing that we would respect middle-class parental autonomy even to the point of refusing lifesaving and suffering-avoiding medical care for an otherwise healthy thirteen-year-old with Down's syndrome, but insist on general in-kind health-care aid to the poor for their children. For such a case, that of Philip Bender, see Will 1980 and Annas 1979.

25. Tighter child-abuse laws and even the revolutionary-sounding idea of "licensing" parents are important proposals to consider for the very same reason. See La-Follette 1980.

3. NECESSITIES AND URGENCY

When people cannot afford health care, we tend to respond with far less hesitation to their call for help than when equally poor people cannot afford the caviar or wine that they may also want. The strength of people's claims on others for assistance apparently depends in part on what the interest is which they want help in satisfying, not just on the importance which they themselves attach to it. If people used cash aid, for example, to build a monument to their god or to buy caviar or wine and did without, say, a decent diet or useful health care, wouldn't we feel they had betrayed their original claim on us? We took that claim to involve some *urgent* interest. The monument, the caviar, and the wine seem to lack that urgency entirely.[26]

The matter may even be worse. If purely subjective preferences ultimately define a person's interest, the moral weight of an interest is determined solely by the importance that that person puts on it. This leaves us open to being "held up" for aid by people who have unusually expensive tastes.[27] "Some people derive great happiness from the simplest pleasures.... Others require the most extravagant expenditures ... before they are moderately happy. A subjective standard makes the first group the hostages of the second" in our moral calculations.[28] Shouldn't we restrict aid to the things that meet a more objective sense of urgency and need, rather than giving it in cash and letting subjective preferences determine its uses? Health care has the requisite urgency and should therefore be provided in kind.

I will criticize this argument in three stages. (1) It relies on the moral relevance of the distinction between subjective preferences and more objective necessities, urgent interests, or needs. Can that distinction carry the moral weight it must if the argument is to work? (2) Even if the distinction is morally relevant, does *health care* have the required urgency and necessity? (3) Even if health care is correctly characterized as a necessity, does it follow that we would be "held hostage" to expandable subjective tastes and desires if aid were given in cash?

26. See Scanlon 1975.
27. Scanlon 1975.
28. Fried 1978, p. 120. Fried, though, does not draw the final inference for in-kind aid from this "held hostage" argument against a subjective notion of preference. Right off he admits that the alternative, a more "objective standard," makes it difficult to avoid what he sees as "the absurdity of giving ... overcoats to people who prefer to go about in the cold in return for an extra ration of wine."

Preferences and Needs

Undoubtedly there is some difference between the desires which form needs or urgent interests and those which do not. But what difference, and how much? And is the difference morally relevant?

We fear being at the mercy of people's mere preferences more than being at the mercy of their needs or urgent interests. Needs are thought to be less voluntary in origin than preferences. People cannot deliberately expand needs to shape demands on us, and they also cannot be held so personally responsible for limiting them. Desires to spend money on religious monuments, for example, are presumably more controllable than needs for health care. What makes the distinction between needs and nonurgent interests morally relevant, then, is the controllability of the latter.

Yet are the interests we *see* as relatively involuntary and urgent perhaps simply the ones that are prevalent in the society? The very example of people preferring religious monuments to health care demonstrates that for *those* people an allegedly urgent need is relatively controllable. After all, they have curbed their desire or need for health care. Why should their interest in religious monuments, voluntarily adopted, have less moral claim on others for aid than an interest in health care that is *equally* voluntarily limited? For society to continue to think that the interest in health care is urgent is for it to have abandoned its neutrality about what constitutes the good life. This neutrality is central to the broad stream of liberalism in our political tradition.[29]

Another defense of the priority of needs focuses on the uneven rationality of preferences. Suppose the people who build a religious monument have correctly ascertained that the monument will satisfy their desires to a greater extent than the increased health care which they have passed over. Defenders of the moral relevance of the preference/need distinction might still call those desires irrational. When a person prefers to satisfy an intrinsic desire that is *not* urgent over an intrinsic desire that *is*, that preference is irrational. Perhaps, in turn, the notion of an intrinsic preference being irrational can be developed: If irrational, a preference does not survive "cognitive psychotherapy"—confront the preference with all the relevant information,

---

29. Dworkin (1978), for example, takes the treating of people "as equals" (not literally equal) as the core of liberal values. Treating people as equals requires that government remain neutral on the question of what is, for each of them, the good life. Each person defines the good life for him or herself; each is equally a chooser of the good.

repeatedly represent the things desired in accurate and vivid ways, and eliminate the effects of any false beliefs, unfortunate experiences in childhood, and so forth.[30] There is, of course, one big problem in using this to defend the urgency of health care: Who is to say that preferences for a religious monument over health will not survive cognitive psychotherapy?

While plausible, the arguments for the moral priority of needs and urgent interests over subjective preferences are far from compelling.

Health-Care Needs

Is health care a need, a necessity, an urgent interest? The surprising thing is that over a range of different countries, health-care expenditures do not show that it is. They even offer evidence that it is not. Newhouse has found that the share of GNP expended on health care rises dramatically with GNP.[31] If medical care were a necessity, one would expect the absolute amount spent on it to rise considerably more slowly than GNP; that happens, for example, with a necessity such as caloric intake of food (but not with the money spent on food—more expensive food is hardly a necessity). Among eleven developed countries with considerably varying GNPs, the ratio of the highest national caloric intake per capita to the lowest was 1.34 to 1. In the same countries, the ratio of per-capita expenditure on medical care from most to least was 6 to 1, virtually the same pattern as for fine wines and foreign travel.[32] A large portion of medical care is intended to save lives by reducing the risk of death, and in our society it is then usually thought to be a necessity. The data on comparative national expenditures throw precisely this line of thought into doubt. Even if in every society some reduction of risk of death or morbidity is regarded as a necessity, the degree of risk which it is a "necessity" to reduce floats relative to national per-capita income. Why should we also not think of the preference/necessity line floating with income levels *within* societies? Much health care, then, would not be a true necessity.

Of course it could be that people in different societies behave as if medical care were not a necessity, while it actually is. Daniels presses this strategy. Strength of preference, he says, "may vary in ways that fail to reflect the importance we *ought* ... ascribe to health care." Health needs are objective, he claims, not determined by sub-

30. Brandt 1979, pp. 111, 113, 156.
31. Newhouse 1976a.
32. Newhouse 1976a.

jective preference; they " 'endanger the normal functioning of the subject of need considered as a member of a natural species.' "[33]

But there is a complication here. While admittedly good *health*
may be a necessity, a great deal of *medical care* may not be. Just because people need to avoid suffering or dying does not mean that they
need all the things which reduce *the chances* of suffering or dying.
How much should we be willing to reduce the risks, and by what
smaller and smaller amount at what greater and greater cost? These
are matters of preference, even if health's good is independent of
preference.

Particular individuals, of course, do find themselves in situations
in which medical care seems to be a necessity. People comment, for
example, that "when a baby needs care, a mother has no choice. . . ."[34]
To be sure, a mother thinks she has no choice. At particular points in
the use of health care, of course, in a sense she really doesn't; care
sometimes is, at least morally, a necessity. We are prone to extend this
impression and mistakenly think that medical care in general is a necessity. Furthermore, while it is often inaccurate to speak of options
and free choice in getting medical care that we need at the moment,
it is perfectly sensible to speak of options and genuine choice in deciding in advance what kind of care to set up for ourselves.

Needs and Access
Nevertheless, let us suppose for the purposes of argument that most
health care is a need, a necessity, an urgent interest. And suppose that
the case for the moral relevance of the distinction between needs and
preferences is sound. Would the argument for in-kind aid then be so-
lidified? Could we be "held hostage" by people's expandable, nonurgent tastes and desires if aid were given in cash and used by some, for
example, for religious monuments? Would we have been tricked by
claims of urgency into giving aid, only to see the recipients themselves
behave as if those needs were not urgent?

To be sure, people should not be allowed to tilt a society's distribution of resources by inserting into the moral calculus a desire for
expensive caviar that is stronger than others' desire for basic food.
Would that happen if cash were the form of our aid? Would we look
to see how much more money some people need than we do to bring
themselves roughly up to our level of welfare, and determine by *that*

33. Daniels 1981, emphasis added. The passage he quotes is from Braybrooke 1968.
34. Fine 1977. Outka (1974) makes the same point in arguing, like Fine, that health
care should not be treated as a market good.

how much cash aid they were to get? Not for a minute. We would still set the level of required cash aid by reference to the general level of desires that most people can satisfy with money.[35] It is a laugh to think that the poor would hold us hostage for more and more cash assistance by their expandable and expensive preferences. The rich might do that, but hardly the poor.

Furthermore, if particular recipients used their cash aid for religious monuments and passed up common health care, should we think we had been tricked into giving them money for entirely nonessential things? I don't see why. Justice presumably requires that an affluent society guarantee that all have the opportunities or means to get the basic goods that are required for people to have a modicum of dignity or equality in that society. On *that* basis we would judge that a certain level of cash aid should be given; it is the same basis that we would use to judge that certain levels of in-kind aid should be given.[36] Then, if particular recipients were to decide that what most of us see as needs are not needs, or that other things which we do not see as needs are needs, or that what most of us think are the greater and lesser needs are in fact the reverse, why should their free choice make us feel offended, tricked, held hostage, or anything of the kind? They presumably have not received enough aid to purchase the usual standards of health care, food, shelter, and other necessities, *and* such things as caviar, wine, and religious monuments. *Surely the point of the aid is not to control recipients. It is simply to make basic necessities affordable to them. Cash aid has already done that,* whether or not they spend it on what we think are, or even what really are, their basic needs.

Undoubtedly critics will still object. We have missed, they will say, the particular role played by specific urgent needs in the argument for in-kind aid. Weale argues that "the reason for making the transfer *in the first place* is that the person is judged deficient in welfare because he does not have access to *certain* policy goods."[37] We do not then try to set any appropriate level of cash aid. Instead we move directly to figuring out what levels of various in-kind assistance to provide so that

35. The level required, say, by the justice-as-equality principle. See chap. 1, n. 46.

36. This point means that Daniels (1981) cannot get any mileage against cash aid out of an admittedly possibly correct point he makes about income distribution: We cannot simply define health-care needs by the preferences people have for this or that much health care once income is distributed justly, because one of the things we need to know in deciding what is a just minimum income is what health-care needs they have. This is similar to the point by Weale which I discuss shortly.

37. Weale 1978, p. 56, emphasis added.

the person will no longer be judged deficient in welfare. We cut off the policy option of cash aid at the start.

This is a different argument. But while at first sight it is more difficult to reject, in the last analysis it too fails. The reason is simple: it misconstrues its very own premise. Are the poor judged deficient in welfare in the first place because they do not *have* certain specific goods? If so, then the argument works; it naturally follows that those goods should be provided. But that is not the precise reason the poor are judged deficient. Even Weale does not state the initial reason for the transfer that way. He says, more plausibly, that the poor are judged deficient in welfare in the first place because they do not "have *access* to certain policy goods" (emphasis added). The natural response then is not necessarily to provide these goods themselves. Instead, it is to make them *affordable*, to give the poor realistic access to them. One way to do that, of course, is to provide these goods free, that is, give the aid in kind. But an equally plausible way is to give the poor the means to buy those goods on the market, assuming or then assuring that the market makes them available. Weale's argument ends up neutral between cash and in-kind aid.[38] Other, perhaps paternalistic arguments cannot be avoided if one is to defend in-kind assistance.

While admittedly we should not let some people's expensive or esoteric tastes hold us "hostage" in our moral calculations, the point simply generates no argument against cash. Then, too, recipients will not have shown an allegedly urgent interest to be a sham if they use the aid for other things; if their needs are independent of their actual preferences, as critics of cash tend to claim, then I would think that the urgency of their interests is not determined by their actual behavior, either. The entire argument against cash from the moral distinctiveness of necessities and urgency is lost.

4. PATERNALISM

The most common reason for providing assistance in kind is probably paternalistic: For the sake of the poor, restrict their choices. In paternalism others interfere with my behavior for *my* own good. They may interfere for the sake of my own good either as defined ultimately by

38. So also does Daniels's argument (1981). He subsumes the right to health care under a general principle of justice guaranteeing fair equality of opportunity. But equal opportunity can justify cash aid as well as in-kind programs. Isn't *access* opportunity? For criticism of Daniels's attempt to derive the notion of a decent minimum of health care from the idea of equal opportunity, see also Buchanan 1982, pp. 34–44.

me,[39] or as defined ultimately by them.[40] If paternalism is thought to be objectionable, it is usually the latter variety which is thought to be more so. To deal with the most persuasive version of the paternalistic argument for in-kind aid, we will only have to consider the former variety. The question for this section, then, is this: In order to prevent the damage to recipients' own ultimately self-defined interests which the freedom of cash would risk, should we restrict their choices by providing aid in kind? If the poor would agree that for them health really is finally more important than some other good on which they would very likely spend cash, shouldn't we provide health care in kind?

The Cycle of Poverty

In one particular circumstance paternalism is especially attractive—if the ill health that recipients allow by spending cash assistance on things other than health care is the very thing that keeps them poor.[41] Then in-kind aid is much more efficient; it is more likely to lift them out of poverty and save the society the expense of future aid. Moreover, it stands in no ultimate contradiction with their autonomy. If restriction of the aid to health care really does alleviate their poverty when cash does not, they will then have even more money—and freedom to spend it—than they would by getting cash.[42]

This argument for interference is persuasive, but it has three conditions, *each* of which must be met for the argument to work. (1) Poor health must be a major determinant of people's poverty. (2) The care provided in kind must improve that health significantly. (3) There must be a significant chance that recipients will pass up *that* care if given cash. The first condition seldom obtains. The second varies widely and depends on our general view of the effectiveness of medi-

39. That is, by my ultimate intrinsic preferences—my final preferences for things in their own right, not as a means to fulfill some other desires I have.

40. At least not as defined by me.

41. This circumstance is suggested by Posner 1972, p. 352. Despite his general sympathy with cash aid, he observes that one of its major shortcomings is that some people get and stay poor because of their poor ability to manage money.

42. It might be said that the freedom thus enlarged by in-kind aid is only one good among many, and one which some people in their freedom will not even knowingly choose. Because of this, interfering with freedom in order to create greater freedom is not justified in the name of freedom alone; the initial freedom includes the freedom to trade at least some freedom for other goals. Surely it is legitimate for people to do *some* of that kind of trading. But it would be very odd to apply this theoretical point in any real-life context. To do so would be to claim that some poor people would freely and knowingly choose to stay in poverty, to forgo their later greater freedom of having more money with which to choose which goods to buy. It is doubtful that they would.

cine. As for the third condition, it is likely to hold only if this care or the insurance for it is very expensive, professional health care has a bad image among the poor, or care for the poor is unavailable in the medical market into which cash aid would feed. It seems unlikely that *all* of these three conditions will often be met.

Classic Paternalism

A more common paternalistic argument focuses on a more general point: Health care has greater final value to the poor than the goods they would probably choose instead. Is not a poor recipient likely to forgo insurance to have more for immediate needs and desires? We all know how this can happen. If all along we have had little for enjoyments, the temptation to forgo investments in future welfare for more immediate gratifications becomes practically irresistible. For health care this temptation is compounded by our perception, when we are well, that insurance is an investment we are not assured of getting even *any* future returns on. Correctly, but undoubtedly foolishly, we keep thinking that we might not get ill.

Several things need to be kept in mind here. For the poor the monetary value of reducing a given risk is less than it is for others, but for them the value of insuring against the costs of truly costworthy care is generally greater than it is for the more well-to-do.[43] That does not cancel out legitimate willingness to take risk, nor does it negate the autonomy that willingness reflects. It only means that the poorer they are, the greater the human welfare costs of that willingness are likely to be, and thus the larger the benefits of paternalistic interference. Clearly, however, that does not allow us to impose *our* aversions to risk on them when theirs are different.[44]

Another factor that influences the relationship of the present benefits of using cash for other things to the benefits of insuring, which largely lie in the future, is the "discount rate." There are very different views of what this rate represents. Generally we think that the value of future benefits is reduced when they are weighed against present ben-

43. See 5.3.

44. Though risk-aversion is one of the ultimate intrinsic desires with which I define my own welfare, it can also be viewed as a way of looking at my other desires. Thus, when others substitute their risk-aversions for mine in judging what is my welfare, they may argue that they are doing the same thing as when they "correct" other of my factually mistaken instrumental desires of one thing for the sake of another. My quarrel with this argument is that the "looking at" one's other desires that risk-aversion involves is not strictly an instrumental desire, that is, a desiring of one thing as necessary to another more intrinsically desired thing.

efits, and therefore they should get discounted. To get people to bargain away present benefits in order to enjoy future ones, the future ones have to be somewhat enlarged at the time they occur. Some economists have thought that this very real, legitimate, current weakness of more distant pleasures largely explains the charging of interest for loans. Others, however, argue that discounting reflects only an irrational, weak ability to imagine the future. Perhaps an intermediate position is the most persuasive: "*To the extent* to which preference for a nearer event derives from inadequate representation of the temporally more remote event, *then it is irrational.*"[45]

Apply this to poor people making choices about whether or not to use their cash aid to buy health insurance. Individuals in various circumstances can have legitimately different discount rates. Poor people will usually discount future enjoyments (and inflate present ones) more than the nonpoor do, due to the real pressure of their circumstances, not necessarily to any weakness of character or irrationality. To the extent, however, that the poor's higher discount rate reflects an inadequate representation of future events, their preference for present consumption is irrational. The press of present needs will undoubtedly make the poor more likely to represent future events inaccurately; to that extent their greater discount rate will be irrational. And to that extent the prediction that they will cause harm to themselves with cash, harm that can be prevented by aid in kind, is well founded. Perhaps, too, we would create relatively little conflict with the principle of autonomy by imposing decisions on others when their own choices would largely be made in ignorance. Probably the extent of that conflict finally depends on how much we think people are responsible for their own ignorance; where apparently they are not, we do not even seem to stand in tension with their real autonomy when we impose our judgments (see 2.6).

This much we can easily grant to the argument against cash. But the major moral question still remains: Doesn't genuine, long-term *respect* for the poor require that they be given the responsibility of cash? Assuming that the poor want to take responsibility for the dangers of making harmful decisions themselves, the moral conflict between autonomy and welfare is especially sharp. There is no easy resolution, and any which is attempted will involve the most basic discussions of moral philosophy on questions of autonomy and well-being. Some object to paternalism on the basis of the intrinsic value of autonomy. Others, for example, J. S. Mill, construct an allegedly utilitarian argu-

45. Brandt 1979, p. 80.

ment for never interfering with a person's private choices when they are free and not grossly misinformed.[46] Once a society has been allowed to interfere to increase the person's own welfare, Mill queries, where has there been a society that has stopped with only helpful interventions? Societies always end up also interfering in many cases in which the person would gain in the long run by being left free and responsible. Thus, a policy of permitting any interventions at all ends up decreasing human welfare. Thoreau's trenchant comment reflects the same point: "If I knew for a certainty that a man was coming to my house with the conscious design of doing me good, I should run for my life."[47]

No matter how reluctant we are here to step into this very large debate, whatever decision we make about the in-kind/cash aid dilemma in the case of health care ought to be consistent with our views on other dilemmas about paternalism in medicine. Suppose we are convinced that people have a moral and legal right to refuse lifesaving medical treatment even when their judgments about the quality of prolonged life are based on flawed if understandable imaginations of its quality.[48] Or suppose we think we should not give placebos even to patients who would benefit from them,[49] or should not interfere coercively with smokers in any attempt to alter their choices and behavior.[50] Wouldn't it then be inconsistent, subtly discriminatory, and blatantly condescending toward the poor if we switched to a paternalistic policy when we considered their health care?

Contracted Paternalism

This conflict between the autonomy and the welfare of the poor would largely dissolve if the poor actually wanted to be restricted to in-kind aid. Their wishes would constitute a kind of "contracted paternalism," paternalism which they contract for.[51] It may in fact be a realistic interpretation of what happens with in-kind aid. People may

46. See Mill 1859/1947.
47. Henry David Thoreau, quoted by Friedman in Friedman and Cohen 1972.
48. White 1975; Engelhardt 1975; Platt 1975.
49. Bok 1974; Brody 1975, 1977.
50. Wikler 1978.
51. It is questionable, of course, whether it has the full ring of "paternalism." Is interference in my life that I myself have requested beforehand really interference with my autonomy, or is it in fact the very carrying out of my autonomous request? The latter, it would seem. There is thus little if anything ultimately "paternalistic" about it. For the sake of convenience, however, I will retain the term. I suppose a better one is simply "contracted interference."

not in fact want a wide range of choice, for fear that they will make foolish decisions.[52] For Robert Ball, former Social Security administrator, whether to have a compulsory system of social insurance is not really "an issue of whether people *ought* to save sufficiently on their own, or even whether theoretically they could." They ought to, and they could. But they don't.[53] Compulsory social insurance is widespread precisely because people know that while they ought to save or insure on their own, they very probably won't. Reasonably, they have taken the immediate decision out of their own hands.

This argument depends entirely on the premise that the poor have in fact consented to their own restrictions to assistance in kind. But have they? In many private arrangements for withholding health-insurance premiums from employees' paychecks, there is little doubt that individuals have consented; *they* chose to remove the temptation posed by wider immediate choice. But is there any evidence that the poor have given this kind of individual consent to government health insurance? They haven't even had the opportunity to show that consent. The opportunity could easily be created simply by offering the poor aid in kind while allowing individual requests to change it to cash for long blocks of time. Nothing like that is currently provided.

Alternately, consent may come not individually, but through some political process. If in this way the poor consent to the restriction of aid, we would then face only a conflict with the autonomy of some individual recipients who still prefer cash. It would now be a different problem—not paternalism, but the extent of political authority of the poor as a group over individual poor people. But in any case, there is little evidence that the poor have made such a group decision through the political process. That is extremely important. One major thrust for cash aid is that health care may well be overvalued for the poor, *given their other needs*. There must be some way for these other needs to be voiced and their provision shaped by the poor; otherwise we will properly remain suspicious that the needs of the poor for medical care have gotten relatively overvalued in our policies.

Since in our present system both individual and group consent of the poor to restricted aid are lacking, "contracted paternalism" cannot resolve anything. We are left with the sharper conflict between autonomy and welfare, the classic form of paternalism, and the need to be consistent with policies that are apparently nonpaternalistic vis-à-vis other conflicts between autonomy and welfare. Paternalistic defenses

52. Fuchs 1979.
53. Ball 1978, pp. 5–6.

of in-kind aid just don't seem to resolve the debate. They only high-light the autonomy of the poor which is at stake in cash.

5. MARKET CHOICES AND THE IDEAL OF JUSTICE

Some societies directly provide health care for everyone at a common, equal, and allegedly minimally decent level. Witness the British National Health Service.[54] One dominant reason for thus providing health care equally and in kind is the vision of a just society.[55] If poor recipients were to take their assistance in cash and spend it on other things, their purchases would reflect the still unjust distribution of income. They would purchase less health care than they would in a society in which income and wealth were distributed more justly. To be sure, people in that more just society would not have completely equal incomes,[56] and in any case they would have varying preferences about how much to spend on health care. Furthermore, that society might itself use cash aid, if it had any need for aid at all. Nevertheless, in our society an equal distribution of health care will much more closely approximate the distribution in a perfectly just society than giving cash assistance and letting the market then distribute the care. Instead of representing society's paternalistic control of the poor for their own good, equal in-kind assistance reflects a commitment to this vision of justice. This is the "ideal-of-justice" argument for in-kind aid.

Initial Injustice
Almost everyone agrees that an effective way to argue against the moral weight of market choices is to find the initial distribution of assets unfair or unjust. Even libertarian defenders of market rights admit that the initial distribution must not be unfair if the results of subsequent free exchanges are to be morally binding.[57] But does that mili-

54. While government provision of care in Britain is designed to be equal, the final distribution of all care is not designed to be. Individuals are allowed, entirely at their own expense, to forgo the free NHS care and purchase other care privately. For discussions of whether such a choice should be allowed, see Telfer 1976 and Steiner 1976.

55. Robert Veatch of the Kennedy Institute of Ethics first articulated this argument to me.

56. See chap. 3, n. 13.

57. For example see Nozick 1974. He and Rawls (1971) agree on this point but then part company in interpreting it. Nozick takes the initial arrangement of unequal natural talents and family inheritances from ancestors' justly earned wealth to be neither unjust nor unfair. Rawls, by contrast, does take it to be unfair in a sense; he constructs the original contracting position for the derivation of subsequent moral principles by effectively removing unequal natural talents and inheritances through his device of the "veil of ignorance."

tate against cash and for in-kind assistance, as the ideal-of-justice argument supposes?

Suppose that the distribution of income is unjust and inequitable. Isn't the proper response either to redistribute income or to reform the social structure so that income gets distributed more justly? The former certainly seems more closely allied with cash than with in-kind assistance. And not even the latter leans toward in-kind aid. It would, if we thought that a justly restructured society would itself distribute health care equally in kind, instead of only producing a just distribution of monetary income. But are there any persuasive arguments that a justly restructured society would do that?[58] If it is merely assumed that a restructured society would include in-kind provision of equal health care rather than justly distributed income, the very question of this whole chapter has been begged.

Political Realities

Defenders of the argument may still persist, citing the fact that in our society greater equality of health care results from providing it in kind than in cash. Providing enough cash aid to approximate a just redistribution of income, it will be noted, is not politically feasible, but we should still try to emulate the pattern of spending on health care in a more just society. Yet this only raises further questions.

Suppose the amount of cash aid that the society is willing to provide is large enough for recipients to prefer it over a greater dollar-per-recipient in-kind aid. Why, then, when we are trying to help and respect the poor, should we give them more of what they do not want rather than less of what they do?[59] Shouldn't we leave to the poor the

58. The only arguments I can readily come up with are the "inalienable-rights," "last-resort," and "fair-burdens-of-the-well" arguments I pick up in the next two sections. I think they are not persuasive, however. The inalienable rights argument, I will conclude, just does not wash. The last-resort argument, while powerful in our society, would surely not be valid in a nearly just society; we could refuse to rescue those who had chosen much less health insurance than they turned out to need without even facing the criticism that unjust conditions had pressed them into going cheap on insurance. The fair-burdens-of-the-well argument, I will explain, also does not finally require in-kind provision of health care.

59. There is obviously a bind here with the principle of autonomy for the poor. Thus Veatch (1979a) at first struck me as inconsistent in defending in-kind provision of equal health care while at the same time remaining "enough of a voluntarist to believe that one has both the right and the power to take such risks" to life and health as smoking or mountain climbing. Privately he has explained away the apparent inconsistency In a more nearly just society, some would smoke and some would not, but all would be roughly equally willing to spend on needed health care. Therefore, restricting the freedom of smokers emulates no ideal of a just society, whereas restricting health-care aid

choice of whether to sacrifice some preference of theirs for the sake of emulating a more nearly just society? If they consent to the sacrifice, then in-kind aid will presumably be justified. But in our own society there is little reason to think they have consented to do that.

Suppose the alternate condition: Political realities push any level of cash aid so much lower than restricted in-kind health-care assistance that the poor themselves would prefer aid in kind. Consent then appears to justify in-kind aid. Even here, however, other serious questions arise. *Why* would a society be willing to provide more expensive aid in kind than in cash? We are driven back either to problematic paternalistic arguments or to the suspicion that society wishes to control the lives of the poor as its taxpayers' prerogative, or to propagate its middle-class values, or to serve the interests of professional providers.[60] If it is aims such as these which drive society's policy, giving political support to a policy of restricted aid hardly seems to be the best way of focusing on the ideal of a more economically just society. On the other hand, if society's genuine concern is to emulate a more egalitarian society, why does it not go to greater lengths to redistribute income itself or to restructure the very processes from which great and widespread economic inequalities emerge?

We should not for one minute criticize a decision of the poor to take the greater in-kind aid under these political realities. In that sense and from their immediate perspective, in-kind aid may be justified. That hardly justifies the society, however, in insisting on in-kind aid and thus creating the very political reality under which the poor consent to the best they can get. There is no argument here for *the society* to think that restriction of aid is justified.

Coerced Choices

There is another interesting argument against cash. Suppose we regard people's poverty as largely and usually not their fault, but due to the way society is organized. Furthermore, suppose that the organi-

---

to aid in kind rather than in cash does. I entirely agree—there is no necessary inconsistency in defending in-kind aid *and* the right of smokers to damage their health. Fried is mistaken in his apparent belief that allowing mountain climbers to risk their lives is the same as permitting cash-aid recipients not to purchase insurance. See Fried 1978, p. 128.

60. Some observers think the society demands greater direct benefits than these before it will support assistance for the poor. The programs must be universal and include the nonpoor, for only then will there be sufficient taxpayer interest in the programs to sustain them at a level of respectable quality. For example, one might argue for a universal social security system by maintaining that "a program that is only for the poor ... is, in the long run, a program the American public won't support." See Cohen and Friedman 1972, p. 55.

zation of income and wealth and their resultant inequalities are largely unjust.[61] Suppose this injustice is largely correctable. Poor people choose to spend considerably less for health care even with cash assistance than do other people, and the reason they do is the pressure of their other needs. These choices might then be called "coerced." Society is really the party responsible for those choices,[62] and providing the poor the opportunity to make them is a merely "coercive offer" to the poor.[63]

A root analogy would be of a person forcibly exposed to deprived conditions in a one-employer town, with the result that the person "chooses" to work for fifty cents an hour. The party responsible for the deprived and monopolistic conditions is the party really responsible for the "choice." An offer is morally objectionable if the situation in which it is received is unjust or unfair, if the party making the offer was responsible for the development of the injustice, and if that party can correct it. Either the choice made by the individual is said not to be free, or it does not carry the usual moral weight which free choices do.

This precisely describes the situation with market choices for health care that obtains in a society with correctable injustices in the distribution of income. Poor people would not willingly spend so little on health care were it not for the unjust inequalities, and society is responsible for the correctable injustices. For society then to give cash to the poor and allow its providers of health care and other services to make offers to them is for society to have coerced the subsequent choices. The freedom of the wider consumer choice which morally drives cash aid is lost. Cash loses all of its even prima facie attractiveness, and in-kind aid rules the day, without any need of a further argument.

This is indeed an elegant defense of in-kind aid. Quite plainly, however, there has to be something wrong with it, for its implications are extreme and unacceptable. If the distribution of income and wealth is injust, and if, as the argument grants, society is responsible for this injustice and could correct it, *every* choice influenced by that

61. To say that poverty is not the fault of the poor and to say that it is unjust are to say two different things. Poverty could be not the poor's fault and still be just. For example, under Rawls's "difference principle" it could be that (see Rawls 1971). The inequality between the poor and relatively well-to-do might provide enough incentives and other benefits to the society that the poor are actually better off with the inequity than with a more egalitarian arrangement.

62. See 3.4.

63. This version of the ideal-of-justice argument for in-kind aid was also first suggested to me by Robert Veatch of the Kennedy Institute. For a helpful, general analysis of the entire notion of "coercive offers" on which the argument turns, see Zimmerman 1981.

background of injustice is coerced and morally invalid. That means, for practical purposes, that nearly every market choice of all the many persons disadvantaged by an injustice is morally vacuous.[64] But why should all these market choices be morally invalid? They are coerced only in a particular sense. People's choices in even much more immediately coercive situations—for example, in prisons—may be free. An at least plausible argument can be constructed for saying that the choices of prisoners to be subjects for risky medical research ought to be honored.[65] To say in general that none of the preferences of disadvantaged persons as expressed in market choices carries any claim to be honored is to deprive these individuals of a large part of the only real life they have. That view is insulting, to say the least.

The ideal-of-justice argument for in-kind aid is thus extremely problematic. Only a sharply conditioned version of it is persuasive: The poor are justified in consenting to greater in-kind aid when the political realities create much less aid in the form of cash. That doesn't justify the *society*, however, in insisting on the priority of in-kind aid to begin with.

6. INALIENABLE RIGHTS

How does health care compare with certain other things which we do not allow into the market but try to distribute equally, for example, voting and other political rights?[66] Suppose we accept a positive right to health care—then society should guarantee, not merely permit, access to health care for all people. The question at the center of this chapter remains: Should people be able to trade off that basic assurance of care for something else? Should they be able to give up—to alienate—their right to health care?

In our society the clearest case of an inalienable right is probably the right to vote. Not only do we not allow people to sell their long-term right to vote; we also do not allow people to sell their particular votes.[67] Are there parallel arguments for making the right to health

64. I imagine some will say, "Well, yes, nearly every market choice of every person disadvantaged by injustice really is coerced and morally irrelevant—so be it, that's what the argument demonstrates." In response to them, I resort to the next argument in the text.

65. Cohen 1978.

66. Thurow (1976) mentions the precedent of equal voting rights for the provision of equal health care and simply accepts it uncritically.

67. People's votes, of course, may in a sense be "bought." But vote buying happens only informally; it is never sanctioned by the state. People do not, for example, advertise their votes to be for sale, nor do buyers openly put out bids for them. Finally, even if you "buy" my vote, *I* still have to cast it.

care inalienable? In both voting and health care we assume that people may not sell their long-term rights, their *access* to health care or the vote. But in voting we also do not allow people to sell their particular votes. If health care is equivalent, we should not allow people to take money in place of insurance for care.[68]

Why do most of us think so strongly that people should not be allowed to sell their votes? The essential reason derives directly from the reason we give people a right to vote at all. Let me borrow from Cohen's justification of democracy.[69] All persons have roughly equal "concern" with the outcomes of the political process; all have a roughly equal potential to be adversely affected by political decisions. All people also have equal "standing" to participate in making political decisions at the *basic* and *voting* level of the political process, though not necessarily at any more final stages of policy formation. There is no equally good way to ensure that their roughly equal concerns will not be ignored.

Now look at vote selling in light of this. One goal of public policies is economic justice. Poor people are more likely than the relatively rich to sell their voting rights to another party. As a result, the people who have perhaps the heaviest stake in policy decisions affecting economic distribution will be precisely those least likely to have a voice even at the most initial, basic level of the political process. That violates the logic of the very justification of democracy itself. Furthermore, as those people who would buy the votes of the poor thereby get more and more political power, they will have a freer hand in engineering the economic policies which keep the poor disadvantaged. The harder they can make it on the poor, the more, and the more

68. The parallel of voting rights to health care may still not be the ideal one to pick for this discussion. A better parallel would be a positive right that the state must pay money to provide. Only in a minimal sense is voting a positive right that the state must pay to provide. Without charge, the state provides the mechanism for voting, counts the ballots, etc., but the state does not save any noticeable amount of money when various individuals decide not to vote. The individual who might not want to vote is not in a position to say to the state, "Why don't you give me the money you save from *my* not voting. If I get some cash from you instead of exercising my right to vote, you're not out any money." Thus cash aid has a realistic financial plausibility for the state in the case of health care that is missing in the case of voting. A closer parallel, perhaps, is the right to legal counsel. I shall keep it in mind in this section. Nevertheless I will retain the more explicit focus on voting rights. Our convictions about inalienability are much more secure for the right to vote than for the right to counsel. The same serious question arises for counsel almost as easily as for health care: If a defendant wishes to have $500 cash instead of a court-appointed attorney for a trial, why should he or she not be allowed to have it? The right to counsel, therefore, cannot serve to *anchor* an argument for the inalienability of the right to health care as well as the right to vote might.

69. Cohen 1971.

cheaply, the poor will be willing to sell votes, and the easier it will be for them to purchase the political power by which in turn they can make it still harder on the poor. The poor will have no hope of getting out of this vicious cycle.[70] Therefore, we disallow vote selling.

But where are the parallels in the case of health care? What is the basic, initial decision-making process of the society, parallel to voting, that forgoing health care or health insurance assuredly cuts one out of? Where is the vicious-cycle character of opting for cash rather than for health care, parallel to the vicious cycle of poor people selling their votes? We have already discounted the significance of the possibility that it is forgoing health care which often keeps the poor poor (see 4.4). Where is the already advantaged group which has an interest in getting poor people to forgo health care? If anything, advantaged groups (at least health-care providers) have an interest in the opposite.

We also do not allow people either to sell their *right* to vote or to buy extra votes. The reasoning here is identical to the reasoning behind not permitting them to sell their initial votes. Again, the parallels with health care begin to break down. They could be preserved by not allowing people to buy extra health care beyond what the state provides equally to all. To be sure, a plausible case can be made for not allowing people to do that.[71] But for various reasons, our society has decided to allow people to buy extra care. Even the British with their National Health Service have decided to. Probably the most important reason is that health care, rather than always being a necessity, is often an amenity. If it is, and if we are going to let stand the differences in income that allow people to purchase amenities and luxuries in general, then we should also allow them to purchase that health care which is more than a necessity. The principles of equality that drive both the ban on buying extra votes and the ban on selling one's own vote do not carry over into health care.

The strongly inalienable character of rights essential to democracy does not carry over to the right to health care. Any case that the right to health care should be inalienable will have to be established independently. Theoretically we could make a case for it with arguments like the ones for in-kind provision of health care that we considered previously in this chapter, but they have been rejected.

70. Unless the price that they got for their voting rights were so high that by selling them they could gain more power in other ways than what they lost by selling their votes. This outcome is unlikely, however. If the market price were that high, it would signal that the advantaged gained a great deal from the sale, presumably enough to enhance their control.

71. Telfer 1976.

7. TWO REMAINING ARGUMENTS

Two of the strongest arguments for in-kind health care aid remain. One is the "last-resort" argument: If a person receiving cash assistance forgoes health insurance and then later urgently needs care, it is unthinkable that we would deny it to that person; yet providing it allows the person unfairly to have cash for other things and now for health care too. A second argument concerns the allocation of costs between the well and the ill. When given cash, the well and likely well are more apt to forgo insurance than the ill and likely ill. Their forgoing the insurance drives up its cost for those recipients who do buy it, the more likely ill. Thus the well escape their just and equal share of the costs of insurance.

The Last-Resort Argument

In its usual version this is an "externality" argument.[72] If I forgo health insurance, I may end up burdening others. They are likely, in the last analysis, to offer me care when I get ill; even if they do not, they at least suffer anguish from having to face the decision of whether to provide me urgent care. The effect my choices about insuring will have on others justifies their restriction.

There is an obvious and sharp reply. Since I have decided not to insure, haven't I shown my willingness to take the consequences of not being provided care if I should need it? Instead of restricting my choice, why don't you just make it clear to me that you will not provide care if I have not insured? If the fact that you will provide me care anyhow is what leads you to change my freedom with cash to restricted, in-kind aid, I will say I even *want* you not to help. Not only do I expect you not to help; I may even want you not to feel anguish about the matter.

This reply seems compelling if we take seriously our consideration for the autonomy and responsibility of the poor, which underlies the entire case for cash. I think even the most dyed-in-the-wool libertarians, however, still wonder how realistic a reply it is. Does it fly in the face of some stubborn facts of life about human reactions? To be sure, when I decide not to insure I may be perfectly willing to go unaided should I need care. It may also be that morally I *should* not be aided, and that we all agree I should not. But, come the time that I actually do need lifesaving or disability-preventing care, won't your virtually inevitable reaction in abstaining from care still be one of an-

72. Blumstein and Zubkoff 1973.

guish, even if I do not finally want you to help, and even if you agree you should not? Your sympathy for me will be accentuated by what you know about the circumstances in which I decided not to insure—poverty, with its competing other needs. Unless cash aid is given at a level to make economic distribution fully just, won't you inevitably feel guilty if you do not now give me the urgently needed care? Won't you feel at least a bit responsible for the choice—even though it was my choice—that led to the present dilemma?

The conclusion that aid should be given somewhat in kind is then imminent. There is, however, a way to avoid it: Insist that *your* anguish is *your* problem. In fact, isn't that precisely what it is? *It* surely isn't *my* responsibility as a welfare recipient who didn't insure myself. Out of respect for my decisions, in fact, you ought not to indulge in your anguish! Therefore you are not justified in restricting my choices. As to your guilt about the conditions which led to the choice that now leaves me in need of health care I cannot afford—again, isn't that *your* problem? I have still made my own choices. Unless I consent somehow to the restriction of choice which in-kind aid involves, why should you feel guilty? And even if you do feel guilty, why does that lead you to give me last-resort care instead of redoubling your efforts to get me a more just income?

Logically this defense of cash seems compelling. Probably, however, all of us still have doubts that our society will ever be steel-nerved enough to be able to take this line in the midst of medical crisis. Suspicions that our anguish and our guilt are not just "our problem" keep creeping back in. Still, what really is the *argument* here against cash? The argument that clearly would work claims that in some way the poor have consented to a policy that would rescue them even when they haven't insured (at the cost to them, of course, of having to pay their fair, prorated share of its cost). But doesn't that consent constitute the "contracted paternalism" argument already discussed and rejected (4.4)?

Furthermore, even if the last-resort argument should be accepted, we would need to add two qualifications to it. First, the argument will restrict the options not only of the poor but also of any *nonpoor* persons who choose not to insure and then cannot pay for certain expensive, urgently needed care. Won't the conclusion of the argument be a *universal* insurance program for financially catastrophic, emergency care? Second, the argument will not entail compulsory insurance for all kinds of unaffordable care—only the most urgent and financially catastrophic.

Sharing Costs

An additional, last argument against cash concerns justly allocating the costs of illness. The well should share the expenses of illness equally with the ill. But those who buy low-option health insurance, or none at all, are more apt to be well than ill. Even banning "experience-rated" premiums (based on prospective need of the person for care) will not resolve the problem; some will still choose not to insure at all. If the reason they did not insure were only lower aversion to financial risk, or greater skepticism about the efficacy of medical care, or a lower value on health relative to other goods that led some cash-aid recipients to choose less or no insurance, we would not object to their absence from the insurance pool. The others who would thereby pay higher premiums would simply be paying for their different values. Such legitimate individual differences undoubtedly explain why some persons will buy little insurance. But since it is undoubtedly impossible to separate adherence to different values from the mere expectation of remaining healthy and not needing much care, we must require all to insure.

It is worth considering other resolutions of this problem, however, before requiring in-kind aid. We could give more cash aid to the likely ill in proportion to the higher health insurance premiums they may choose to pay. Cash aid would be adjusted by people's actuarial health-care expense category. Then we could permit people their choice about insurance without creating greater burdens on the ill.[73] Undoubtedly people will object to this suggestion as administratively impractical, but perhaps it is not. If it has administrative costs, they might be warranted by the moral resolution it permits: We preserve the autonomy of cash aid without financially burdening the ill more than the well.

8. CONCLUSION

We have considered an array of diverse arguments for in-kind aid. Externality arguments emphasize the positive effects on others of designating aid for health care.[74] Necessity and urgency arguments criticize cash aid for mistaking the very basis of a society's initial decision to

73. See 6.2 for a similar point about health insurance options for everyone, not just the poor. Also, some inequity will still result if actuarial categories are less accurate an indicator of likely wellness than people's own sense of their health is. The most-well people may still be less likely to insure than the less-well in the same actuarial category. Premiums will then be higher for those who do insure than if all insured.

74. See 4.2.

assist the poor. Paternalistic arguments restrict aid for the poor's own good. The ideal-of-justice and inalienable-rights arguments focus on basic equalities of a just society. The last-resort argument blends humanitarian, paternalistic, and fairness considerations. Furthermore, these arguments are often complex, making subtle distinctions and presupposing other positions of social philosophy. Amidst all that, I have added to potential confusion with a mixture of evaluations, usually refuting arguments for in-kind aid, but occasionally accepting them. The need for a summary is urgent.

Several considerations run against restricting the aid to health care. (1) The externality arguments for generally providing health care in kind dissolve if the basis of assistance is justice for the poor, not the largesse or preferences of others. There are two exceptions: the maternal and child health-care portion of health care, and the circumstance in which taxpayers will contribute enough extra restricted aid that the poor will prefer it to the lesser cash. (2) The most persuasive version of the necessity and urgency arguments implies only that we should make minimally decent health care *accessible* to the poor. That, in turn, is neutral as between cash and in-kind assistance. (3) Paternalistic arguments against cash stand in tension with popular and apparently nonpaternalistic ethical policies in other areas of health care. There is little evidence of consent, on either the individual or political group level, to paternalistic policies that would dissolve the conflict with the autonomy of the poor. (4) Ideal-of-justice arguments generate policies of general social reform or income redistribution, not policies of restricted aid; if mistakenly used as arguments for in-kind aid, they deny poor persons a major part of the only real life of choice they have. These arguments work for in-kind aid only given the political reality of society's willingness to fund more in-kind aid than cash. Political realities, however, are no justification of *society's* restricting the aid, but only of the poor's self-interested preference for in-kind aid *given* those unfortunate realities. (5) The arguments for inalienable political rights do not transfer into arguments for restricted aid for health care. (6) The last-resort argument reflects our own inability, psychologically, to stick by the logical arguments against it. Even if it did work, it would justify only provision of minimal, low-style, catastrophic and emergency care. It would also require a program that is universal, not just for the poor. (7) If we would apportion cash assistance by actuarial health-insurance-premium category, the costs of illness could be borne equally by the well and the ill without the need to resort to in-kind restriction. (8) Even if some particular arguments do finally favor restricted aid, the principle of autonomy still tugs toward cash. The burden of proof should fall on the defenders of restricted aid.[75] Only a coerced character to the poor's choices with cash can remove this presumption.

Only two arguments for restricting aid to health care are persuasive, and they are sharply qualified. (1) Maternal and child health care is required as long as we give greater weight to the protection of innocent children than to the autonomy of adult recipients of cash. Ideally, however, such a program should be universal rather than only for the poor. (2) Though the society is not justified in giving general health-care aid in lieu of cash, political realities may not permit as much aid in cash as in kind. In that case it is the prerogative of the poor to take the best they can. But we must always remember: The society is not thereby justified in being unwilling to give equal cash to begin with.

If no such political realities lead the poor to choose in-kind programs beyond the universal maternal and child health care just mentioned, several things will need to be emphasized. Both the principle of autonomy of recipients and the fact that ultimately only they can determine what care is costworthy lean heavily toward casting the maternal and child care program in *voucher* form, not as direct government insurance for or delivery of the care.[76] Beyond this maternal and child coverage, the government might need to take a very active role in stimulating low-style plans to aid recipients, plans that are geographically accessible and genuinely costworthy to the poor. Undoubtedly there are barriers and disincentives against that kind of care in the outlook of providers. These need to be overturned or compensated for, or else the poor will get shortchanged by the market in using their cash aid. For example, one characteristic of plans most costworthy for the poor might be a greater emphasis on preventive care, but there may be few incentives for private providers to deliver it. Costworthiness considerations for the poor may not so much demand lesser amounts as different styles and kinds of care.

If, on the other hand, political realities lead the poor themselves to prefer more across-the-board in-kind aid, then as faithful an attempt as possible must still be made to keep health-care programs in balance with other needs. "In balance" must be ultimately determined

75. Even Thurow, who otherwise defends in-kind aid, acknowledges this burden of proof. See Thurow 1976.

76. For further discussion of voucher arrangements, see 4.2.

by the poor's own intrinsic preferences. The middle class's desire for tax advantages for health care and its presumptions about the effectiveness and costworthiness of particular levels of care must not skew priorities. If recipients are unable to influence allocation nearly as directly as they can with cash aid, a skewing of priorities may be difficult to prevent. Vouchers for health care may be of some help in this respect.

Undoubtedly there will still be a tendency to regard a morally equitable distribution of health care as one in which no group receives substantially lower levels of service than the average. The delivery of lower levels of health-care services to the poor, however, is not necessarily any sign of inequity. We are very apt to feel that it is, because of an association of "lower levels of care" with practices in which health care for the poor has been provided as "charity" at austere and humiliatingly low levels. Defending legitimately different levels of care for rich and poor has nothing in common with that patronizing view. Also, choosing cash does not at all ignore the perhaps persuasive arguments for more fundamental reform of a system that produces great economic inequalities. Providing lower levels of care for the poor out of recognition of their other needs may in fact keep our eyes focused on the fundamental problems of social justice more effectively than any commitment to equal levels of health care for all would. We need to see it not as a moral heresy, fracturing our fundamental commitment to equality, but as an old respect for the equal moral worth of each person's freedom.[77]

The arguments for comprehensive and equal in-kind health-care aid, then, largely fail. That failure preserves and reflects a role for variations in the monetary value of life and health care with income. The model of willingness-to-pay is one that is neither morally corrupt nor impotent for evaluating reductions in risk.

77. For an interesting exchange on the question of equality in health care, see Gerber 1975 and Cazort 1975.

CHAPTER FIVE

The Value of Insurance

In important respects the culprit in escalating health-care costs is insurance. Once they have insured for care, patients have little incentive to refrain from using it, though its benefits may be small, its costs high, and its contribution to rising insurance premiums clear. Insurance gives physicians a freer hand to do all that they can regardless of cost, as of course they are inclined to do anyway. As insurance becomes more extensive they may also raise their fees. Furthermore, the more comprehensive the insurance, the more quickly hospitals adopt technologies whose benefits are often small or unproven.[1]

At the same time, however, insurance is an indispensable aid to making costworthy decisions. Aren't we able to weigh the value of care more honestly and accurately when we do not have to pay for it all at once? We are often able to make rational decisions about whether to incur the cost of a certain procedure only when, because of insurance, we can spread its cost over a period of time longer than the illness itself. Here, instead of disrupting costworthy decisions which patient and provider would otherwise make, insurance makes them possible. Insurance also has other important functions—providing financial security and reflecting a prior commitment not to let immediate financial strains deflect us from needed care.

Now suppose that in fact insurance has enormously raised the total cost of care and encouraged a great deal of care that has only slight benefits. If, nevertheless, the value of insurance outweighs these bad results, then the care made possible by insurance will indeed still be costworthy. Of course we have to ask seriously whether its value does

1. See Feldstein 1973 and Russell 1979.

outweigh its bad results. If so, is that less true—and how much less?—for first-dollar expenses than for catastrophic ones? As true—or more—for the poor as for the rich?

In this chapter I will discuss these values and costs of insurance, make some observations about their relative weight, draw some implications for first-dollar as compared to catastrophic coverage, and reflect on the implications of that entire discussion for the poor as compared to the rich. Finally, I will apply the previous observations to current political debates about the relative merits of various health insurance plans, those that offer relatively comprehensive coverage and those that cover financial catastrophes only.

1. BENEFITS AND COSTS

Insuring ourselves for health care has three major benefits. It gives us financial security. It spreads the costs of illness more fairly between well and ill. And it assures that we will get care when we need it.

Financial Security

There are various things we can insure for in relation to illness. We can insure against the costs of medical care we will want and need if we get sick, and we can insure against the loss of income stemming from illness. These fall under our concern for *financial* security: If we become ill, we may incur sizable expenses for care or a significant loss of income, and we want to reduce our attendant financial liability. Another possible aim of insurance is less directly concerned with financial security: We might insure to compensate ourselves for the loss of comfort we experience when ill.[2]

Why do we want this financial protection? Part of the answer has to do with diminishing marginal utility. As the income and wealth available to us increase, the value of an extra dollar to us decreases; conversely, as our available wealth and income fall, the value of each additional dollar we lose increases. Thus, in order to maximize the overall value of financial assets, then, we will forgo some of our own earnings in good times in order to have more in bad. This benefit of insurance is more than enough to make up for its administrative cost. Not to be adequately insured, then, is to take a welfare loss.[3] Our aversion to financial risks is rooted in a rational assessment of diminishing marginal utility, not just in fear or cowardice.

2. Arrow 1963.
3. Arrow 1963.

In addition to spreading out our assets over time to maximize utility, security has a less financially calculated dimension, one whose attraction may be even more powerful. It not only focuses on increasing the value of our money if we should need care; it is also security for us *now*. If we are insured, already now we need not worry about having to shell out a lot of money for care. There is a more subjective sense of "contentment" here than what is connoted by the principle of diminishing marginal utility. While this contentment may have some of its roots in that principle, it operates somewhat differently. The fact of diminishing marginal utility implies that we should *give up* some present satisfaction that we derive from spending money on consumption now, so that we will lose less later. But also, right now we gain the contentment of security, *whether or not* we ever fall ill and need our insurance to help us avoid actual financial losses. Immediate gratification, not just rationally controlled saving, lies behind the financial security of insurance.

Spreading Costs among Well and Ill

Not only does insurance disperse the costs of illness over the lifetimes of the ill; it also disperses the costs of illness among the well and the ill. The ethical principle of justice as equality of net benefits between all persons makes this morally significant. To be sure, insurance per se does not fully equalize the total burdens of the well and the ill. For example, private insurance premiums are often not equal for everyone, and then the likely well still carry a lower financial burden than the likely ill. And illness itself, not just its cost, is a burden the ill still bear and the well do not, even if they all are comprehensively insured. Still, insurance itself takes a bigger step toward a just equality between well and ill than any other single later refinement. (It may, of course, do little to remedy injustices between rich and poor.)

Pre-commitment to Care

While *insuring* focuses on these two cost-spreading functions, *health* insurance realistically has another function. It not only insures against medical expense, but *assures* us that we will use needed health care.[4] The purchase of insurance represents a kind of "pre-commitment": Since we know now that we do not want financial considerations to

4. Ball 1976.

influence our later choices to use or not to use health care, we insure.[5]
Insurance becomes our "assurance" that money won't get in the way.
It may be very rational for people to deal with their potential later
weakness or miserliness in this way—certainly, it seems, as rational as
borrowing on an installment loan at high interest while keeping
money in a lower-interest savings account.[6]

The need for pre-commitment may vary significantly with individual personalities. With the same income and health needs that I have,
you may be much more likely than I to keep your commitment to pay
out-of-pocket for health care when it is needed. You may not place
any greater value on the care than I do (certainly ahead of time I
might value it as much); it may only be that my resolve to get needed
care when I later face the financial pinch of actual expense is weaker
than yours.

Costs

Just as there are many different benefits to insurance, there are also
many different costs to financing health-care expense in this way:

(1) The insurer incurs administrative costs in trying to sell policies, in having people buy them, and in processing claims.

(2) The insurer is taking some risk in assuming individuals' financial liability for health-care expense. In large insurance pools that may
be miniscule. Still, it is understandable that private insurers want
some small return for their willingness to take that risk.[7]

(3) Total dollar costs for care rise when people are insured. Insured people have no incentive to forgo care which, if they were uninsured, they would even all agree wasn't worth its price (see 1.2).

(4) With insurance, care rises in price above and beyond its increase in sophistication. Unless the number and training of providers
can immediately be expanded or there are special outside controls,
the increased demand for care created by insurance raises the price

5. There is an interesting reason why a person may want to avoid this influence:
People insure just so they can then avoid the mental agitation of thinking about the costworthiness of given health-care services. Insuring is valuable to us precisely because we
hope to forget about the costworthiness issue. If I am right in my general line of thinking
in this book, however, insurance has really made the costworthiness considerations all
the more urgent, intriguing, and complex. It does not offer a way of avoiding them, as
this reasoning would claim.

6. Fuchs 1979.

7. The term economists use for the first and second of these costs is "loading,"
the deviation from the "actuarially fair" price under which benefits paid out for clients'
losses are exactly recouped by the premiums. See Ehrlich and Becker 1972.

of care. Even if supply catches up to demand, that usually takes long enough that prices are driven up in the meantime. The increase usually gets sustained thereafter.

(5) The widespread availability of care that insurance makes possible dampens some of our natural incentives against neglecting and abusing our own health.[8] The prospect of having to pay out of pocket for later illness creates some incentive to keep ourselves well, which insurance largely removes. To be sure, there is undoubtedly some of this psychological, "bail-out" effect even in uninsured medical care; Rene Dubos remarks that "it is part of the doctor's function to make it possible for his patients to go on doing the pleasant things that are bad for them—smoking too much, eating too much, drinking too much—without killing themselves any sooner than is necessary."[9] Removal of financial incentives to avoid needing or using care, however, magnifies that effect. If in the long run preventive self-care is more significant than medicine in improving health and extending life, and if the freedom from out-of-pocket medical expenses enhances sufficiently our culture's orientation toward relying on the prospect of medical care instead of reducing the likelihood of illness ourselves, it is conceivable that insurance could even create a less healthy population.

2. EXCESSIVE INSURANCE

How do we weigh these costs against the benefits? Obviously it is an immensely complex matter. It is also ultimately a judgment heavily dependent on some subjective and probably individually idiosyncratic preferences. We all easily concur in the value of financial security that is rooted in diminishing marginal utility, and we often think it outweighs the insurer's administrative costs. Yet even here, how *much* the marginal utility of money diminishes—and therefore what costs of insurance are worth paying—is somewhat a matter of individual prefer-

8. Under certain conditions, however, the availability of insurance may enhance these incentives; see Ehrlich and Becker 1972. Suppose, for example, that my premiums are higher if I engage in a dangerous behavior like smoking. The opposite and more usual effect of insurance—weakening the incentive to avoid future losses—is called "moral hazard." See Arrow 1963; Arrow 1968; Dickerson 1963; Ehrlich and Becker 1972; Marshall 1976; and Pauly 1968. I assume that the term has its roots in the observation that insurance may weaken our moral resolve to avoid accidents or illness. Moral hazard explains why certain hazards, like failure in business, are not insured by the market.

9. Anderson 1972, p. 142.

ence. Immediate satisfaction is a dimension of financial security that is probably even more individual and subjective. How rational it is to pre-commit myself to health care by insurance will depend on just how inclined *I* am to forgo needed care to save immediate money. The value of insurance varies with individuals.

Nevertheless, several general observations may be made about the rational weighing of the costs and benefits of insurance. The more elastic the demand for medical care is—that is, the greater the increase in my demand for care created by a drop in its out-of-pocket expense to me—the more it encourages utilization of disputably or minutely beneficial care. The less people are willing to pay for such increasingly sophisticated and expensive care, the higher the overall cost of the extra and decreasingly beneficial care which insurance stimulates. The actual dollar costs of insurance will rise the more that the price of particular health services is sensitive to changes in demand. In turn that sensitivity will partially depend on how elastic is the supply of providers and how monopolistic their control of entry.[10]

If we are to stand any chance of rationally weighing insurance's costs and benefits, we must be aware of these effects. But they provide no secret formula, either. We cannot conclude that insurance has excessive costs just because we know, for example, that the demand for health care is sensitive to out-of-pocket expense and that its total price is sensitive to demand. Costly and apparently wasteful insurance will still be costworthy to an individual purchaser if to him or her the benefits of financial security and pre-commitment are great enough. But right here we come back to willingness-to-pay again: What those benefits are worth to a given individual will presumably be indicated by how much that person would pay for them if he or she were knowledgeable about all the particular effects that I have already mentioned.[11]

Feldstein's Calculation

It is precisely this last thought which leads Feldstein to his well-known argument that insurance with little or no patient cost sharing

10. See Feldstein 1973 and Pauly 1968.

11. We might also ascertain in this way the degree of another benefit of insurance to an individual, that is, that it spreads the risks out among the well and the ill. That we should, however, is debatable. In terms of justice, the equalizing of costs among well and ill which insurance accomplishes may be considered the costs and the "waste" that insurance creates. And equalizing may be worth those costs even when few individuals would be willing to pay for them. Justice and its moral value themselves are not, I assume, ultimately matters of subjective preference. In that respect they differ from utility.

constitutes a welfare loss.[12] The amount of money that security is worth is indicated by the maximum premium a person would pay to avoid the mere uncertainty of a given expenditure. This can be expressed as a coefficient of risk aversion. It is easiest to understand by considering a simple bet. If a man is willing to participate in a bet in which there is an even chance of winning and losing $1,000, he has a risk-aversion coefficient of zero. He would also place no value on insurance. If, on the other hand, he requires a side payment of $150—that is, he is equally indifferent between no bet and an even chance of winning $1150 and losing $850—his risk aversion is what Feldstein considers normal.

Using this allegedly typical degree of risk aversion, Feldstein now calculates the value of insurance. He comes to a striking conclusion: In making insurance more comprehensive by lowering the average proportion of health-care expenses paid out-of-pocket from 50 to 33 percent, Americans lose the welfare equivalent of $4 billion in 1971 dollars.[13]

Feldstein's reasoning cannot be faulted on the grounds that he has ignored either the immediate satisfaction of greater security from lower cost sharing or the value of security attributable to diminishing marginal utility. Because his argument is grounded in willingness to pay to avoid financial risk, he already includes those factors. He takes little account, however, of the greater pre-commitment benefits and the spreading of costs among well and ill in more comprehensive insurance. In that respect, Feldstein's estimate of the total benefits of full coverage would appear to be low. Yet he also takes no account of a possible long-range cost of insurance, the increasing neglect of self-care and the greater reliance on being bailed out by modern technological medicine that it fosters. Thus his overall point remains compelling: We may indeed be creating an aggregate welfare loss when we increase insurance coverage without simultaneously taking steps to hold down prices and utilization.[14]

12. Feldstein 1973.

13. This assumes three conditions: the moderate willingness of patients to pay for the increased quality and sophistication of care which is stimulated by the more comprehensive insurance, the low elasticity of patient demand for care with respect to its out-of-pocket price, and the relatively high sensitivity of health-care prices to the extent of insurance.

14. There is a corollary: Arrow (1963) is wrong to take the presence of risk-averse people who do not have insurance to be a sign of market failure, requiring some kind of collective intervention. The welfare losses from insurance may make insurance a bad buy even to the significantly risk-averse. See Cullis and West 1979, p. 69.

That is still not the end of the story: Perhaps such a welfare loss is morally acceptable. It will be, if the more comprehensive insurance that created it distributes the burdens of illness more equally among well and ill. In purchasing that insurance and encouraging health care with declining marginal benefits, we may admittedly be purchasing gains for the ill so slight that overall there is a welfare loss when we consider everyone who pays the higher premiums. But maybe we *should* purchase those slight gains at that high price. Don't patients whose burdens from illness are already unjustly heavy deserve it? Feldstein's "excess insurance" is excessive—that is, it generates a welfare loss—only from the perspective of the *whole group's aggregated* benefits. That includes the perspective of the insurance purchaser willing to take some risks. On the other hand, the person who does get ill probably suffers no loss from such insurance. And it is precisely that latter person whom we are concerned to compensate for the burdens of illness.

Of course we might be able to transform the potential savings from cutting back on excessive insurance into aid for the ill that would be of greater value to them.[15] Furthermore, isn't the claim of the ill on us for the slight benefits of extra insurance weak when that insurance eliminates only first-dollar expenses, not the devastating out-of-pocket payments for the upper end of expense?[16] Feldstein's warning that the waste of excessive insurance may be morally objectionable is still well taken.

First-Dollar Coverage
Feldstein develops his general point into a criticism of "high option," "first dollar," low cost-sharing insurance in particular.[17] Tax breaks

15. A recent employer plan in California illustrates the extent of this saving (*Newsweek*, 25 August 1980). The Mendocino County Office of Education switched from a $105 per month first-dollar coverage to a $65 per month $500 deductible plan. It set aside the $40 per month saving in individual accounts for each employee. They could each, as needed, draw on their accounts to cover the first $480 of their medical expenses in a given year, and they could collect whatever of that was left at the end of the year. No one could lose more than $20 per year by the switch, and many gained $480.

16. I suspect it is just this point that drives Feldstein's larger position on health insurance. While he is a strong defender of cost sharing, his proposal for national health insurance is "major risk insurance." It completely covers expenses above a certain percentage of income (10 percent is suggested). See Feldstein 1971.

17. Feldstein's attack on excessive first-dollar coverage rests on the premise that copayments and deductibles will significantly reduce demand for medical services. The empirical question of how much reduction they actually bring about is a matter of some dispute. See 5.4.

aside,[18] why don't people who can seemingly afford cost sharing rest content with catastrophic insurance? Why do they also want *much* more expensive first-dollar coverage?[19] Are they ignorant of the potential welfare loss of overinsurance? Or do they see some value in first-dollar coverage which critics like Feldstein have overlooked? Suppose the expenses that annually total less than 10 percent of a person's income are the significant majority of aggregate health-care expenditures; they become the field for the greatest potential aggregate gains in costworthiness. If they are relatively predictable expenses that can in some sense be budgeted, why do people still demand more complete insurance?

The puzzle may be strikingly illustrated. In 1980 a typical annual premium for a family of four with a $100-per-person annual deductible was roughly $1,200. For a $500-per-person deductible, the premium was roughly $600.[20] An extra $600 for premiums brought the maximum family deductible down from $2,000 to $400. But is it worth $600 to avoid $1,600—assuredly no more than that—of unlikely expense? Viewed another way, the financial risk may even be less. Shouldn't I risk paying $1000 more, counting *combined* premiums and out-of-pocket expenses, than what I risk paying if I buy the more complete coverage, all the while standing a good chance of saving $600 in

18. Clearly, tax breaks provide greater incentives for first-dollar coverage, at least that portion purchased by employers, than for coverage for catastrophic expenses. I will defer the main discussion of tax breaks until chap. 6. Only a brief description of them is in order here. Though the relative predictability of medical expenses in first-dollar coverage would seem to make it a bad bargain as "insurance," those expenses are entirely excluded from taxable income only when they are paid as premiums by employers. If they are uninsured, first-dollar, out-of-pocket health-care expenditures, they are not likely to be tax deductible for the individual, while uncovered *catastrophic* expense almost always will be.

19. Perhaps I should not assume that catastrophic coverage is the higher priority for them. In a study for Pracon, Inc., of Fairfax, Va., Stephen Sudovar and Patrice Hirsch Feinstein found that only 29.4 percent of the population had catastrophic coverage, defined as that which paid at least $250,000 for a long and protracted condition and guaranteed that out-of-pocket costs would not exceed 30 percent of annual income (*Washington Post*, 18 January 1980). While we do not know how this figure compares with the percentage who have first-dollar coverage, and while the latter percentage is probably lower than 29.4 percent, it is still surprising that protection against catastrophic losses as defined by this study is not more popular. It is especially so since the same study showed that 85.3 percent of the population was protected for 80 percent of hospital room-and-board costs for medium-expense stays over fifteen days, and nearly two-thirds were covered for maternity-care provisions. Two explantions come readily to mind: Many people do not realize their lack of truly catastrophic coverage, or more people than I would have expected are willing to gamble on the very low probabilities of very high losses.

20. This example is adjusted to 1980 dollars from the one in 1971 dollars in Krizay and Winston 1974, p. 29.

lower premiums not canceled out by later expenses?[21] Consider also the fact that 20 percent of the extra $600 for the more complete insurance never gets back to me as reimbursed medical expenses—it goes to administrative costs. Isn't, then, the extra $600 a truly exorbitant fee to pay an intermediary for reimbursing expenses as predictable as many common household expenditures?[22] Not only are those expenses predictable; aren't they in the long run also affordable for middle-income families?

In looking so askance at first-dollar coverage, however, we may have failed to consider one of the important values of insurance, pre-commitment to care. First-dollar coverage may be popular because people want to assure themselves now that out-of-pocket expense will not deter them from the care that they may need later.[23] The health of our bodies seems to demand this assurance and commitment. Still, what is the value of such assurance? It is an assurance that I will be more likely to use care, and care from which I will really benefit.[24] But while much of it is care whose benefits are worth the cost, some of it undoubtedly is not. Without other controls on costworthiness, first-dollar coverage not only assures me that I will not be deterred by expense from seeking care that is beneficial, needed, *and really worth the money*; it *also* assures me that I will not be deterred by expense from seeking some care that is of so little benefit relative to its expense that it is not worth its cost. Generally invoking "pre-commitment to our health" to justify first-dollar coverage hides this fact—the pre-commitment is really to noncostworthy as well as to costworthy care. Perhaps it is even a commitment not to give serious consideration to the costworthiness of care at all.[25]

---

21. These figures may be a confusing implication from the stated premiums. A clear explanation gets rather lengthy. First look at the range of combined annual premium and out-of-pocket expense for the low-option plan: It is *$600* (the premium—we do not have any medical expenses in this year) to *$2,600* (the $600 premiums, plus the $2,000 deductible). Next look at the range of combined annual premium and out-of-pocket expense for the earlier-dollar coverage: It is *$1,200* (the premium—no medical expense that year) to *$1,600* (the $1,200 premium, plus the $400 deductible). If every family member gets sick enough to surpass our deductibles in a given year, we will save $1,000 by having chosen the high-option plan. If, on the other hand, none of us incur any expenses, we will save $600 by having chosen the low-option plan. This last $600 saving of the low-option plan will also be gained if each of us incur anywhere up to, but not more than, $100 of medical expenses that year; the higher-option plan's more comprehensive coverage is still not of greater help to us in that case.

22. Krizay and Wilson 1974, p. 29.

23. Fuchs 1979.

24. Ball 1976.

25. See n. 5 of this chapter.

What different reactions to this now-complicated state of affairs are plausible? (1) We could put up with the extra cost and the waste generated by first-dollar coverage in order to assure that we would get all the care we needed. (2) We could try to avoid being deterred by high deductibles from necessary and costworthy care by accruing (in this case) $1,600 of savings for health-care contingencies. (3) We could look for first-dollar coverage, but only from plans that tried to control our tendency to use unnecessary or marginally beneficial care. To many people it will seem that the second and third courses of action are more likely to maximize their welfare. That will not hold for everyone, however. Some people may evaluate the matters of assurance and pre-commitment and the perhaps objectionable nature of insurer-applied controls and then choose the first course. Which one is best may ultimately be a matter of personal, subjective preference, even for the perfectly knowledgeable agent. In any case we must be well aware of what we are buying with the much higher premiums of complete coverage.[26]

3. VARIATIONS WITH INCOME

How is this consideration of the value of insuring for health care affected by the level of income and wealth of the person insured?[27] If there is any correlation between economic status and the monetary value of insurance, how does that compare with the correlation be-

26. Throughout this discussion of the advantages and disadvantages of first-dollar as opposed to catastrophic coverage, I have ignored an aspect of the cost of catastrophic-only coverage which bothers some people a great deal. It is one of the major arguments against catastrophic-only national health insurance: When catastrophic expenses alone are fully covered, the care associated with that magnitude of expense tends to come to occupy a larger share of the medical economy compared to other types of care. This can happen at the level of research and development, hospital and physician orientation and emphasis, or patient decisions. Once they have paid out all the deductibles, people get more quickly into the catastrophic range of expense, or stay there longer, in order to "get their money's worth."

27. We are concerned to compare the value of insurance to one person who is rich with its value to another who is relatively poor, or to compare its value to one person when he or she is rich with its value to the same person when poor. We are not concerned about the effect of a change in a person's *expected* income on his or her present demand for insurance. If in the future my real income is expected to decrease, my present demand for insurance for the future will be higher than it would otherwise be; and if my future real income is expected to increase, my present demand for insurance will decrease; see Ehrlich and Becker 1972. Presumably these changing demands for insurance say something about its changing value to me. If my future income is expected to increase, the largely future risks I insure against are just smaller financial threats, and committing myself in advance to care will seem less necessary.

tween income and the value of health care itself? For poor people, is insurance a better (or worse) buy than health care?[28] Is it an even better buy (or even worse) than it is for the rich? The answers will directly bear on what type of socially provided insurance policies—first-dollar, catastrophic, etc.—will represent the best use of scarce resources for the poor.

In chapter 3 we concluded that the monetary value of risk-reducing health care was less to the poor than to the rich. The main fact accounted for by this conclusion is the greater value to the poor of competing uses for money. This fact is morally significant: It draws our attention to competing needs and desires, which have higher priority for the poor than they do for the rich. Monetary pricing of life and health care is a notion that may be grossly misused, however, if pricings are aggregated over individuals and then used as evidence that scarce health-care resources can generate more value by being allocated to the rich. We need to relate all that to the present discussion: Does the claim that health care has lower monetary value for the poor extend to insurance for health care? It might not.

An initial, obvious fact is that family spending on health insurance clearly increases as income goes up.[29] That by itself tells us little about whether insurance is a better buy for the poor than health care itself is—the uninsured poor spend less on health care than the uninsured rich do. With income differences in mind, we need to take another look at the various benefits and costs of insuring for health care.

The Benefits of Insuring

(1) Financial security. As my income drops, the risk of a given proportion of my income being lost to actual health-care expenses increases and the value of insurance rises.[30] The value and satisfaction to me of knowing *now* that I am insured against these risks is also undoubtedly greater if my income is low. Furthermore, the higher my income the more I can myself provide the same things that insurance provides. I myself can spread out the costs of illness over a longer period of time—when sick I just use up some of my assets, leaving fewer assets to cash in at later times.

Another factor leans in the opposite direction. As my income

28. I am not assuming that either one is a good buy, or a bad one. I am asking whether insuring for health care is a *better*, or a *worse*, buy for the poor than paying out of pocket for it.

29. Mitchell and Vogel 1975.

30. Feldstein 1973.

drops, my demand for medical care and its relative value to me also drop. Therefore I have less actual expense to insure against. Richer families, by contrast, have greater dollar expenditure risks against which to insure, since marginally beneficial health care which is not costworthy to the poor is still a good buy for them.[31]

There is no evident, accurate way to weigh these competing observations against each other. We do know that when I am poor instead of rich, I find less care costworthy. There is therefore less care for which I want to insure. Nevertheless, it would seem that this drop in the value of insurance when I am poor is more than offset by the increased value of insurance as security and protection against higher proportion-of-income financial risk. Though relative to their other needs the poor need and want less health care than the rich do, the poor are *much* more vulnerable to the financial disasters of illness. They are particularly vulnerable to the middle range of expense, which bankrupts poor families but leaves middle-income families only tightly budgeted for several years.

(2) Distributing costs among well and ill. Unlike financial security, this benefit may seem to fall to rich and poor equally. A poor ill person, however, has a greater need than a rich ill person to have the well help bear the costs of illness. To be sure, involuntary illness can throw rich as well as poor into unjust relationship to the well, but the poor have a greater and more urgent interest in ameliorating that injustice. Furthermore, the very injustice between the well and ill that is created by illness seems greater among the poor; the financial burdens of illness are greater for them.

(3) Pre-commitment to care. As a poor person, I have greater reason than a rich person does to fear being later tempted to forgo necessary care because of its expense. The poorer I am, the greater the benefits which insurance buys in the form of care that I would never have used had I not insured. I have greater need to protect myself against both my miserliness and my inability to pay.

Yet this greater value of insurance for the poor may be offset by other factors. First, pre-commitment assures care that is only marginally beneficial and possibly noncostworthy, as well as that which is clearly costworthy. Since the ceiling of noncostworthiness is lower for the poor, insurance will lead to care that is for me less and less costworthy the poorer I am. We can sense this every time the insured poor get cared for in very expensive American hospitals. Second, although the value of assuring myself that I will not be deterred by expense

31. Feldstein 1973.

from using health care becomes greater and greater to me the poorer I am, I will probably also be more and more inclined to gamble that I will not need care. At the same time as I am increasingly aware of the importance of assuring myself of care, I am less and less willing to pay for that assurance. My other needs for the money may make me more willing to gamble about less than catastrophic levels of expense. My willingness to gamble here is not necessarily irrational. I am not necessarily drawn to do it out of an addiction to any Las-Vegas-like excitement at the prospect of great gains. I may be knowledgeably drawn to it because of my financial needs. While the monetary value to me of the assurance that is cashed in when I need care may be greater the poorer I am, that value assessed now before I need care may be less.

Thus the value of insurance as pre-commitment may seem to be equal for rich and poor. Probably, however, it is still greater for the poor. The bulk of care assured by insurance is necessary and costworthy in the eyes of rich and poor. While gambling is more attractive to me when I am poor, I stand so much more to lose by letting the out-of-pocket expense of care stand as a barrier to my using it that, on balance, pre-commitment seems all the more important the poorer I am. At the same time, of course, the more important it becomes to control the cost-escalating pressure of this pre-commitment.

The Costs of Insuring

(1) Administrative costs, insurer risk, and increasing reliance on medical care rather than prevention. With these costs, no variations with income are apparent.

(2) Increased expenditures caused by incentives to use noncostworthy care. Here, as mentioned, the poorer people are, the greater the costs that insurance will create.

(3) Rising health-care prices from the increases in demand that are induced by insurance. Here, too, the costs of insurance are higher for the poor. Because insurance cuts the patient's out-of-pocket expenses, the poor are more likely than the rich to seek extra care once they are insured. If insurance thus increases demand for care more for the poor than for the rich, the attendant change in prices will also be larger for the poor than for the rich.

Thus, while the three major benefits of insurance are greater for the poor, so, too, are two of the five costs of insurance. It is hard to see how these factors will balance out without knowing several things more specifically. First, *how much* of the care which is noncostworthy

to the poor is generated by insurance, compared to that which is generated by insurance in the case of the rich? Second, *how great* is the
increase in prices stimulated by increased demand? Third, *how much
more* value do the poor put on financial security, on spreading out
the costs of illness among the ill and the well, and on securing care in
advance? To most of us it will seem that the balance of insurance's
benefits over costs is probably greater for the poor, but new data could
easily lead us to reverse such a loose, subjective judgment. In any case
the poor will undoubtedly not be willing to pay nearly as much for
insurance's benefits as the rich; just as with health care itself, their
monetary valuations of insurance will be less. Nevertheless, insured
health care seems to be a better buy to them than the same care
uninsured.

Implications

All this reveals something very important. As we focus on the poor in
shaping our public health policy, we should be insistent on providing
insurance. At the same time, we should be more insistent than ever
that insurance's expense-inducing effects be controlled. Even though
the poor consider *marginally beneficial* health care to be not such a
good buy as the rich do, they are likely to find that insurance for care
that *is* costworthy to them is an even better buy for them than for the
rich.

What does this implication mean for the respective points at
which the rich and the poor will find comprehensive insurance becoming "excessive"—that is, creating a welfare loss? In particular,
what does it mean for the relative values of first-dollar coverage for
rich and poor? The lower one's wealth and income, the greater one's
vulnerability to the financial disasters of illness: To the poor, this statement implies that coverage that is first-dollar, not merely catastrophic,
will then have greater value. For one thing, as we go up the ladder of
incurred expenses, the level at which the poor find illness financially
"catastrophic" is much lower than for the rich.

Let us go back to the example in the previous section. Suppose to
a relatively rich person it is not worth $600 to buy first-dollar coverage
and avoid $1,600 of extra liability. Will it be worth $600 to a poor person? It is not a simple matter. Avoiding the $1,600 liability has much
greater value to me if I am poor, but the extra $600 premium is a
much higher real price for me to pay. As a relatively poor person I
might well think it a good bargain to gamble on not incurring the
$1,600 of expense in forgone deductibles in order to save $600 in pre-

miums. (Can't we imagine a rich family saying, "Six hundred dollars? We'll hardly notice that. But $1,600, should we get sick? We would probably notice that, even though we could afford it. So we'll pay $600 for the extra first-dollar coverage"? At least *that* is a rationale for first-dollar coverage that I would never utter if I were poor.) Perhaps, however, the poorer I am, the lower the odds are that I will incur the $1,600 expense, and the more I should be willing to gamble in order to save $600. That gamble may look objectively more foolish for the poor than for the rich, yet the first $600 which I hope to save is worth so much more to me if I am poor. We just can't be sure that first-dollar coverage is a better bargain for the poor than for the rich.

There are other considerations. Although it is exorbitantly expensive, I may find first-dollar coverage attractive because it is a pre-commitment not to let expense deter me from later needed care. The poorer I am, the more necessary and valuable such a pre-commitment seems. On the other hand, the first-dollar coverage rooted in pre-commitment also assures me the use of a greater amount of marginally beneficial, even unnecessary, care. And the poorer I am, the less of that care will be costworthy.

Earlier we noted three likely reactions to any observed welfare loss of excessive first-dollar coverage (5.2). (1) I will put up with the waste in order to assure all my needed care. (2) I will accrue savings to minimize being deterred from getting needed care by its expense. (3) I will keep first-dollar coverage, but use a plan that tries to control for me the use of marginally beneficial care. The poorer I am, the less plausible the second option becomes, and the more wasteful the first becomes. The third, by contrast, has more advantages for the poor than for the rich. *Insured-applied costworthiness controls will seem to be a better bargain to the poor than to the rich.* No wonder some prepaid plans were initially designed especially to meet the needs of the poor. If in fact they have not met those needs, it is not the fault of the prepaid idea itself.

Compared to the rich, the poor find less health care itself a good buy, but first-dollar insurance for whatever care is costworthy a better buy. This is certainly true if we implement effective controls on care that isn't costworthy.

4. COST SHARING AND ITS GRADUATION

Discussion of first-dollar coverage would be incomplete without a more detailed consideration of the merits of cost sharing as a device to contain health-care costs. In the last decade cost sharing has been prominently and notably pushed as a means of containing costs.[32]

It has three common forms: (1) Deductibles—in which I pay, for example, the first $100 in a year before any insurance takes effect. (2) Coinsurance—in which I pay 20 percent of the total bill, for example (I am the "co-insurer"). (3) Copayments—in which I pay, for example, $3 for each prescription, $10 for each office visit, $300 for delivery of a newborn, etc., while insurance pays the rest.[33] These can be combined in various ways, for example, a $100 annual deductible, 20 percent coinsurance on the next $2,000, 10 percent on the next $50,000, full coverage above $52,100, with drugs treated separately throughout by a $3 per prescription copayment.

These are deliberate cost-containment devices. By eliminating small claims, deductibles greatly improve the ratio of administrative expenses to claims paid, and all three kinds of cost sharing give patients some immediate economic incentive not to make unnecessary use of medical services. In this respect they are obviously not ideal; even with 20 percent coinsurance, for example, I will want to use care whose benefits to me are worth only one-fifth its total cost. Since insurance is ideally a way both to equalize the costs of illness between well and ill and to avoid discouraging needed care, cost sharing is a compromise.

Does Cost Sharing Actually Reduce Costs?
Two different major controversies surround cost sharing. The first one is factual, the second moral. Factually, does cost sharing really reduce health-care costs as much as it promises to? In discussing "excessive insurance," we have already seen that Feldstein relies on the contention that it does. By contrast, Enthoven's well-known plan for strengthening competitive forces in the medical economy supposes that the patient is not the best agent to instill cost consciousness.[34] While cost sharing does give patients an incentive to conserve, that incentive is largely impotent; it is usually the physician who determines what services are used.[35] To be effective, cost-control measures must first attempt to change providers' and insurance buyers' incentives to use noncostworthy care.

32. Especially by Feldstein 1971.
33. Sometimes the terms "coinsurance" and "copayment" are used to cover this whole field of cost sharing, but usually they are more specific. "Cost sharing" is the broader term.
34. Enthoven 1978a.
35. Ball 1978.

Probably there is some truth on both sides in this controversy. Undoubtedly cost sharing reduces *some* expenditures. One study has found that 25-percent coinsurance reduced per-capita physician visits by 24 percent in the first year after previous full, first-dollar coverage.[36] Another study has shown when insurance buyers went from full coverage to 25-percent coinsurance, their use of ambulatory services declined by 25 percent, while their use of hospital services declined by approximately 5 percent.[37] There may be one coherent viewpoint in all this: Use of hospital services is not reduced much by cost sharing, while use of physicians and ambulatory services is. This is attributable to the dominant role played by physicians in using hospital services, and the greater role that patients play in seeking ambulatory care. Only insofar as *ambulatory* services account for a significant portion of noncostworthy care should cost sharing be seriously considered as a cost-control device.

Is Cost Sharing Just?

The moral issue in cost sharing is this: Since cost sharing more strongly discourages poorer persons from using care than it does richer ones, can it be just? Cost sharing, to be sure, has its moral as well as its practical defense: While incomplete insurance works great and unjust hardships on the ill, cost sharing puts back on the patient only the relatively affordable expenses that people can bear.[38] But the problem then becomes clear: These expenses are not so affordable for the poor. And even if the poor can in the strict sense afford particular levels of expense, these costs are *harder* on them than they are on wealthier persons.

Thus, to be just and morally tolerable, cost sharing must be progressively graduated with income and wealth. After, say, 10 percent of annual income, all expenses could be covered, and for some of the earlier expenses of lower-income persons, government and employers could guarantee loans.[39] Former senator Schweiker's bill for national health insurance before the 1979-80 Congress limited its cost sharing

36. Scitovsky and Snyder 1972; Klarman 1977.
37. I derive these from the slightly different estimates of Newhouse, Phelps, and Schwartz 1974. Their estimates differ from mine because theirs were made in reference to a different starting point from which to measure the percentage of change. More generally, see Beck 1974 and Helms, Newhouse, and Phelps 1978.
38. While deductibles and copayments on a series of medical bills are generally affordable, coinsurance may not be. A 20 percent portion of a $250,000 bill will bankrupt many people.
39. Feldstein 1971.

to 20 percent of family income.[40] While a graduated system of cost sharing has usually been thought to pose great administrative problems, in a more universal, integrated national insurance system it would be perfectly feasible. The identity of some patients as poor would not be revealed to providers if all people had the same health-care card. Providers would send bills to a payer who would reimburse them in full but then bill patients for various shares according to their incomes. Even deductibles and copayments, not just total annual liability, could be graduated with income.[41] If such a system makes graduation administratively feasible, cost sharing is morally acceptable. If cost sharing is not graduated, then we should refuse to entertain it as a just means of controlling total expenditures on health care.

Some will scoff at this argument. In chapters 3 and 4, they will note, I argued that because less care is costworthy for the poor than for the rich, it is perfectly acceptable, even optimal, that the poor use less health care. Ungraduated cost sharing leads the poor to do without care when they need or desire the money it would cost for other things. How then can we argue against cost sharing by simply describing it as working a greater hardship on the poor? Doesn't that hardship discourage precisely the kinds of care which the poor's choices reveal are not costworthy to them?

That line of criticism misleads. We need to ask first whether a health-care plan with cost-sharing provisions is a shrewd choice for the poor. For their own self-interest, would the poor choose, among various options, a health plan with cost sharing? From their perspective, cost sharing is probably one of the worst ways to discourage the use of noncostworthy care. It is especially bad if it is ungraduated. We have already seen that while less health care is costworthy for the poor than for the rich, the poor are likely to find *insuring* for whatever care *is* costworthy a better buy than the rich will. Furthermore, that is as true of first-dollar as it is of catastrophic coverage. While the more well-to-do may choose either a cost-sharing or a first-dollar plan for

40. See Butler 1980. Senator Durenberger (S. 1968) and Representative Ullman (HR. 5740) did not graduate the cost sharing in their 1979 bills. So also in 1979 the Senate Finance Commitee spearheaded by Senator Long did not graduate a good share of its catastrophic coverage bill; while it limited the family deductible to 25 percent of income, its $3,500 fixed-dollar maximum meant that for a high-income family the deductible would be a far lower percentage of income. See Butler 1980; U.S. Senate, Committee on Finance 1979a, p. 1. It is appalling that so many major proposals for national health insurance by congressmen and administrations in the last fifteen years have relied on ungraduated cost sharing. Former senator Schweiker's 1979 bill (S. 1590), by contrast, limited total cost sharing to 20 percent of adjusted gross income.

41. Ball 1978.

expensive "high style" care, *the poor are likely to find plans for less (or lower style) care without cost sharing a better buy*. At least we can say that *cost sharing in any government or employer arrangement in which people do not have a choice of plans will meet the needs of poorer recipients less than the needs of richer ones*. In ungraduated form, especially, it will ignore the needs and preferences of the poor. If we are going to resort to cost sharing at all, we must face the necessity of graduating it.[42]

What Degree of Graduation?

What, then, is a fair degree of graduation? Two options theoretically suggest themselves.

(1) Design cost sharing to represent roughly the same proportion of all persons' income. As popular as this approach is, however, it is very doubtful that it is correct. Ten percent of income, for example, is still much harder for the poor to pay than it is for the rich.

(2) Devise whatever graduation leads to equal use of care by rich and poor, once we have adjusted for any actuarial illness differences between economic groups. This, too, is incorrect. (a) The perception of illness which triggers people to seek services undoubtedly increases with income.[43] Should we "erase" the effect of this perception by using a formula for graduation designed to make the actual use of services equal between rich and poor? Such a graduation of cost sharing will effectively take away any benefits that would accrue to individuals from being more perceptive about their health. (b) If the best use of the poor's resources involves less health care than the best use of the rich's resources does for the rich, it is simply inconsistent to judge the equity of graduated cost sharing by how equally care is consequently used by different groups. The kinds and styles of care that are delivered in a plan for the poor ought to be more limited, though then the poor should not be discouraged from using *that* care any more than wealthier enrollees are.

Are any other formulas for graduation essentially more correct? Perhaps at this point we should confess: We face a radical and theoretical ambiguity in what is the right formula for determining a just graduation of cost sharing. Since graduation is still essential for cost

42. If we were discussing a society with a distribution of income and wealth that was perfectly just though still somewhat unequal, it might well be perfectly acceptable to leave any cost sharing ungraduated. I would think, however, that in such a society any cost-sharing provision would not be mandatory. In fact there would not be any required health insurance programs for cost sharing to be part of.

43. Anderson, Kravits, and Anderson 1975, pp. 266–67.

sharing to be just, perhaps we should try to *avoid compulsory cost sharing entirely in any plan which enrolls people of significantly different income levels.* At least we should try to avoid it if it is not graduated.[44] This conclusion holds for private place-of-employment groups as much as for widespread public programs.

Time-Cost Sharing

But if health care is not rationed somehow and somewhat by price, won't it get rationed some other way? This will likely be by queue, it will be said, as has already happened to a considerable extent in Britain. So, for example, Wildavsky coins his "Axiom of Inequality": All systems ration care, so decreasing the inequality in one dimension (financial access) will simply increase it in another (the waiting time that is necessary to get care).[45] Yet if charging some out-of-pocket price for care unjustly discriminates against the poor, does charging none unjustly discriminate against the rich? When care is "free," demand increases and the total time necessary for an individual to procure care in the consequently overloaded system rises. This discriminates against the rich. In earning power their time is more valuable; "waiting" costs them more and discourages them from getting care.

This argument is seriously mistaken, however. Though the time of the rich is worth more in dollars, a $100,000-a-year lawyer's waiting cost of $50 is undoubtedly less of a sacrifice than is a $10,000-a-year custodian's waiting cost of $5. (Look at what the lawyer has left.) The only ones who will sacrifice less in *real* temporal costs than the rich will be the *unemployed* poor. Furthermore, *what does it matter if the rich are charged more for care in terms of time than the poor are? That is simply a kind of graduated cost sharing.* Will it be any less justified than the more ordinary graduation of cost sharing that is morally required if we are to use cost sharing at all? If significant time-cost sharing is necessary in the delivery of health care, we should graduate it. In fact, when we compare the case of the $100,000 lawyer with the $10,000 custodian, progressively graduating the *real* sacrifice involved in time costs may require the lawyer to spend, say, five hours for the same care that is delivered to the custodian in one. That our health-care system often does something closer to the opposite is only a

44. By "compulsory" I mean not only the situation in which people are required to take some plan and have no option of refusing to take any of them, but also the situation in which employees, for example, have choices, yet the variety that they have to choose from is not wide enough to include some with little or no cost sharing.

45. Wildavsky 1977.

mark of its injustice. We should note again the exception: Real time-costs are already very progressively graduated in a comparison between the lawyer and an *unemployed* poor person. Waiting probably costs the unemployed person very little at all, while it certainly costs the lawyer something significant. But unless the $10,000-a-year custodian has ample sick leave which he can use to wait for care, waiting will cost him or her the most of all.

We can conclude, then, that unless it is graduated with income, cost sharing in any government or employer arrangement in which people do not have a choice of plans will meet the needs of poorer persons less than the needs of richer ones. We are at something of a loss, however, about what the theoretically correct formula for a just graduation might be. We should probably entirely avoid compulsory cost sharing in any plan which enrolls people of significantly different income levels. The greater waiting costs on the rich in the resulting demand-saturated delivery system with first-dollar coverage are acceptable as a kind of graduated cost sharing of their own.

CHAPTER SIX

Some Cost-Cutting Proposals

The current talk about health-care cost containment is not all theory. Four specific proposals have been recurrently and vigorously pushed: increasing patient cost sharing, eliminating the federal tax breaks for medical expenses and insurance premiums, creating truly competitive forces in the health-care economy, and encouraging prepaid health plans, one form of which is the health maintenance organization (HMO). These four proposals have been intimately linked in some package recommendations for controlling costs. A fifth suggestion, a national health service, seems less prominent of late in the U.S., but it is still very important in the panorama of organizational structures devised to control costs.

It is not just inefficiently delivered care which these measures hope to contain; it is also noncostworthy care. One issue then always arises: Who is to bear the loss of benefits that will result from restraining the use of care, and who will get the monetary savings? Since the losses and savings will not always accrue to the same people, we have to ask whether these measures will fairly and justly allocate their costs and advantages. That question has already been asked in the previous chapter in regard to cost sharing. This chapter will evaluate the other four cost-cutting proposals primarily in terms of this question.

It is important to insert the question of fair and just allocation into the larger context of costworthy health care. A proposal which keeps care that is noncostworthy in the narrow sense to a minimum might not finally be regarded as the best buy if it also creates injustices. Justice must be worth something in terms of money; moralists, too, have to put their money where their mouths are. Moreover, instituting cost-cutting measures has a more positive connection with justice. Many people presently are un- or underinsured for health care.[1] Any correction of that inadequacy will increase what our society spends on health care, raising the pressure to recoup these increases with cost-control savings. Politically it may simply not be feasible to expand coverage to those presently uninsured, unless costs for those presently covered are contained.[2]

1. TAX EXCLUSIONS AND DEDUCTIONS

Because the law allows them to subtract many health-insurance premiums and medical expenses from their taxable income, U.S. taxpayers in fiscal 1979 paid $17 billion less in taxes than they otherwise would have. Since premiums paid by employers are totally untaxed, in 1979 the taxpayers were able to save $8.25 billion in federal income taxes, $4 billion in Social Security payroll taxes, and $2 billion in state income taxes. In addition, taxpayers can itemize a certain portion of individually paid premiums and actual medical expenses as individual deductions: (a) one-half of premiums, or $150, whichever is less, and (b) any portion of the sum of the other half of such premiums and actual medical expenses in excess of three percent of adjusted gross income. This practice saved taxpayers $2.89 billion in federal income taxes.[3]

These tax advantages go back to the 1940s. In 1943 the Bureau of Internal Revenue ruled that the amount an employer paid in premiums on group insurance policies was to be excluded from taxable income.[4] In 1954 Congress made the exclusion statutory and extended

1. While Medicare covers almost all people over sixty-five (all who receive any kind of Social Security), it pays less for the poor than for the relatively rich. The poor cannot afford its ungraduated coinsurance as easily as others, and they more often live in underserved areas. Medicaid does not cover many of the near poor at all. In the mid-1970s, half of those under sixty-five with less than $5,000 family income had no hospital or surgical coverage whatsoever. Ironically, sometimes those who are covered by Medicaid were initially made poor by inadequate earlier insurance. Furthermore, most insurance is financed by employers for their employees. That means that the bulk of even the adequate coverage that people have is regressively financed. If the government does not require employer-financed insurance, unionized and better paid workers are much more likely to get better coverage, but if employer-financed insurance is required, then lower paid workers still in effect pay a higher proportion of their wages for it, and marginal workers are more apt to go unemployed. See Enthoven 1978a and Sidel and Sidel 1977,p. 37.

2. McClure 1978.

3. Hoffman and Steuerle 1979; Mitchell and Vogel 1975.

4. "Exclusion" here means not that the premiums can be deducted, but that they are never even declared as income. Excluded earnings are then not subject to Social Security or state income taxes.

it to all employer-paid premiums. In 1942 Congress added the personal deduction for individually paid premiums and actual medical expenses beyond 5 percent of income, subject to a $2,500 maximum deduction. In 1954 Congress changed the floor to 3 percent.[5]

Two concerns are commonly voiced about the resulting, and current, arrangement: (a) It contributes to escalating health-care costs by subsidizing noncostworthy care, and (b) it unjustly benefits the rich more than the poor.

Subsidizing Care

The $17 billion reduction in taxes is equivalent to 14 percent of gross private medical expenses. Health care is thus 14 percent cheaper to the average consumer than its true cost—a subsidy.[6] The extent of the effect on health-care costs, however, is barely apparent from this figure. The reduction in the price of care to the insured which is created by an extra unit of insurance is greater still. The marginal federal income tax rate for the average employee is 22 percent. If instead of receiving an extra dollar in wages, a taxpayer gets an extra dollar of employer-paid premiums, he can also avoid state and local income taxes, plus Social Security taxes, on that dollar. One very plausible estimate is that the final saving from an extra dollar spent on health care in the form of employer-paid premiums is 35 percent. For a $25,000-a-year employee, the saving is over 40 percent.[7] Since 10 percent of a premium is usually sufficient to defray the "loading costs" of insurance (administration and profits), the average employee will get back 25–30 percent more in benefits with a given extra dollar of employer-paid insurance than he will by first taking it home as income.[8] The extra insurance will still be purchased even if the monetary value of its benefits is 25–30 percent less than they cost.

Furthermore, the exclusion adds greatly to the attractiveness of

5. Hoffman and Steuerle 1979. There are other tax breaks for medical care. Contributions to hospitals are "charitable" and therefore deductible. Nonprofit hopitals can sell bonds whose interest to their holders is tax-free, and these hospitals themselves are tax-exempt. See MacLeod 1980 and Bromberg 1975.

6. Many writers do call it that, for example, Feldstein 1976 and Enthoven 1978a. In the more general economic literature about tax deductions and exclusions, the term with similar connotations is "tax expenditures"—tax revenue which the government forgoes and therefore really "pays" to people by allowing deductions and exclusions. Later I will consider the objections to using either of these terms to describe the medical exclusion and deduction.

7. Hoffman and Steuerle 1979.

8. Hoffman and Steuerle 1979. The 40 percent figure is calculated from Enthoven's figures on the saving in Federal income taxes, adding in my own estimate of 6 percent Social Security tax and 5 percent state income tax. See Enthoven 1978a.

first-dollar coverage. Under the exclusion, first-dollar coverage "enables the employee to finance *regular and expected* annual medical costs ... out of untaxed income. The insurance is in effect a form of tax-free installment payment for relatively predictable costs. Catastrophic costs, on the other hand, are a very low risk for any single employee...."[9] Most out-of-pocket catastrophic expenses will be tax deductible on individual returns, while out-of-pocket first-dollar expenses will likely not be. *If* first-dollar coverage without cost controls is more likely to encourage noncostworthy care than coverage with deductibles will, the exclusion of employer-paid premiums is the cause of even more noncostworthy health care than the previous estimate of 25 to 30 percent connotes. In any case, why should health insurance and health care be subsidized in such open-ended fashion?

Unjust Breaks for the Rich

Suppose, however, that there is reason to subsidize care, for example, the hidden externalities that we cited in favor of in-kind as opposed to cash aid (chapter 4). Critics of the income exclusion and tax deduction will still object. Both provide a discount which rises with income. Deductions and exclusions generally do that in a progressively graduated income tax system.[10]

The direct and obvious way this happens is inherent in the progressive tax rate itself. Indirect effects may be even more important. People with less income are statistically less likely to have employer-paid premiums, with their greater tax break than personally deducted premiums or actual expenses. And despite the proportional three-percent-of-income floor, savings from the personal deduction still rise with income: Medical spending increases as income rises, and high tax brackets increase the amount one saves by deducting expenses. Thus, even for all returns, not just those which itemize, the average 1978 tax saving for people under $5,000 was zero; for $5,000–$10,000, it was $10; for $10,000–$20,000, $28; for $30,000–$50,000, $105; and for $100,000–$200,000, $365.[11]

9. Butler 1980, emphasis added.

10. This is true for the tax breaks for health care even if the apparent "progressive" look of our overall tax system is illusory, and rendered so partly by the effect of deductions. In 1966, for example, taxpayers in every income bracket between the 10th and 97th percentiles paid roughly the same proportion of income in all taxes combined. See Klarman 1977, citing Pechman and Okner. Nevertheless, every marginal dollar of finally taxable income is taxed progressively. The tax break from the exclusion and deduction for health insurance and medical expenses is thus greater for those with higher incomes.

11. Hoffman and Steuerle 1979.

There is another unfortunate effect of the tax laws. Because they lower the net price of insurance and increase the use of care, they increase demand for it and thereby raise its price. But poorer persons already benefit less from the subsidies. *If they also end up paying higher prices for what care they do get, poorer people may finally actually lose from the subsidies, not merely gain less than the rich!*[12]

The least drastic suggested change in the present law is to limit the exclusion. Feldstein has proposed, for example, that it be limited to the equivalent premium for catastrophic, high-deductible coverage, or even more effectively, to an amount 30 percent below that.[13] These proposals aim primarily at controlling the inflationary effects of the exclusion. A suggested reform which directly attacks the exclusion's unfairly distributed benefits changes it to a tax credit. That could be either a flat amount which everyone who bought insurance could claim, or a percentage of what people spend for insurance and care that decreases with income. Both would stop rewarding people for choosing the most costly coverage, and both would equalize the rewards which rich and poor respectively receive from the tax laws. Enthoven has proposed further adjustment of the credit by actuarial risk category—by the likely expensiveness of one's insurance. His proposal to graduate the credit to reach 100 percent of the likely insurance premiums of the poor for minimally decent, presumably "low-style" health care would make the credit into a kind of national health insurance program.[14] Need, not what is spent on insurance and care, would determine the size of the credit.

Income Refinement, Not Subsidy of Care

By now this case against the present tax laws may look definitive: They apparently encourage excessive and noncostworthy insurance, and they subsidize the rich far more than the poor. Yet so far the entire case has been subtly one-sided. *If* "subsidizing" care is what the

12. Hoffman and Steuerle 1979. In the Social Security system such hidden and surprising effects also benefit those with higher incomes more than those with lower. High-income persons will likely receive more benefits relative to Social Security taxes paid than low-income persons will; they start paying at a later age and have higher life expectancies, and thus they collect more benefits, gain more from the tax exclusion of employer-paid contributions, and gain more from the tax exemption of Social Security benefits. See Friedman, in Cohen and Friedman 1972.

13. Feldstein's testimony before the Health Subcommittee of the Senate Finance Committee, 15 March 1979, is cited by Butler 1980.

14. Enthoven 1978a. To be a true government health insurance program, the credit would have to be arranged so that refunds would be provided if people's credit exceeded their tax liability; see Jensen 1954.

exclusion and deduction are doing, then instituting tax credits instead would be unquestionably preferable. But "subsidy" may be the wrong term for a perfectly legitimate method of reducing taxes. Some tax laws are meant to *refine a person's income base before it is taxed, not to subsidize anything.*[15] Deductions and exclusions look like subsidies only because we too easily assume that a person's gross income before paying for health care is really all income. That assumption begs the very questions which those defending exclusions and deductions press to our attention: What is the income which represents ability to pay? Isn't it income which a person can use to consume and accumulate, and isn't that the person's income *after* medical expenses? To be sure, an income tax is not the direct tax on consumption and accumulation that a sales tax is; you would be taxed for your income even if you threw it away and consumed or accumulated nothing. Still, it is a tax on *ability* to consume and accumulate.[16]

Examples make this strikingly clear. If people earn $30,000 a year, have accidents or serious illness, and spend $20,000 on necessary medical bills, they have only $10,000 left with which to consume or accumulate anything. Their "real" income has simply dropped to $10,000. While they may still have the financial ability to pay the medical bills, their ability to consume and accumulate is surely more accurately represented by the $10,000 figure than the $30,000. Therefore only $10,000 should be subject to income tax. The labels "tax subsidy," "tax expenditure," "tax preference," and "tax incentive" are all misnomers. An equally bad misnomer would be to call deducting an expense that is indisputably business-related a tax expenditure or subsidy. Such an expense surely ought to be subtracted from gross income to get real, taxable income.[17] Likewise, income spent on health care ought to be deducted.[18]

15. Jensen 1954.

16. Andrews 1972; Simons 1938.

17. We might wonder whether this general argument for deductions is applicable to interest payments. Andrews (1972) suggests that it is. Money spent on interest, he says, is more like medical care than like consumption; it is not spent on bread, wine, travel, etc., and thus if it is spent in a sense on "nothing," it should not count toward the ability to consume and accumulate, which is what we want to tax. It astounds me that this argument is seriously proposed. Surely enjoying a pleasure now rather than later and paying interest to do it is a kind of consumption. Driving a car, unlike breathing air, is a kind of consumption; to drive a car is to take resources away from something else. Spending now instead of later is likewise using something scarce and desired, and it takes that away from someone else—someone *else* has to give up spending now (loan me money) so I can spend now.

18. Abel-Smith 1976, p. 39. In some "progressive" developments in the delivery of health care at the turn of the century, in fact, health care for workers was looked at in

Reforms

Suppose this defense of the present deductions is persuasive. Minor reforms, however, would still be required in the tax laws. If income refinement is the proper logic of medical deductions, why have any percent-of-income floor for personal medical deductions?[19] The disparity between full exclusion of employer-paid premiums and partial deduction of individually paid premiums should also be reconciled.

More importantly, the logic behind income refinement seems to demand that deductions be given for *illness itself* instead of for the costs of its *treatment*. After all, what is the reason for using ability to consume and accumulate as the criterion for determining ability to pay, the intended base for taxation? It is the well-being constituted by ability to consume and accumulate,[20] for then the principle of justice as equality can come in to justify the progressive income tax. Now note: Illness itself, not only necessary medical expense, subtracts from that well-being. The principle of justice as equality is reason for directly compensating for illness instead of only deducting medical expenses—illness is a loss of well-being.

The suggestion may, admittedly, sound wild, but perhaps it could be implemented by tax credits (or by payments if a person's tax liability were lower than this credit).[21] If some of the ill want to spend their compensation on medical care, they may. Others will see what they think are better uses of the money, or part of it. The Christian Scientist who gets sick but uses no medical care would get the same tax advantage as the equally ill person who spends $10,000 on care. Of course the medical profession would oppose this. But its moral logic is powerful. Basing taxes on ability to consume and accumulate is driven by the principle of justice as equality, but that principle also demands some kind of compensation for illness, not only the exclusion from taxation of money actually spent for treatment.

---

precisely this way. Frederick Gates of the Rockefeller philanthropies successfully persuaded many businessmen to take a greater interest in preventive health care because healthy workers are more profitable. In 1909 he calculated that it took 25 percent more laborers in the cotton mills of those counties of North Carolina heavily infected with hookworm to secure the same production. In the early twentieth century the American Association for Labor Legislation, an alliance of business and labor leaders, won considerable business support for compulsory national health insurance. The National Association of Manufacturers supported it against voluntary employer-provided insurance, saying it wanted to eliminate some corporation presidents' foolish temptation to sacrifice long-run profits for the current year's gains. See Brown 1979, pp. 112–17.

19. Hoffman and Steuerle 1979.
20. See Andrews 1972.
21. Posner 1972.

Such a tax credit with its "compensation" logic avoids a nasty problem of deductions. In deductions the larger tax "saving" which accrues to those with higher incomes does not necessarily indicate greater medical need. To be sure, "need" is an elastic concept, but can it possibly be so elastic that *everything* medical which a rich person spends money on (and can deduct), and *no* care which a poorer person *forgoes* (and cannot deduct), is a medical necessity? Poorer people monetarily value health care lower than rich people do, but that hardly means that what is a necessity to a rich person is never a necessity to a poor person. Nor does it mean that for the poor, doing without care is less of a sacrifice than it is for the rich. It means only that other needs of the poor are more urgent than other needs of the rich. But then what could be the basis for allowing a person with a $50,000 per year income to deduct $5,000 of actual medical expenses, while allowing a $10,000 per year person with the same health problem to deduct only $1,000? *Actual medical expenditures do not accurately indicate the degree of welfare loss from an illness. They are the wrong thing to subtract from gross income to get the relevant ability to pay.*

In conclusion, the present system of tax exclusion and deduction is a relatively unjust and waste-encouraging way for the government to support people's decisions to insure and compensate for the financial ravages of illness. A limited tax credit adjusted by risk category, and possibly reversely graduated by income, would seem to be more just; it would also encourage less noncostworthy care.

2. STIMULATING COMPETITION

To some

> it is inconceivable that high-quality, efficient care can be provided for all without welding all ... health care institutions and programs into a single system. And yet there is a continued demand for pluralism in the development of a national health care system. Imagine how silly it would be to demand pluralism in telephone communications.[22]

Yet to others health care is regarded as a market good, a service offered by a variety of different providers competing for the choices of consumers. Health care fails to share with the telephone precisely many of those characteristics which tend to make telephone service, or roads, or national defense either natural monopolies or public util-

22. Rutstein 1974, p. xxi.

ities.[23] Pluralistic competition, it is claimed, will give consumers of health care more for their money than public ownership or extensive public regulation will.

The claim is directly about efficiency. But the claim is also, though secondarily, about costworthiness: Different plans and providers emphasize different types of care and arrangements for paying for them, and only individual consumers can match these variations to their own values. Some want chiropractors, others do not; some do not want psychotherapy covered, others do; some prefer one prepaid network of providers to be responsible for delivering all care, while others insist on wider immediate choice of physician; and so forth. By increasing competition in health services, total costs for health care will decrease, and even if costs do not decrease, greater consumer satisfaction will result.

Presently there is little competition. Physicians generate most of the demand for services, services about which patients are usually ignorant. Hospitals are paid at rates set simply to reimburse the costs they incur. Physicians rest content that insurers will pay patients' bills. Insurers are seldom in a position to dispute physician or hospital charges, and in fact they have a long-run interest in total health-care costs being as high a proportion of GNP as possible. Physicians limit their own supply, and even in oversupplied areas generate their own demand, target their incomes, and work and charge accordingly. Medical fees, even hospital rates, are rarely advertised or even publicized. Employees get no savings from choosing a lower-cost plan than their employer offers.

Concrete Proposals

Various strategies for stimulating competition are aimed directly at changing these noncompetitive aspects of the medical economy. (1) While patient demand for health *care* is relatively independent of the prices of competing providers, consumer demand for health *insurance* or health care plans is more elastic. Patients ("pre-patients") do shop around at the point of purchasing insurance or subscribing to a plan. Here physicians and hospitals cannot simply create demand for their services.[24] (2) Employers must give employees a wide choice of plans and pay no greater premium for one plan chosen by an employee than for any other. Only then will employees have an interest in

23. Enthoven 1978a.
24. Phelps 1973; Enthoven 1978a.

choosing the most costworthy plan. (3) Exclusion of premiums from taxable income must be limited so that the subscriber pays the full extra cost of less efficient or costworthy plans. (4) To assist employees and others in choosing intelligently, all competing plans need to be described in simple and succinct language in clearly comparative publications.[25] (5) The effect of competition will probably be felt by hospitals and physicians most if they belong to plans which already give them an incentive to practice cost-consciously.[26] Any plan with a closed panel of providers who are accountable for the costs they generate will create this incentive. Ironically it is not "free choice of physician" which generates cost competition.

Some of these conditions for increased competition are already present in the Federal Employees Health Benefits Program. At specified intervals, Federal employees choose from among a large number of approved carriers, plans, and benefit packages. The government pays the same amount regardless of the employee's choice, an amount less than the full premium for one of the least expensive low-option plans; the individual employee makes up the difference.[27]

This same sort of arrangement could be legislatively expanded into a requirement for all employers in the society. It could also be made by government into a kind of national health insurance scheme, as in Enthoven's Consumer Choice Health Plan: Vouchers to be used toward the purchase of health insurance could cover the poor for the full expense of the cheapest no-cost-sharing plans and cover those with higher incomes progressively less.[28] Various legislation intro-

25. To be consistent, we might also want to publish facts about the quality of care provided. Perhaps, for example, mortality statistics for coronary bypass operations in different hospitals ought to be published if they are not too misleading—that is, more misleading than not knowing them at all. The whole idea behind competition is to enable the consumer to make an intelligent choice about health-care costs, but an intelligent choice requires knowledge of the quality of care, not just costs alone.

26. They may not even have to belong to such plans to feel this competition. Other providers will feel it if they have to compete with such plans in their locale, that is, if such plans have achieved a high enough level of enrollment to exert pressure on all providers in the area to be cost-conscious. For a description of such a level of competition in Minneapolis-Saint Paul, see Christianson and McClure 1979. For an extreme and interesting example of the reverse pressure—on prepaid plans by open-panel providers, and upward on costs—see Goldberg and Greenberg 1977. Havighurst and Hackbarth (1979) argue that medical-profession-sponsored plans which include more than a certain percentage of physicians in an area, even closed-panel plans, should be banned. Otherwise the profession itself can effectively eliminate competition. Even an HMO can dampen competition if it gets too large.

27. Somers and Somers 1977, pp. 133–35.

28. Enthoven 1978a, 1978b, 1979a, 1979b, 1980.

duced in Congress has aimed at increasing competition, though it has generally been less comprehensive than Enthoven's plan.[29] Schweiker's bill required employers to rebate to individual employees, as tax-free income, any savings from their choice of the less expensive plans.

Two questions about proposals to stimulate competition are crucial: *Is* competition more likely than government regulation to contain costs and satisfy consumer preference? Can a competitive free market provide *equitable* care for all segments of the population?

Will Competition Contain Costs?

Medicare's refusal to pay for body scans until the CT scanner was shown to be effective has been cited as an example of successful, cost-controlling government regulation.[30] But the government only required that *some* benefit be shown for the procedure and that it be proven *safe*. Its initial refusal to pay was not made in order to restrain expensive care with too few benefits to justify the cost. Decisions of that harder sort are likely to be made only by individual consumers

29. See bills introduced by former senator Schweiker, Senator Durenberger, and former representative Ullman in the 1979–80 Congress. I have not included Senator Kennedy's 1979 Health Care for All Americans Act (S. 1720) in this list. While it is far more complex a proposal for guaranteeing universal, comprehensive coverage than Enthoven's Consumer Choice Health Plan, it incorporates several features of the competitive strategy. As in competitive proposals, private insurers are kept in the act; except for those presently covered by Medicare, the government is not the insurer. The government only subsidizes the program and oversees the collection and allocation of premium money to different plans in proportion to the number and risk-category of their subscribers. Enrollees of more cost-conscious plans get either rebates from their plan or additional services beyond those required in the basic coverage. The bill is not, however, as thoroughly competitive or pluralistic as Enthoven's CCHP. It does not make rebates tax-free unless they are taken in the form of additional services. By setting fees for all regional physicians, it discourages physicians from underbidding each other, a practice which would hopefully occur in more competitive plans. The total health-care budget is restricted to a certain percentage of GNP. Thus individual consumer choices are not allowed to determine indirectly what a costworthy percentage would be. Similarly, Kennedy's bill sets budgetary limits on the total spent for preventive-care services. It also excludes certain things from the basic package for everyone (e.g., chiropractic care) and mandates inclusion of other things; it does not permit individual consumers to fashion their own basic packages. In general, its "consortia" method of collecting and allocating funds for premiums and its state health-care budget limitations require bureaucratic arrangements far in excess of those supported by the proponents of competition.

30. Ball 1978. A better example might be the Health Care Financing Administration's 1980 rescission of its previous decision to reimburse selectively for heart transplants. Thereby HCFA allegedly saved $500 million. HCFA's justification, however, made its decision seem to concern, not really costworthiness, but only efficiency—it claimed that paying for the transplants would prevent it from paying for other more cost-effective health-care procedures. See Warner and Luce 1982, pp. 190–91.

for themselves: Any democratic body politic will find it very difficult to impose such choices more universally on all. Even government regulation of providers merely aimed at making them more efficient is unlikely to be effective. Since a regulator will usually use provider's costs as a starting figure, cost reimbursement will naturally become the operating if not the official formula. But of course that puts no brake on costs at all. In effect regulators, understandably, are captured by the regulated. As a claim about hospital regulators in particular, the "capture" critique seems persuasive; the regulators just depend too much on the professional expertise of the regulated.[31]

Even specific attempts at regulating costs, such as Certificate-of-Need (CON) requirements for hospital expansion and Professional Standards Review Organizations (PSROs) for physician practices, seem to have failed. Special circumstances of a hospital, instead of real community bed needs, have usually dominated CON decision. CON legislation may actually have escalated hospital costs by driving capital expansion away from beds and into advances in technology.[32] While PSROs were originally aimed in part at cost containment, they quickly became largely occupied with quality control. Made up entirely of physicians, whose orientation is naturally toward improving the quality of care regardless of price, PSROs, ironically, may have actually contributed to cost escalation. Even the less critical commentators grant that any of their savings have been offset by their administrative costs.[33]

The apparent futility of this kind of regulation is illustrated strikingly by a 1980 development in New York state. It ended up in the absurd situation in which the more empty beds hospitals had, the larger the state subsidies they received! To discourage excess bed capacity, earlier regulation had penalized hospitals for not filling at least 85 percent of their beds. The president of the Greater New York Hospital Association explained the cost-escalating effect of that earlier, only apparently sensible, approach: "If you continue to pay hospitals for filling beds, then they are going to be filled"—filled, that is, with patients who only marginally need to be there. So you switch to the opposite policy and reward empty beds. "If you ... pay hospitals ... for empty beds, then ... you're going to get ... empty beds." The empty

31. Enthoven 1978a; Enthoven and Noll 1979; Salkever and Bice 1978; Havighurst 1973; Alford 1975, pp. 203–04.
32. Luft and Frisvold 1979; Salkever and Bice 1978.
33. Blumstein 1976; Anderson 1976; Donabedian 1978.

beds still cost money, of course, but less, and it is disguised by being spread onto the average charge per patient day.[34]

The critics of regulation conclude that any regulation will be largely circumvented, new regulations designed to correct the circumvention of earlier ones will be frustrated, and so forth and so on. A less futile and costly strategy, they claim, is for the government to regulate only so as to stimulate competition and change the incentives within the market itself. Some areas, most notably Minneapolis-Saint Paul, have shown promising results using competitive strategies.[35]

Suppose we agree that regulative strategies will not likely restrain costs in the long run. Which policy—direct regulation or stimulating competition—is most likely to maximize the satisfaction of consumer preferences? Both, theoretically, lay claim to doing that. Obviously, competition claims to satisfy consumer preferences. But public regulation does also: The standard of reference for determining what regulation is justified is a market of *reasonably informed* consumers.[36] The preferences of such informed consumers are essentially unobservable; a priori, we cannot say they are revealed any more by a competitive market than they are by public policy decision and consequent regulation. Public regulators try to stimulate the choices of informed consumers, and the health-care marketplace will not work well to reveal consumer preferences if physicians themselves create most of the demand for medical services.[37] Defenders of competition, of course, will claim that at the point of choosing an insurance policy or plan, consumers, not physicians, create most of the demand. It might be argued that even there, physicians have an indirect influence on most

34. Sullivan 1979.

35. Christianson and McClure 1979.

36. Newhouse 1976b. Are reasonably informed consumers needed as a reference point? It might be claimed that consumer choices have moral weight even when they fall far, far short of being reasonably informed, for two reasons. (1) The autonomy of even a relatively uninformed choice needs to be respected. In many walks of life people should have to take responsibility for their uninformed choices. (2) We do not measure the morally relevant utility or welfare of real, actual individuals by reference to some hypothetical, knowledgeable persons they will never be. In this respect there is, to be sure, a huge theoretical ambiguity in subjective preference versions of utilitarianism: Should the ultimate, intrinsic preferences in reference to which we define one's welfare or utility be disregarded if one is not highly knowledgeable? If we were to require a background of complete knowledgeability for preferences, we would end up regarding as morally relevant only what people would prefer if they had comparatively experienced all the relevant life-styles in question. Surely we would make utilitarianism into a very paternalistic position if we were to define morally relevant utility only by reference to such fully informed persons. Analogously, to argue against the medical-care marketplace because consumers are not all that informed may also reflect paternalism.

37. Fuchs and Newhouse 1978.

demand by what they say about the quality of care in those plans. How, for example, are most health-care consumers to know whether the use of intensive care units to give only slight benefits to 90 percent of their patients is a good buy? People will ultimately take their cue in choosing plans from what physicians have to say about the costworthiness of a plan's use of resources. The sufficiently knowledgeable consumer doesn't often exist.

But neither does the reasonably knowledgeable voter. That's the catch. Regulators lack critical information about consumers' preferences. Furthermore, regulators cannot accede to a variety of different consumer preferences at the same time. The *pluralism* of options, not consumer choice per se, of a competitive health-care marketplace is what makes it appear to fit consumer preferences better than public-policy decisions are likely to.[38]

Equity for the Ill

There is a nastier problem which competitive models must deal with. Can they be fair to the ill? Without restrictions on what providers and insurers can offer, a completely free market clearly puts the ill at a disadvantage. Low and high risk individuals will not remain pooled together. The history of Blue Cross and Blue Shield illustrates this. The Blues had to abandon their original community-rating of premiums once private commercial companies began to experience-rate theirs to particular individuals. Any insurer who community-rated quickly lost healthier clients to plans which experience-rated. The remaining, more likely ill, people pushed premiums up for Blue Cross and Blue Shield, causing even more of the relatively healthy people to leave for other plans. Thus, any insurer who refuses to experience-rate ends up with the most likely ill people, paying more for their insurance. The only way out is to prohibit experience-rating completely.[39]

Not even prohibiting experience-rating, however, will stop the more likely well from gravitating to the less expensive plans. To attract them as its predominant subscribers a plan has only to fashion or de-

38. See Brock (1982) for a sensitive and careful assessment of competitive strategies in terms of both consumer welfare and liberty.

39. Krizay and Wilson 1974, p. 40; Schelling 1976. Here, for purposes of simplicity, I am assuming that the likely ill are not likely ill because of their own freely adopted habits or life-styles. Of course, if they are, then it may be fair indeed to charge *these* likely ill people higher premiums, or to tax them and devote the proceeds to government subsidies for others. For a comprehensive discussion of this complex question, see Veatch 1980. At this point my claim is that if we do decide that it is fair that the voluntarily unhealthy pay more, this is the *only* sort of experience-rating that should be permitted if the well and the ill are to share costs equitably.

liver its benefits to appeal to them. It could, for example, use significant deductibles and coinsurance. It could also cover certain categories of benefits which appeal more to statistically healthy groups, or
exclude certain categories which are likely to be needed more by
groups with a higher incidence of illness. Thus, many prepaid plans
have been very shrewd to cover maternity benefits, thereby attracting
a younger clientele; despite the higher cost of covering maternity benefits, having a younger, healthier clientele has allowed these plans to
offer better coverage for a lower total cost. Or plans could locate their
primary-care facilities in nonpoor areas to attract fewer of the poor,
who are statistically more likely to need care.[40] Apparently, then, a fair
competition-stimulating approach must prohibit the use of most cost-
sharing arrangements, mandate a basic coverage package, and prohibit additional coverages which appeal to involuntarily healthier
groups.[41]

But by now the competitive approach begins to look as though it
protects a lot less pluralism than at first it claimed to. Is conflict between the just sharing of costs among well and ill, on the one hand,
and individual consumer autonomy and cost control, on the other,
ineradicable? Since excessive insurance may be a significant contrib-
utor to rising costs, and since the larger strategy within which we are
operating is to stimulate the competitive market in order to restrain
costs, it seems particularly ironic that in the end a competitive strategy leads to preventing less risk-averse consumers from choosing
cheaper plans. It is not, of course, clear that justice should always win
the day when it conflicts with autonomy or welfare. Nevertheless, it is
plausible to require even consumer-choice-oriented competition strategies to incorporate basic coverage requirements and restrictions on
cost sharing.

Perhaps, however, this makes the dilemma between justice and
consumer autonomy sound sharper than it is. For one thing, the market for health care quickly evolved group insurance by itself; employees *voluntarily* pooled themselves to equalize the premiums for the
well and the ill.[42] Autonomy did not need to be sacrificed. Perhaps the
dilemma can also be blunted by using less restrictive measures than
banning cost sharing and standardizing basic coverage. The first step

40. These examples were suggested to me by Harold Luft (Health Policy Program,
University of California Medical School at San Francisco). An excellent review of this entire set of problems is presented by Rushefsky 1981.
41. Senator Kennedy's 1979 bill (S. 1720) does the first two of these things, and Enthoven's plan does the second.
42. Ball 1978.

of a less restrictive approach would simply be to have open enrollment at required regular intervals, as long as the additional cost of
more expensive premiums was picked up by a greater tax credit. Or
people who have been refused twice by community-rating plans could
be distributed across all plans statewide in proportion to the size of
each plan's business. These persons would even be given their first
choice of plan, unless that plan's quota of high-risk subscribers was
already filled.[43] Another suggestion is to fill half the places in any plan
which has a surplus of applicants by a lottery among them.[44] Most of
these steps are administratively cumbersome, and it is doubtful
whether any combination of them could put a stop to the leakage of
healthier people into cheaper plans as completely as more drastic restrictions would. Nevertheless, they demonstrate how far a bit of crea-
tivity and imagination on the part of policy planners might go in making competition fair to the likely ill.

There is one dimension of distributive justice between well and
ill in which competitive models may even have advantages over direct
governmental regulation. Suppose we wonder, for example, how a future society will allocate expensive, implantable, artificial hearts.[45] Governments will find it difficult to limit the diffusion of such technologies, even for people for whom the benefits of such technologies
would be slight. It will be almost impossible to get any political consensus on what technology for whom to forgo, and without such a
consensus the pressures on government to underwrite the use of a
given technology will be nearly impossible to resist.[46] The beauty of
the competitive market is that no consensus is needed. Certain plans

43. Former senator Schweiker's bill incorporates this last provision; see Butler
1980. Enthoven (1978a) requires open enrollment in all plans; he allows different premiums for persons in different actuarial categories, but proposes that tax subsidies pick
up the difference for the consumer. McClure has made all these suggestions privately to
the author.

44. Christopher Jencks proposes a similar lottery as a final safeguard against unjust movement of easier-to-educate students to the better schools in a system of educational vouchers. See Jencks 1970. On educational voucher plans in general, see Maynard 1975 and Stevens 1971. There are many parallels between the voucher plans for
health care and for education. Many people do not realize how seriously the educational voucher strategy for making the public schools face competition has been proposed. It has even tried experimentally under Federal Office of Equal Opportunity funding in the Alum Rock Unified School District, in San Jose, California. In Gary, Indiana, a
similar proposed experiment met with vigorous opposition from the public school
teachers' union. Competition with equally funded "private" schools may cost public
school teachers dearly in power and security. One can muse over the parallels in health
care.

45. Annas 1977.

46. Schroeder and Showstack 1979.

exclude certain services from coverage and others do not, but they all
then put themselves out for sale. Are those who are "committed to un-
constrained financial commitments to all life saving as a moral imper-
ative ... entitled to have their preferences supported involuntarily by
persons who are not like-minded"? Furthermore, isn't an exclusion
only a contractual agreement adopted for economic reasons, not an
offensive judgment that you and your body don't really need this
care?[47]

Still, the competitive market is not yet off the hook. Plans that
cover lifesaving and death-delaying procedures without regard to expense will attract people who are likely to need them. Only if every
plan excludes some such expensive services (though each plan excludes different ones) will the premiums for people likely to need a
certain service not be higher than the premiums for others. We could
require that insurers loan members the money to purchase excluded
services,[48] but that only moderates, rather than alleviates, the injustice.
Unfortunately, we cannot distinguish two morally different groups—
those who legitimately choose the cheaper plans because they think
that even if they should someday need the excluded service, it isn't
costworthy, and those who choose the cheaper plan simply because
they are unlikely to need the service in question. While competition
may "solve" the problem by avoiding the need for the difficult-to-get
political consensus, it generally does so at the cost of injustice to the
likely ill. Government's technologically permissive decisions to expand
the category of mandatory basic coverage and not allow individuals to
go their separate ways will understandably creep back in.

Equity for the Poor
There is another important question about competitive models for
health care: Can they be fair to the poor? Their assistance to the poor
will take the form of either cash aid or a national insurance scheme
like Enthoven's voucher plan. Any vouchers would be graduated to
cover the full expense of low cost-sharing, relatively comprehensive
plans for the poor while covering much less for others. Even then, the
nonpoor are likely to have great enough purchasing power to attract
providers to meet their needs, and the poor will remain at a disadvantage. And, for cultural reasons alone, members of a profession earning
incomes far higher than the societal average are not likely to locate
close to the poor.[49] Even if physicians are present in excess supply,

47. Havighurst, Blumstein, and Bovbjerg 1976; Havighurst and Hackbarth 1979.
48. Havighurst and Hackbarth 1979.
49. Anderson 1972, p. 164; Sidel and Sidel 1977, pp. 300–01.

they can still target their practices to the upper and middle incomes, since they are largely able to create their own demand.

The problem is crucial. The poor probably prefer less-than-equal, low-style, thrifty health care with access to the resultant savings. That preference argues in the direction of competitive models. But the poor have a grievous complaint if providers are then not accessible to them. Moreover, not just any accessibility will do, only accessibility to the care *which fits the poor's standards of costworthiness.* While they don't want "Medicaid mills," they do want relatively low-cost, low-style care, even if medically speaking it is not the best. In a society that is heavily middle-class and highly technological, health-care providers are not likely to offer those options. *For competition to succeed in providing adequate and costworthy care for the poor, either their government-provided vouchers will have to be very large, providers will have to be willing to deliver the level of care they want, or the government will have to coerce or entice providers to do that.* That is a tall order indeed. A competitive approach must involve either very large programs of societal assistance to the poor, a medical profession genuinely able and willing to imagine itself in the shoes of the poor, or considerable cajoling of providers.[50]

Despite these problems of justice for a competitive model, we should not forget its likely advantages of pluralism and consumer autonomy over direct government insurance or delivery. We should also note, however, that a fully competitive, consumer-autonomy-oriented system would use not vouchers but cash. For one thing, some people will not want to spend much money on medical care at all; witness Christian Scientists. And any voucher system will inevitably impinge on consumer autonomy in defining the health care for which the vouchers count. Does health care include laetrile? "Holistic" health care? Care from naturopaths? From Gurus? Tribal medicine?[51] And so

50. The latter will be objectionable to those who think the standards of health care for low-income persons ought to be as high as those for wealthier people. Arras (1981) apparently thinks that. Because of their deprivation, he says, the poor are "unable to appreciate either their own health needs or the potential benefits of medical care." Especially with a voucher system with cash rebates for those who find a health plan cheaper than the value of the voucher, the poor will be "compelled to buy plans . . . [that] fail to meet their greater than average health care needs." My reasons for generally rejecting this paternalistic viewpoint have already been developed in chaps. 3 and 4; see also the reply to Arras by Lomasky (1981). If, of course, Arras's viewpoint is not rejected, we will either have to insist on rigidly high standards for all plans for which the vouchers can be used, or abandon the competition proposals entirely as inequitable for the poor.

51. I am told, for example, that the Navajo tribe was refused its request for coverage of tribal medicine in the United Mine Workers' health insurance policy that covers union members in the tribe.

on. The moral thrust behind vouchers logically pushes toward aid pre-dominantly in the form of cash, though with universal maternal and child care and perhaps minimal emergency care (see 4.2). Equity con-siderations may not stop this push. If the inequity between well and ill can be alleviated reasonably well in a voucher system by graduating the vouchers by actuarial health risk, inequity between well and ill in a system of largely cash aid can be handled in the same way. Of course, in either case, cash or vouchers, government will probably have to be called in to entice, cajole, or require providers to make their services more accessible and qualitatively more appropriate to the poor.

In any case, we should temper any enthusiasm for competitive models with more qualifications than just the last one. A major threat to the cost control and consumer autonomy which drive competitive proposals is the potential for collusion among large corporate health-care providers. They may come to dominate health-care provisions as much as they do some other sectors of the economy. Especially with hospitals, we may need the sharpest watchdogs to keep things truly competitive. Even then the effort might be futile. The "capture theory" (of the regulators by the regulated) that was used initially to dismiss the effectiveness of more government regulation and argue for com-petition may come home to haunt the proponents of competition themselves.

A concluding quotation from Victor Fuchs is apt: "I value freedom *and* justice *and* efficiency.... I may have to give up a little of one goal to insure the partial achievement of others. Moreover, ... the best way to seek multiple goals is through a multiplicity of institutions—the market, government, the family, and others."[52] I suspect he is right. There are no panaceas.

3. PREPAID PLANS

Prepaid plans are distinguished from ordinary insurance in that they merge the roles of provider and insurer: We prepay the provider to give us the care we might later need. Thus, when we do need care, we cannot pick our provider, but must choose from a closed panel of providers—this is the "closed-panel" character of prepaid plans.

New varieties of prepaid plans require us to use the latter char-acteristic as the defining feature of "prepaid," rather than the merging of provider and insurer. In addition to the usual health maintenance

52. Fuchs 1979.

organizations and prepaid group practices, closed-panel arrangements now include "independent-practice associations," "foundations for medical care," and "primary-care networks."[53] In these arrangements the provider and the insurer are not always one and the same institution. In other ways, too, they are hybrids. Their physicians are sometimes paid on a fee-for-service basis, and there is no essential reason why they cannot involve significant patient cost sharing.

The Savings

The ways in which these various, new, closed-panel arrangements give providers an incentive to be cost-conscious are diverse. Sometimes providers own the plan, and other times their salaries are linked in some way to the plan's annual surplus or deficit. In a fee-for-service "primary-care network," each member primary-care physician gets reimbursed according to a schedule that is slightly affected by whether that physician's patients have exceeded the average annual medical expenses that they would actuarially be expected to accrue. In independent practice associations, incentives may be less direct; physicians are not kept in the plan if they are judged by the plan not to be practicing cost-consciously. All these arrangements hope to give physicians an incentive to keep people healthy, not just to prescribe expensive services for them once they are ill.

The cost savings of prepaid plans have often been impressive. In Western areas, for example, Kaiser-Permanente comes in 33 percent below commercial plans and Blue Cross and Blue Shield in total expense per patient.[54] A 1975 study showed annual hospitalization rates for Medicaid patients to be 356 hospital days per 1,000 patients for HMOs, compared to 936 days per 1,000 patients for fee-for-service providers. Prepaid group practices in the U.S. have half the surgery rate of Blue Shield fee-for-service providers. CT scanning and gastrointestinal endoscopy use is significantly lower in HMOs. Some of these studies have tried to control for differences in the initial health of the enrollees.[55] In any case, with their typically very low cost sharing and comprehensive coverage, prepaid plans will likely attract their share of likely ill subscribers. We are reasonably safe, then, in viewing prepaid

53. Lewis, Fein, and Mechanic 1976, pp. 220–40; Moore 1979.
54. Luft 1978. That may not show up as *premiums* that are 33 percent lower for Kaiser than for the other plans, since Kaiser may have had either less cost sharing or broader coverage than the others. It is only that total individual health-care costs for people who subscribed with Kaiser were 33 percent lower than for subscribers with other plans.
55. Gaus et al. 1975; Rice 1977; Schroeder and Showstack 1979; and Blumberg 1980.

plans as a cost-restraining development in American health-care delivery.

But is this restraint a function of their closed-panel and insurer-is-provider characteristics, or of some other associated factor? Couldn't it largely be a function of tighter hospital-bed supply? Lower hospitalization rates account for most HMO savings, and the larger, better established HMOs have their own more tightly controlled hospitals.[56] Or could it be the fact that most prepaid plans pay physicians on a salary rather than fee-for-service basis?[57] It could also be the competitive environment that surrounds a new form of delivery that has to prove itself to the public. In fact, without competitive pressures to keep their rates down, prepaid plans could easily show a surplus even with exuberant use of care. If we imbued the whole system with competitive pressures, perhaps equivalent savings might occur with other delivery arrangements.

Dangers

A crucial point about the lower costs of prepaid plans remains unclear. Is it costworthy or noncostworthy care that is being cut? Traditionally the medical associations have alleged it is the former. A 1962 AMA editorial unconditionally pronounced that "in the interest of good medicine and the public health, the principle of fee-for-service must not be set aside."[58] Third-party insurance paying fee-for-service tends to direct the physician's loyalty to the patient, not to the plan or the insurer. While fee-for-service physicians may tend to "overdoctor," prepaid physicians may tend to "underdoctor."[59] This is a significant moral issue, one which prepaid plans cannot dismiss simply be-

56. Klarman 1979; Luft 1978, 1980.

57. Redisch 1978.

58. Ward 1975, p. 13. The AMA's opposition is long-standing. In 1943 the U.S. Supreme Court upheld the conviction of the District of Columbia Medical Society for antitrust violations in trying to stop the formation of the Group Health Association. See Rayack 1977, pp. 414–16, and *AMA v. U.S.*, 317 U.S. 419 (1943). Many other examples of similar opposition can be found; see Goldberg and Greenberg 1977; Rayack 1977, pp. 416–19; and Kessel 1958. More recently physicians have tried to halt new prepaid health plans by denying certificates-of-need for capital facilities; see Kingsdale 1979.

59. There is a much more damning explanation of the reason for the medical association's opposition. In a brilliant essay Kessel (1958) argues that the basis for the opposition to prepaid plans is not any principled objection to the danger of underdoctoring, but simple economic self-interest. Price discrimination—charging low- and high-income patients different fees—reflects the monopoly power of physicians, which enables them to charge high-income patients whatever those patients feel they can afford in the psychologically pressing circumstances of a threat to their health. It also spills over into charging insured patients more than uninsured ones. Prepaid plans then "represent a means of massive price cutting to high income patients."

cause fee-for-service medicine has been so narrowly self-interested in its war against them.

Each side here probably has some of the truth. Clearly, conflicts of interest are inherent in both methods of delivery. At their worst, fee-for-service physicians either prescribe more unnecessary or noncostworthy service or increase their fees when a patient is insured.[60] At their worst, prepaid physicians are motivated only to minimize their members' need for medical care, not to prevent death or the kind of disablement which does not call for expensive care. It has been suggested that ideally a prepaid plan would make providers responsible not only for the medical care of subscribers, but also for their morbidity, disability, and life insurance payments.[61] Above all, it would seem that physicians should be precluded from owning a plan.

Nevertheless, in the context of contemporary American medicine the greater, more realistic dangers seem to lie with fee-for-service, open-panel insurance. Since the bias of American medicine already probably lies with overdoctoring, prepaid plans are a natural antidote. With competition from fee-for-service physicians, who will quickly stigmatize any prepaid plan that underdoctors, only plans "with very secure reputations or explicit subscriber acceptance of their policies will be able to take even the most appropriate gambles with the health and lives of patients."[62] Furthermore, if a board of subscribers agrees with provider-imposed restraints, underdoctoring loses its morally suspicious character. If people want to control their costs, why shouldn't they freely associate in a way that they realize restricts their services?

Nevertheless, it is clear by now that two conditions are absolutely crucial: *The plan must be a free association,* and *subscribers must somehow be aware of cost restraints.* The first may require competition from other plans, including open-panel ones. The second also points to this requirement. Above all, prepaid plans should have some kind of system for registering complaints about inadequate care, and other subscribers should have access to what these are. (For example, a subscriber-provider board might hear complaints at open meetings.) The kind and amount of monetary interest that individual physicians have in holding down costs should be publicized in a plan's public relations literature. In the case of physician *refusals* to perform surgery, second opinions from providers outside the plan should be cov-

60. See Schwartz 1978 and Barker 1980.
61. Luft 1977.
62. Havighurst, Blumstein, and Bovbjerg 1976.

ered; that stipulation is fair only if in traditional insurance a second opinion should be provided when surgery *is* recommended.[63] One of the greatest irritations to patients in prepaid plans is not being covered for a different but no more expensive kind of care from another provider. Here independent-practice associations and primary-care networks have distinct advantages over prepaid plans with a smaller range of personnel.

Whether these dangers of prepaid plans outweigh their advantages is properly a matter for subscribers to decide. Having a choice among a range of plans is essential. It is also crucial that competition between these plans be fair. Very often it has not been. Taxable-income exclusions for unlimited premiums hide part of the real extra cost of traditional insurance. Medicare has done the same, paying as much as 76 percent more for fee-for-service beneficiaries than for HMO recipients.[64] And unlike open-panel insurers, HMOs have been required by the government to community-rate and maintain open enrollment.

As long as there is fair competition, prepaid plans have a crucial role to play in making health care more costworthy. They reflect prospective patients' right to associate freely with others in order to control costs. If any ill subscribers get somewhat worse care than they would in the better non-prepaid plans, they have no complaint—in subscribing, they have freely chosen the bargain.

4. A NATIONAL HEALTH SERVICE

A national health service (NHS) is essentially a single, exclusive, government-owned prepaid plan for the whole population. Like prepaid plans it is a way for people to control the escalation of costs without leaving themselves less insured. Through the political process people set a maximum budget limit for spending on health care. Unlike present prepaid plans, however, an NHS has a virtual monopoly on care. It gives *individual* prospective patients little room for choice about the level of service they want, think they need, and are willing to pay for.[65]

This restriction of consumer choice may be as objectionable as a medical association's attempt to confine patients to open-panel arrangements is. The poor may prefer to spend less on health care than

63. Schwartz 1978.
64. Enthoven 1978a.
65. Neuhauser and Lewicki 1976. For the rich, of course, the NHS may not look as though it monopolizes care. In Britain, for example, care can be bought outside the NHS by those who are willing to pay for it entirely by themselves.

NHS services reflect and use the "savings" on other things. The relatively wealthy may prefer to spend more, but not to pay fully again (in addition to what they pay in taxes for the NHS) for the alternate care they feel is costworthy. Then, too, Christian Scientists have little use for NHS services, as pacifists have little use for the Pentagon. But defense is hardly a good parallel, since most health care, unlike defense, is not a "public good."[66] Thus the Christian Scientist disavowal of health care is logically more bothersome to an NHS than the pacifist disavowal of violence is to the Pentagon.[67] Education is not a good parallel for an NHS, either. The arguments for discouraging a pluralstic, competitive choice of schools at the early levels of education—the importance of minimizing separatism and the influence of parental prejudices—do not apply to health care.

A monopolistic NHS may also reduce one's sense of personal responsibility for one's own health and health care. A person's preferences about health care "can no longer be expressed in a large number of separate decisions.... They must all be reduced to a single decision expressed through the election ballot."[68] Furthermore, in an NHS a decision to forgo expensive and only slightly beneficial care will usually be disguised. Individual voters will hardly ever feel they are making those decisions. Even at higher levels of the political process, these decisions will be hidden by speaking of "operating within an already fixed budget." While those who set the size of the budget think they are only setting an overall total, they are actually deciding to trade lives for money. But in an NHS, individuals do not trade their own lives for money; some individuals do it for all.

In another respect, however, an NHS may increase one's sense of responsibility for health care. One student of the British NHS comments: "Everytime I had scratched through the mud and moss of the overt and vocal signs of unrest, I came down to a solid bedrock of support at all levels."[69] People feel an NHS is *theirs;* it is not just someone

66. See 4.2.

67. To be sure, the pacifist objector is also logically bothersome to a defense of the Pentagon. Still, defense is a public good. Unlike health care, it cannot be provided for some without being provided for all, and it cannot be provided at one level for some and at another for others. If a majority of citizens want defense to be supported at a certain level, how can they get it without giving everyone the "benefits" of the decision? Thus everyone should pay for it, to avoid free-riders. Even if it is argued that not everyone should pay for it because some vigorously deny it gives them (or anyone) real benefits, should the majority that supports it be denied the prerogative of establishing the particular level of spending? None of these things can be said about health care in the face of the Christian Scientist's objection.

68. Steiner 1976.

69. D. Nowlan, quoted by Cullis and West 1979, p. 219.

else's plan which they choose among others. No matter how small and indirect a role they have in shaping it, they are members of the group (voters, taxpayers) that is finally solely responsible for what that service is. This responsibility of persons in an NHS, however, should not be overrated. In a truly competitive pluralistic model, enrollees are also ultimately responsible for what happens—by choosing to keep particular plans in business.

The clear control of health-care institutions by nonprofit and nonmedical parties has made an NHS much more attractive to general critics of a capitalist economy than any other arrangement, including any kind of national health insurance. All physicians would be paid by salary or capitation, the government would own hospitals and control the education of health professionals, insurance companies would be eliminated, and local policy could be subordinated to community-based boards.[70] But if businesses producing for the military can dominate a Pentagon, what would stop physicians producing for the government from dominating an NHS? After all, they are viewed so much more clearly than the military businesses as "good guys." There is certainly no a priori reason physicians would not dominate an NHS.

There is also no a priori reason for critics of capitalist medicine not to embrace more competitive, pluralistic models. One might, of course, prohibit private and especially physician-dominated ownership of plans, making them all like the subscriber-owned cooperatives that constitute a significant portion of present prepaid plans. Diversity and competition would remain crucial, however. Even subscriber-owned cooperatives probably get smug and self-serving when they become too large and securely established. Competition, of course, would need to be tempered with restrictions to ensure justice for the ill and the poor, keeping in mind that justice does not mean equal levels of care regardless of income.

Neither an NHS nor competition is a panacea for effectively containing noncostworthy care and simultaneously distributing benefits and costs justly. Yet isn't the problem of justice for pluralistic competitive schemes less intractable than the moral problem of individual autonomy for an NHS? Practical, historical experience may tip the final judgment the other way, but until such time as truly competitive models are given a sustained chance to operate, we will only be guessing.

70. Brown 1979, p. 216.

CHAPTER SEVEN

Prevention or Treatment?

1. SOME FACTS, AND THE ISSUE

Overwhelmingly, health-care expenditures today go for the medical treatment of health problems after they have arisen.[1] In the last decade, only 1 percent of U.S. health-care dollars were spent on prevention and control.[2] The total Public Health Service budget for 1976–78, for example, was equaled by just the *increases* in Medicare and Medicaid spending in those years.[3]

At the same time the old adage, "an ounce of prevention is worth a pound of cure," seems more apt today than ever before. We are entering a stage in the development of health care in which, many believe, the only noticeable improvements in national health statistics will come from better prevention, not better rescue medicine.[4] The dis-

1. The terminology has not been standardized. "Treatment," "medicine," and "medical care" are often contrasted with "prevention," yet some uses of what we ordinarily call "medicine" are preventive—we even talk of "preventive medicine" and "preventive treatment." "Curative care" is incomplete; it does not include an important part of the care that is not prevention—ameliorative care which does not cure. See 7.2 for expansion and clarification of these terminological problems. I will continue to use the term "treatment" and the terms "medical" and "curative" care to designate the entire category of care for preexisting problems, though undoubtedly "curative/ameliorative care" would be the most accurate term.

2. This does not include the at least $4 billion spent annually for research and development; see Fain, Plant, and Milloy 1977, p. 490. Much of this research is for developing medical and curative, not preventive, care.

3. U.S. Public Health Service 1976, p. 1.

4. One of the many instances of this claim is the U.S. Public Health Service's *Forward Plan for Health, 1977–81* (1976), p. 15. Another is a similar plan for 1979–83 of the U.S. Health Services Administration (1977).

tribution of contemporary illness among disease categories tells much of the story. In the mid-1970s ischemic heart disease, cancer, and stroke accounted for 54 percent of the lost expected years of life; if respiratory infections, bronchitis, asthma, accidents, and suicides are added, the figure reaches 72 percent.[5] Cures for all of these remain partial, problematic, or very expensive, but often they are preventable.

Even some dramatic technological breakthroughs in medicine can be made obsolete by prevention—for example, *in vitro* fertilization. In 1979 the birth of Louise Brown, the first baby conceived in a test tube and reimplanted in her mother's womb, received immense attention. If the fallopian tube disease which makes women unable to conceive naturally were prevented, the sophisticated procedure of fertilization and embryo reimplantation used in her case would be rendered largely obsolete. And prevention is realistic; the main causes of fallopian tube disease are defective IUDs, pelvic inflammatory disease, and gonorrhea.[6]

Armed with facts like these, anyone concerned to get the most for our health-care dollar is likely to advocate increased emphasis on prevention. Already in the mid-1970s the cost of a life saved by coronary-care units was $70,000, and in 1981 the cost of a year of life saved by kidney dialysis was over $30,000.[7] By contrast, some preventive programs for cervical cancer have been passed over that were estimated to cost as little as $2,200 per life saved.[8] For a developed country like the U.S. such figures indicate that significant cost savings or improvements in health will result from switching some resources away from treatment and toward prevention. However, they pale by comparison with figures for less developed countries. In Morocco, for example, the cost of a life saved by new health programs ranges from 120 dirhams for tuberculosis prevention and 190 dirhams for vaccination for diphtheria, tetanus, and whooping cough, to 11,000–15,000 dirhams for hospital care.[9]

To be sure, we should not get too enamored of the cost savings of prevention. For one thing, there are many health problems for which preventive steps still are unknown. For another, effective preventive care will increase the average length of life. Then, this older population is likely to suffer from new or more frequent types of morbidity

5. Gray 1979.
6. Streeter 1980.
7. Rich 1980.
8. Carlson 1975, pp. 125–26.
9. Cullis and West 1979, p. 284.

and mortality, imposing new costs for disease care.[10] Money spent on prevention may gain more life years than an equal expenditure on medical care, but it will still not get us to the ideal of "dying young, as late as possible."[11] Also, screening programs often have hidden costs of follow-up care for those who show up falsely positive for a disease.[12] Despite the problems, however, the evidence seems to indicate considerable cost savings from many preventive programs. One critic maintains that we probably could eschew much of our costly chronic and crisis care, use some of the savings for increased prevention, statistically leave people just as healthy and long-living, and have enough left over to "guarantee each member of society one bottle of good claret a day...."[13]

And yet, in our society a flood of donations will flow from publicizing the picture of one small child suffering from a serious accident or illness, while the same population will probably refuse to fund the school crossing guard who would save several children per year.[14] We seem to revere physicians most when they are prepared to move heaven and earth on behalf of one suffering individual; often no one is prepared to move things far short of heaven to prevent the same illnesses. How can that attitude possibly be justified?

There are, of course, many explanations of our society's relative emphasis on treatment, but they often only make it more suspicious. One is the self-interest of the medical profession, which can keep costly curative care more easily under its control than it can preven-

10. Gori and Richter 1978.

11. This quotation is a remark of John A. Gronvall, dean of the University of Michigan School of Medicine, at the annual meeting of the American Association of Medical Colleges, 6 November 1979, in Washington, D.C.

12. An interesting case is described by Phelps 1978. Imagine a $10,000 total cost for a 10¢ screening test on 100,000 people. Suppose the cost of early treatment of those detected by the test is $500 per patient, and that this $500 alleviates the need for $1,000 of later treatment. The test turns up 99 of the 100 people who actually have the disease, saving $49,500 (99 × $500). But suppose there are 100 false positives (those whom the test shows to have the disease but who do not). The test will appear to be "even a more stunning success to the uninformed doctor, because he ... believes he has cured 199 patients for a savings of $99,500. ... In fact he has wasted $50,000 on the false positives," and the test is financially a loss ($10,000 plus $50,000 of extra costs, minus $49,500 of benefits). If the patient has full insurance coverage for the early care, "both the doctor and the patient will agree to proceed with the screening test and to follow up on the results.... When the disease being screened has low true frequency in the population screened, the false positive results often dominate the desirability of the outcome." Phelps claims that this kind of problem is not fanciful. Many not uncommon tests have false positive rates of 20 to 90 percent.

13. Engelhardt 1980a.

14. Williams et al. 1976.

tion. Another is insurance, which directly encourages medical care while indirectly dampening the motivation to use preventive care. Insurance alleviates our worries that medical bills will later leave us destitute. Another is the protection of a capitalist economy. High medical technology may divert our attention from the political and economic causes of illness—alienation in the workplace,[15] occupational diseases, environmental pollution, aggressively advertised and highly profitable unhealthy foods, and so forth. The low priority given to prevention protects the capitalist economy from being seen as responsible for disease.[16] Still another explanation is a political fact: When push comes to shove, rescue medicine can more easily mobilize actual victims for its appeal than preventive care can mobilize its merely potential beneficiaries. Then, too, perhaps we put greater weight on treatment than on prevention simply because our imaginations are foolishly and irrationally anesthetized until such time as harm strikes.

The Essential Moral Question

Still, possibly, isn't there a more defensible factor behind the overriding emphasis in our culture on crisis care? Isn't there a *moral* difference between helping to rescue people already in trouble and helping to prevent their getting in trouble in the first place? Even when prevention appears to be more efficient, don't those already in trouble still have first claim on our resources? Is the current predominance of medical care irrational, wasteful, and just protective of special interests, or is it finally costworthy? The answer will depend on what moral weight this distinction between rescue and prevention ought to have. In this chapter our business is to determine whether rescue and prevention are morally different.

15. A special report to the secretary of DHEW found work satisfaction to be the most important factor in longevity. See Navarro 1976, p. 211.

16. Brown 1979, p. 231; Navarro 1976, p. 207. In calling our attention to this aspect of prevention, these authors do not mean to say that capitalist institutions do not have any interest in preventive care. Brown himself details the important role played in the early years of this century by Frederick T. Gates, chairman of the board of the Rockefeller Institute of Medical Research, in getting employers to see the value of preventive medicine. Gates cited one report that 20 percent of the employees of large companies were sick each day. A zoologist convinced Gates and John D. Rockefeller, Jr., that hookworm was one of the most important diseases of the South and the cause of "some of the proverbial laziness of the poorer classes of the white population." It was said that in countries with hookworm, textile mills needed 25 percent more laborers to produce the same product. See Brown 1979, pp. 113–16. Their perception of the importance of preventive medicine was undoubtedly one reason the otherwise conservative National Association of Manufacturers explicitly supported compulsory and opposed voluntary health insurance in the first decades of this century.

We can label the first of the two contending views *moral equiva-lence*: If treatment and prevention both generate the same results for a given dollar spent on them, then neither has moral claim to be at-tended to first; if treatment costs more per dollar than equally produc-tive prevention, however, money should first be spent on the more ef-ficient preventive measures before spending it on treatment. The other view is *moral priority*: If treatment and prevention are equally cost-efficient, then resources should be used for the treatment before the prevention; if treatment costs somewhat more than equally productive prevention, money should still be spent on the treatment first. How much more can the treatment cost and still warrant investment of re-sources before spending on prevention? That will depend on how great a priority is being claimed. This priority can be quantified: A 3:2 moral priority of treatment, for example, means that as long as the ra-tio of the cost-effectiveness of treatment to that of prevention is no less than 2:3, treatment should receive attention first.

Between these two views our intuitions pull us in sharply differ-ent directions. On the one hand, to deny a person's plea to be rescued seems more of an affront to individual human dignity than to deny the request of a not-yet-failing person for prevention. On the other hand, when we focus on the health and lives affected, we come out strongly for a policy of equivalence in order to maximize the lives we save and health we preserve with our limited dollars. Dramatic plead-ing, too, is not always on the side of rescue and treatment; while we may rush to rescue people from a preventable tragedy and spend far beyond what we were willing to spend earlier for prevention, the pre-ventable loss of a few lives often leads to urgent and strident demands for more investment in prevention.[17] We keep wondering: Why should the lives preserved in prevention be worth less than those saved in medical rescue? We are pulled toward the charge that it is just bad medicine for a doctor who treats patients for rat bites, for example, to send them back to the tenements without working hard to get rid of the rats.[18]

Moral Weight

Some philosophers might see an easy resolution of this puzzle: There really is a moral distinction between rescue and prevention, but it only gives *weight* to allocating more per life saved to treatment than to prevention, and that weight is sometimes smaller than the value of the

17. Weale 1979.
18. Sidel and Sidel 1977, p. 273.

greater number of lives which prevention can save. This, however, is inadequate. It incorrectly represents the moral intuitions on the side of prevention—even if the *same* number of lives were to be preserved by prevention as by treatment, we keep wondering, why aren't those lives equally deserving of care? Also, we are told nothing about *how* weighty a factor the prima facie distinction between rescue and prevention is. How much greater must the number of lives preserved by prevention be for them to outweigh the prima facie priority of rescue? And does that priority always have the same weight?

The better approach on all these counts is to clarify as sharply as possible what factors might explain any moral weight which the distinction has. This will enable us to make a more rational decision about whether the moral urgency of prevention is as great as the moral urgency of rescue. It will also enable us to make an educated guess about *how much* moral weight the distinction between rescue and prevention has when it does have weight. It will help us do that not just in general, but also in particular, and particular sorts of, cases. If the good reasons for the distinction are much less present in one case than in others, we would need to cite smaller advantages in lives saved or health preserved to justify prevention than the distinction would usually require.[19]

2. CLARIFYING THE MORAL ISSUE

In assessing the distinction between treatment and prevention, several misinterpretations can mislead us. They need correcting at the outset.

Treatment or medical/curative care is usually defined as an intervention upon an ill person in order to *restore* health, while preventive care or preventive medicine is an intervention or precaution taken in order to ensure *continued* health. The "in order to" dimension of these definitions keeps us focused on health care: Some acts which affect health are not preventive health care, for they are not done in order to preserve health (zoning laws, or reducing the length of the work week, for example).[20] And prevention covers both "promoting health" and "preventing illness." The latter is more disease-specific,

19. The strategy espoused in this paragraph is similar to the one I have used in assessing the moral relevance of the distinction between killing and letting-die. See Menzel 1979.

20. Freedman 1977. Ambiguities may arise with things like sanitation, where purposes are multiple (aesthetic, say, as well as health). There is nothing in a proper definition of preventive health care which would require the purpose of some measure to be *only* health in order to be preventive care.

unlike, say, better general nutrition, which, even if it is intended to affect health, is not usually pursued with any specific diseases in mind.[21]

There is no sharp line between treatment and prevention. Those who are more likely than others to get a specific illness but do not yet have it may already be said to have a kind of "illness," yet by convention it is said to be preventive care which they would undergo. We could stretch our terms on the one end and call more ordinarily curative care "preventive" because it prevents people from getting worse (that is, dying). Or we could stretch our terms on the other end and refuse to call ordinary preventive care "prevention" because the *likely* ill person allegedly already has a latent form of the disease. Perhaps, in the last analysis, the best we can do is to define preventive care as whatever keeps you from getting worse, and curative care as whatever makes you better—except when you are already very bad off and the worse state that you are kept from is something extreme like death or total disability. In that case we still have a case of rescue or treatment, not prevention.

That, however, suggests a third branch to the distinction: There are forms of treatment which do not cure but only assuage, comfort, or prevent things from getting worse. Prevention contrasts with rescue or treatment, and "curative" care is a subdivision of the latter. When prevention is thought to have lower priority, it is the broader category of treatment, not just *curative* care, which has higher priority. "Medicine," on the other hand, is broader than "rescue" or "treatment"— technically it includes preventive medicine, though we frequently contrast "medical" with "preventive" care. Thus both the "prevention/ cure" and "preventive care/medical care" contrasts are clumsy in labeling the essential distinction. "Rescue/prevention" or "treatment/ prevention" seem more accurate.

One connotation of "rescue" is nevertheless misleading. While rescue is "saving life," it would be odd to speak of prevention that way. In prevention we do not even "possibly save" a person's life—we do not save at all.[22] Doing something that has a particular likelihood of averting another probability of death is not "saving" unless someone is *already* in big *enough* trouble to be "saved." Then, since rescue is "saving life," while prevention isn't "saving" anything, some will im-

---

21. Schweitzer 1974.

22. Freedman 1977. He acknowledges that this terminological move has no argumentative power unless "saving a life" can be shown to be more praiseworthy than "preserving health."

mediately think that rescue has moral priority. But in fact that begs the question. Critics of the moral priority of rescue will only have to rephrase their claim: Saving lives is not morally more urgent than preventing deaths.[23]

Another clarification is important. We can distinguish two moral questions about the relation of prevention to cure: (1) Would anyone's moral *rights* be violated by a policy of equivalence? (2) Is it morally *wrong* to adopt such a policy?[24] Now suppose that at the moment we are asking the narrower, first question. And suppose what seems at least plausible, that only if society was obligated to prevent illness, and can now be blamed for my needing to be rescued, does society violate any *right* of mine to be rescued if it later leaves me uncured and opts for more efficient prevention.[25] Yet this is puzzling: Can it really be the case that it is just when we are as obligated to prevent

23. Another distinction is similarly impotent. Some will think they can demonstrate rescue's priority over prevention by distinguishing a right to health care from a right to health. If we focus on results, rescue and prevention look morally equivalent. Doesn't that focus shift any alleged right to health care toward a right to health—that health which care is supposed to produce? Haven't advocates of prevention then cut their own throats? If a right to care is problematic because it leaves the degree and amount of care undetermined, a right to health is many times more problematic. Just look at the impossible amount of resources we would have to invest to implement that right.

This argument against equivalence is simply a logical fallacy. A right to health would imply that prevention was morally equivalent to rescue. But the argument needs the reverse implication. Only the denial of a right to health together with the claim that prevention's moral equivalence to rescue implies a right to health—*not* the reverse implication—logically generates the conclusion that rescue is more than equivalent to prevention. And we cannot say that making prevention morally equivalent to rescue implies a right to health. To be sure, if people do have a right to rescue care, and if preventing harm is as morally obligatory as rescuing people from it, then people do have a right to the health that can be feasibly preserved by prevention. But a right to health in *that* sense can be defended. The argument in question, however, is driven by the premise that a right to health cannot be defended because the health in question cannot feasibly be created or preserved.

For a defense of a right to health which is precisely also a ringing defense of prevention over medical and curative care, see D. Beauchamp 1976. For sharp criticism of D. Beauchamp, see T. Beauchamp 1978. For a cautious defense of a right to health, see Siegler 1979. In general, see Beauchamp and Faden 1979.

24. Equivalence could be wrong, though it might not violate the rights of the ill; violating someone's rights is one way, but not the only way, to do something wrong. Violating someone's rights is also not always finally wrong. Even if regarding prevention and rescue as morally equivalent did violate some people's rights to be rescued, that might still be outweighed by other result-producing advantages of equivalence. That weighing, however, may not simply be a matter of balancing the values of the results. Rights do cut off at least some kinds of balancing. See Dworkin 1977, pp. 193, 197–200. For a stronger, more absolute prohibition on overriding rights with the value of consequences, see Nozick's defense of moral "side-constraints," 1974, pp. 28–35.

25. Engelhardt 1980a.

illness as to rescue people from it that we are most obligated to make any subsequent necessary rescue first priority?[26]

The contradiction, however, is only apparent. We have missed what precisely is the larger question at issue: While society may be obligated to provide preventive care, is it morally *more* important to treat a given harm than to prevent the same harm? Suppose it is; that does not say that we are not obligated to prevent. In this chapter we focus entirely on this *comparative* question about treatment and prevention.

With this last point in mind we can see something else: Whether treatment (or prevention) is finally worth the money it often costs is not directly our question. Instead, the issue concerns trade-offs between prevention and treatment: By virtue of its greater efficiency alone, should prevention be said to be *more* costworthy, or less non-costworthy, than treatment?

3. STATISTICAL AND IDENTIFIABLE LIVES

Another, and lengthier, clarification is also necessary. How does the distinction between rescue and prevention relate to the distinction between statistical and identifiable lives?

The debate between prevention and treatment is often traced to this latter distinction. In treatment, the persons we are helping are known, identifiable individuals. To many it seems morally more important to help identifiable individuals than to do what we perceive will only statistically avert some harm to people whose identity we do not yet know. It seems more important to help identifiable hostages, for example, by acceding to a kidnapper's demands than to help potential, statistical victims of future kidnappings by refusing to meet the demands. While critics of treatment's priority over prevention typically deny that the wider distinction between statistical and identifiable lives is morally relevant, the advocates of treatment typically claim that it is.

A Puzzling Example
The precise relevance of the statistical/identifiable lives distinction for treatment and prevention, however, is less than clear. Suppose a crowded hospital discharges most of its appendectomy patients a day

26. "We" here can mean any group that decides somewhat collectively to use resources for this much preventive and that much curative care. It could be a group of employees or a family, for example, and not the whole society.

earlier than usual to make room for a much smaller number of heart-surgery patients who would otherwise be turned away at the door. Even though there would be fewer deaths from not treating heart patients than from releasing appendicitis patients a day early, the hospital releases them, because their individual chances of dying are so much lower than that a given untreated heart patient will.[27]

Yet how can the hospital argue that the deaths from the early release of appendectomy patients are only statistical? The patients released are all perfectly identifiable persons. But note: Then it looks as if the statistical/identifiable distinction is irrelevant to the issue of treatment versus prevention. If the appendectomy patients who may later lose their lives are said to be "identifiable" merely because we now know who they are, even though we cannot tell which of them will be actual victims, we will also have made most preventive care to involve identifiable individual patients. Though water sanitation and certain other kinds of public-health measures would not be aimed at such identifiable individuals, the recipients of most preventive care would be identifiable.[28] With prevention, just as with treatment, at some point we know who gets the care.

There is another, obvious interpretation. Perhaps what the "statistical" half of the legitimate statistical/identifiable distinction calls attention to is only the fact that the actual individual *victims* of going without the care are not known. Then discharging the appendectomy patients a day early risks only statistical lives, and the distinction between identifiable and statistical lives is again relevant for the choice between prevention and rescue.

But then an even more bothersome problem is forced upon us: We will have turned most curative treatment into the saving of lives that are only statistical. Though the persons who are put into intensive-care units, for example, are certainly identifiable individuals, we can seldom identify which of them will actually benefit from the care. Even after "successful" treatment, only rarely do we know that a given individual has benefited. We may know the person is alive, but do we know that *this* individual would not have lived had the treatment not been given? And if treatment is forgone and the person dies or takes a turn for the worse, do we know that the same thing would not have happened to this individual even with treatment?

By now the conceptual problems seem impossible. How do we retain any significant match between the statistical/identifiable and prevention/treatment distinctions? If we focus on the people *receiving*

27. Fried 1970, pp. 207–08.
28. Childress 1981.

the care and note that they are identifiable individuals, we will have made most preventive care to involve identifiable lives. On the other hand, if we focus on knowing who are the individuals who *benefit* from the care, we will have made most medical treatment into care which affects statistical, not identifiable, lives. Both options are distinctly unsatisfactory.

Three Component Distinctions

This all points to dispensing with the distinction between statistical and identifiable lives per se. We can use it only as dissected into several other, component distinctions: (1) Between cases where the care is given to identifiable individual recipients and instances where the care itself goes to a group. (2) Between relatively high risks to individual recipients and low ones. For example, discharging appendectomy patients one day early does not subject any one of them to nearly as high an increase in risk as that to which an individual heart-attack victim is subjected by being turned away at the hospital door.[29] (3) Between future perils and present ones. Usually it is the lives of known individuals which are also the ones in present peril, and the people who are helped statistically who are saved from future perils. Sometimes, however future perils may be avoided for individual, known persons.[30] We can also conceive of cases where present perils are avoided for statistical, not identifiable persons; we might not know which individuals among a very large group in present peril will benefit when we treat the whole group.[31]

29. In other cases the presence of equal probabilities of harm leads Morillo (1976) to argue strongly against the moral relevance of any identifiable/nameless distinction itself. She compares rigging a machine with a 75 percent chance of killing a now nameless person with shooting a person in the face with a 75 percent chance of death. Morillo claims that we should regard both as equally blameworthy actions. Now suppose she is right about the equal blame in these two cases. The example only shows that the identifiable/nameless recipient distinction in itself is not morally relevant. It does not show that the statistical/identifiable lives distinction is irrelevant where it is used to indicate that one of two equally nameable recipients has a higher chance of harm (a less "statistical" chance) than the other. Her example might also show us nothing at all about the moral equivalence between preventive *aid* and rescue. At most it strictly shows only some equivalences between two kinds of active harming, not between two kinds of aid or failure to aid. It is conceivable that the identifiable/nameless distinction is relevant in cases of active harming but not in cases of failure to aid.

30. Fried 1969, pp. 1430–31. He illustrates this: The commander of a small force of individually known persons may decide to avert future peril for all of them by sacrificing one of them now.

31. Suppose something in a water supply is making many people ill. The substance cannot be removed, but its effect can be ameliorated for many of these individuals by adding something else to the water. The peril is present, but the individuals benefited are statistical and the treatment is not even given to them as individuals.

Really, then, three distinctions are at work in the difference between statistical and identifiable lives: identifiable individual recipients of care as distinct from group recipients, the high as distinct from low risks to which these would-be recipients are exposed, and the present as distinct from future perils which threaten them. Allegedly the former part of each pair is morally the weightier.

In some specific cases, prevention represents all the less morally compelling halves of these distinctions and is posed against treatment that represents all the more compelling halves. Contrast high-school education for aerobic fitness, for example, with emergency-room care of heart-attack patients; care for identifiable individual recipients at high risk of immediate harms contrasts with care dispensed not even individually to patients at low risk of distant harms. Here the case for treatment over prevention is the strongest it ever gets.

In most cases the allegedly more morally compelling halves of the three component distinctions do not all line up behind treatment. (1) Often we do know who the individuals are who will receive the preventive care we might choose as a matter of policy to emphasize; at least *at some point* it will be *dispensed* to them as individuals. For example, we may know who the individuals are to be screened for hypertension as much as we know who the individuals are who will need any coronary-bypass surgery. (2) In some cases the odds that a certain treatment will actually save people from harm which would otherwise have come about are no greater than the odds that some competing earlier preventive care will avert the same harm. (3) Almost always, however, treatment does avert harms that are temporally less distant than those averted by prevention.

Now we can greatly sharpen our central question. Most cases of the treatment/prevention dilemma can be captured with this question: *Should we give relatively inefficient treatment to identifiable individuals at relatively high risk for relatively immediate harms, rather than more efficient preventive care to equally identifiable individuals at lower risk for more distant harms?* Hereafter I will assume that prevention, like treatment, has identifiable recipients (though not necessarily beneficiaries).[32] I will also assume that the harms alleviated by prevention are

32. Certain "personalist" arguments for the priority of treatment are thus rendered inapplicable to the issue I have focused. Fried, for example, notes that only with known individual lives do we enter into relations of love and friendship; even if the identifiable person is a perfect stranger, we still relate as potential friends only because we face each other as particular individuals; see Fried 1970, pp. 222–24. In any case this personalist argument may fail, even if it is not avoided by the stipulations I have made. Weale (1979) claims that the argument does not support priority of treatment; even in medicine we do now know the individual victims of forgoing treatment when the choice gets shoved

more distant in the future.[33] Realistically, then, we will have only one
further variable to keep in mind, one departure from the confines of
the question above: The risks to ill patients from not being provided a
certain treatment will not always be greater than the risks to not-yet-
ill persons from not receiving preventive care.[34]

We now can proceed to the debate itself. I will take up what I
think are the weak arguments first, and then present two much
stronger ones.

4. WEAK ARGUMENTS FOR THE PRIORITY OF TREATMENT

Psychological Difficulty

Only a stoic society, it will be said, could always give priority to prevention whenever it was more efficient. In such a society, for example,
we might invest money to prevent end-stage renal failure, enjoy the
resources saved, but then pay the penalty of dying in uremic coma
when our kidneys fail.[35] But in our society we just aren't that stoic.

By itself this is hardly even an argument. It might be *difficult* to
opt for preventive care whenever it is more efficient, but why *shouldn't*
we opt for it? Some of us, for example, "believe it is morally permissi-
ble to kill and eat chickens" though we "find it psychologically difficult to wring a chicken's neck, cut out its guts, and then cook and eat
it." Surely this difficulty shows not that it is wrong to eat chickens, but
"only that we have weak wills or stomachs."[36]

The argument may take a more persuasive form. If we resonated
as much to the claims of the future ill as to the pleas of those who are
ill right now, wouldn't we immobilize ourselves? We would be
swamped in claims to prevent all those possible ills in all those future
years. It is much more difficult to carry out a duty to prevent future

---

back to the more important *policy* stage. Fried is less persuasive in his rejection of the
argument. He correctly notes that it does not explain our preference for people in present perils over those in future ones, but I do not know why the failure of an argument
to explain a preference for one thing (people in present perils) implies a failure to explain a preference for a quite different thing (known, identifiable persons).

33. Among other things, this last assumption captures the fact that prevention is
for not-yet-ill people, while curative care or treatment is for already-ill persons. I am
aware of the tenuousness of this already-ill/not-yet-ill distinction (see 7.2).

34. "Greater risk" here denotes the product of multiplying the probability of a
harm eventuating by the degree of the harm (length, severity, etc.). A risk can be lower
in probability but for sufficiently greater harm, and thus it can be a greater risk overall.

35. Engelhardt 1980a.

36. Bayles 1978.

illnesses than only to treat present ones. It would take more time and attention, and distract us from most of the rest of our pursuits; perhaps it would not, realistically, be humanly possible at all.[37] George Eliot describes the emotional side of this point:

> We do not expect people to be deeply moved by what is ... usual. That element of tragedy which lies in the very fact of frequency has not yet wrought itself into the coarse emotion of mankind, and perhaps our frames would hardly bear much of it. If we had a keen vision and feeling of all ordinary life, it would be like hearing the grass grow and the squirrel's heart beat, and we would die of that roar which lies on the other side of silence.[38]

But here, too, the argument fails. To be sure, to accomplish the *same* good, we are more obligated to do any relatively easy duty than a more difficult duty. Nevertheless, we need other, more debatable premises to arrive at the conclusion that we should perform our easier duties to produce less benefit before our harder duties to produce more. What proportion of ease of duty to drop in benefit absolves us from our harder duties? Even if this were specified, in some cases we would still have abandoned the priority of treatment over more efficient prevention. Furthermore, prevention that really is more efficient than treatment is not always more difficult for a society to emphasize. We need not pursue all possibilities of prevention, no matter how unlikely they are to succeed or how costly they are for their benefits. We would be as immobilized if we pursued with equal relentlessness all the possibilities for curative and ameliorative care of those already ill.

Avoiding the Need for Allocation

The moral argument for treatment over prevention might be the same as that for the use of lotteries to allocate scarce kidney dialysis facilities: Human beings should not adjudicate the competing claims of persons in dire need.[39] If prevention is morally equivalent to treatment, we will have to cut the resources devoted to treatment. We will

37. This is the "dischargeability" difference between certain duties that is discussed by Trammel 1975. He uses it to defend the priority of negative duties not actively to cause harm over positive duties to aid someone to prevent harm, and in turn to defend the moral relevance of the distinction between killing and letting die. For qualified criticism of the moral relevance of the latter distinction in medical contexts, see Menzel 1979.

38. Eliot 1964, p. 191, as quoted in Morillo 1976.

39. Childress 1970.

then be faced with more frequent and harder decisions to allocate curative care. But we should minimize those sorts of decisions.[40]

Unless we devote nearly unlimited resources to treatment, however, we are allocating by human judgment anyhow. Suppose, however, that we do devote nearly unlimited resources to treatment of the presently ill. This still avoids only one kind of allocation decision, and it makes another: We still have to decide to sacrifice the less identifiable, more distant, less highly risked lives of those who might have been helped by the very preventive measures which our singular devotion to treatment precludes us from pursuing.

Maybe, however, that misses the argument's central point. If prevention is morally equivalent to treatment, and if therefore we have cut our spending on treatment, won't we be faced with fiercer competition between the already ill for the remaining resources? Admittedly, unless we devote unlimited resources to treatment, some difficult allocations will have to be made even if treatment has priority over prevention. But won't *fewer* have to be made than if prevention is considered morally equal to treatment?

Yet that begs the question. We will have sacrificed a finally greater number of less known, more distant individuals who are each exposed beforehand to admittedly less risk. Is that morally defensible? That is precisely one of the larger questions at issue. Citing the need to "avoid allocation" only assumes that allocating resources away from the "statistical" beneficiaries of prevention, and toward the presently ill, is less onerous than other allocations.

Avoiding the Survival Lottery

Some critics of equivalence worry about the precedent it would set for the rest of our thinking. In regarding prevention as equal to treatment, we are willing to count the number of deaths we avert as more important than the manner and circumstances in which we avert them. How far will we be willing to carry that consequentialist logic? Critics worry that we will be inclined to endorse, for example, the "survival lottery." In this piece of medical science fiction, the success of vital organ transplants from living donors sets the stage for an intriguing arrangement: One person would be chosen by lot to be the donor of various organs that would be distributed to several people who were in desperate need. Such a lottery would raise average life expectancy, and no one could tell beforehand whether he or she would turn up as the unlucky donor. All would thus find it in their interest to con-

40. Freedman 1977.

sent to the arrangement. Yet isn't such a lottery still morally unacceptable, and isn't any maximizing strategy that morally equates prevention with treatment equally so?[41]

Suppose, however, that the survival lottery is unacceptable. The lottery involves killing a person; to defend it we would probably have to claim that killing people is no worse than letting them die. If, however, we think that killing is prima facie worse than letting die, we can reject the lottery for that reason, without abandoning the strategy of maximizing the number of people we save when *no* killing/letting die difference is present (as in the dilemma between prevention and treatment).[42]

In fact, the matter is even worse than this for the priority of treatment. Ironically, the threat of having to end up endorsing the lottery may actually be more ominous for defenders of priority than for defenders of equivalence. Suppose that killing is prima facie worse than letting die; that will tilt the scales against accepting the lottery. If the statistical/identifiable lives distinction is also relevant, it will tend to support the lottery: One statistical death by killing (statistical at the time when lots for who will be killed are drawn) would save several identifiable persons who would otherwise be allowed to die. While defenders of prevention need to distance their use of the maximizing strategy from the lottery, those who favor treatment over prevention need to do the same.

An Analogy: Exposing Others to Risk
Another ingenious argument fares no better. Suppose, as seems plausible, that it is worse to kill one person than to give twenty people their first cigarettes, when statistically three of them will die prematurely from the hazards of smoking. Analogously, Freedman claims that it is better to cure one dying person than to prevent twenty from

41. For the initial discussion of the lottery, see Harris 1975. For other arguments about whether it is morally acceptable, see Singer 1977 and Trammel and Wren 1977. For its connection to treatment and prevention, see Weale 1979.

42. The "numbers-counting" issue has broader and narrower forms. Whether to avoid letting several die by killing one and whether a statistical life is less important to save than an identifiable one are instances of the numbers-counting question in the broad sense. In the narrower sense of that phrase, however, they are not. In the narrower sense the issue is whether letting two persons die is worse than letting one die, whether killing two is worse than killing one, whether not saving two statistical lives is worse than not saving one, whether letting two identifiable persons die is worse than letting one die, etc. It is this narrower issue of counting "sheer numbers," which is the focus of 8.3.

smoking, and that this is the case regardless of whether smoking is somewhat voluntary. Then, he says, "it is better to save lives than to preserve health"; it is better to treat when lives are now threatened than to prevent similar threats from developing.[43]

Freedman couches the point in a series of moral equations. "It is worse to kill than to cause pain, and it is *therefore* better to save than to prevent pain." Suppose the relation of saving life to killing is a relation of x to $-x$ ("not x"), and the relation of preventing illness to causing illness a relation of y to $-y$. Suppose also that killing is worse than causing illness, that is, that $-x$ is worse than $-y$. Then x is more right than y, as, for example, if -5 is less than -2, then 5 is greater than 2. Conclusion: "Saving life is greater, more praiseworthy, than preventing illness."

In syllogistic form, the argument is this:

1) $-x < -y$ (killing is worse than causing illness)
2) if $-x < -y$, then $x > y$

3) $x > y$ (saving life is better than preventing illness)

But the argument is simply wrong. Suppose that killing is worse than causing illness and saving life is better than preventing only illness. That does not show that saving life is better than preventing *death*. If $-x$ is killing (causing death), then x is preventing death, *whether by "prevention" ahead of time or by "saving life" already threatened*.[44] Preventing death is better than preventing illness, and preventive medicine may prevent death, not just illness. Furthermore,

43. Freedman 1977.
44. Freedman has privately indicated to me that the crux of our difference may be right at this point. He intends his argument to show that saving from death ("saving life") is better than only preventing death, not just that saving from death is better than preventing illness. And the proper contradictory of killing, he thinks, is not preventing death but saving life. That raises the complicated issue, of course, of what the logical contradictory of some of these natural-language expressions is. I have said that the contradictory of killing is preventing death, broadly construed to include, but also to extend beyond, saving life. Perhaps he would say that killing is causing death by action when the person is *not* already in great danger, so that its contradictory is preserving life by action when the person *is* already in greater danger, i.e., saving life. Analogously, he might take preventing death to be preserving life by action when the person is not already in greater danger, and its contradictory to be causing death by action when the person is in great danger—in our language, still killing, but of a person who may very well have died anyway. I am not at all sure that that is correct, but in any case I am doubtful it will help his argument. He will still have to say that killing a person already in danger is not as bad as killing a person not already in danger, an admittedly plausible but to me not persuasive claim. Otherwise his x/y, $-x/-y$ argumentation will not work.

"treatment" may only save from further illness. It may not save life—suppose that health, not so much life, was threatened.[45]

The Symbolic Value of Rescuing Life

Perhaps a moral distinction between prevention and rescue symbolizes and thereby demonstrates the value we place on human life. By spending much higher amounts per life saved on rescue than on prevention, it will be said, we *symbolize* our belief that life has no price—or nearly none—without bankrupting ourselves by a general policy to that effect.[46]

But what an odd dilemma that creates. On one hand, we see our efforts for rescue as representing what life is really worth. Yet to be consistent, shouldn't we then spend the same (per death avoided) on prevention? How can there be a difference between the worth of an identifiable, presently threatened life and a more statistical, future life? The "symbolic value" argument is no argument for treatment over prevention unless there is a difference. But then it is no *separate* argument. We could, of course, spend more on identifiable, presently threatened lives and regard what we spent as *more* than they are worth. But then we would have violated our desire "to symbolize the value of life as it [really] is, that is, one value out of many, having certain relations to other values."[47]

Nonetheless, this unpersuasive argument may point to a more successful one. We would need to argue that the value of a less identifiable, more future life really *is* less than the value of a more identifiable, more presently threatened one. We will next consider that. Somewhat surprisingly, it harbors a much stronger argument for the moral priority of treatment.

---

45. In his larger argument Freedman may also have jumbled two arguments together. He starts from the premise that killing is worse than causing pain or illness. He next observes that saving life stands in an $x:-x$ relationship to killing. He then concludes that saving life is better than preventing illness. This is one argument; I have argued above that it is invalid as an argument for the priority of treatment. His other argument starts with the premise that it is worse to kill one person than to cause twenty people to contract an illness which has a 5 percent chance of killing any one of them (i.e., than to cause what is statistically one death among twenty people). It concludes that prevention is less than morally equivalent to treatment. To start with that premise, however, begs one of the important issues in the debate—whether the distinction between identifiable and statistical lives is morally relevant. If Freedman takes the moral relevance of the statistical/identifiable lives distinction to be a basic axiom, he has begged one of the essential questions in the whole discussion.

46. Calabresi 1965.

47. Fried 1970, pp. 217–18.

5. PRIOR CONSENT

Suppose the health-care budget has been fixed, at whatever level you want it to be. Won't it be prudent for you to vote for a long-run policy of morally equating prevention with treatment? As long as we ask you in advance of serious illness, you will vote to distribute care between prevention and treatment so as to maximize the number of lives saved.[48]

To be sure, this "prior-consent" argument for prevention's equivalence contains an important truth: From an early vantage point of being well we will value treatment over prevention less than we will from a later vantage point of being ill. Yet, as persuasive as it is, this argument for equivalence can be stood on its head to support precisely the opposite view—some priority for treatment over prevention.

Different Pricings of Life

People generally price life lower in low-risk situations than in high-risk ones (see 2.3). Suppose that you *know* you do that, and that you are now choosing between a policy of priority and one of equivalence. *Though you are not yet ill, won't you even now consent to spending more on saving your life in higher-risk situations?* These are precisely the circumstances that obtain when you are ill and need treatment, and the present circumstances of possible preventive measures are relatively low-risk. Asking you in advance will yield precisely the priority on treatment which the initial prior-consent argument claims to refute.[49]

To be sure, right *now* the lowest risk to you is from a policy of equivalence. How, then, can it be rational for you to vote for a policy of priority that will actually increase your chances of suffering or dying from an illness? Though you now know that you will price life more highly in later, higher-risk, treatment-warranting situations, why should you let that influence you *currently* to vote for a policy of some priority?[50] Look, however, at what we should always be doing when we vote for a policy. We should not vote to create the results which constitute the maximum value only from our *present* vantage point.

48. Weale 1979.
49. The rudiments of this argument are suggested by Weinstein, Shepard, and Pliskin 1976 and by Jones-Lee 1976, p. 150.
50. I am indebted to Charles Marks (University of Washington) and William Talbott for pressing this objection.

When we vote for a policy, shouldn't we realize that we may value its results differently in the future? If we know what those changes will be, shouldn't we vote for the policy that will maximize the value we will put on events when they eventuate? After all, we do that all the time in making policy decisions. *We look into ourselves as future evaluators of events, not just as future subjects of them.* We in fact know now that we will put a higher monetary value on life if we ever do fall ill. Prior consent generates treatment's priority, not prevention's equivalence.[51]

There is another, more drastic way of putting this entire argument: The value of a presently less threatened life saved in the future by prevention just *is* less than the value of a more immediately and highly threatened life saved by treatment. That may sound crazy— after all, the two sorts of lives may both be *the very same person's* life. Yet how else are we to interpret the *monetary* value of people's lives— the value of saving lives compared to doing other things with the resources—than in reference to what people prefer to have these resources used for? Once we ground the pricing of life in preferences, we must face what seems to be a plain fact: People *are* generally more than proportionately willing to take a chance of losing their lives when they are choosing from low-risk situations, as opposed to high-risk ones. Once we realize that whatever monetary value we do put on lives is a subjectively based value, not an independent characteristic of the object (life), we can readily accept this argument.

Qualified Priority

Nevertheless, we should qualify the argument. The appropriate conclusion is not that *all* treatment has a moral priority over prevention. Two elements have so far been mixed together. Part of our willingness to pay for care which generates higher monetary valuations of life in

51. Other considerations of prior consent may also tilt the scales toward priority. A policy of equivalence will lead to more illnesses for which you cannot get treatment. Call these "untreatable" illnesses, in a very practical sense of that term. By voting for equivalence, you decrease your chance of getting ill, but you may increase your risk of getting an untreatable illness. This will lead you to modify your vote for equivalence into one for mild priority.

I have not included this as a prior-consent argument against equivalence that is separate from the main argument which I have developed. The reason is this: It can already be taken into account in a sensitive calculation of the respective benefits and losses of treatment as compared to prevention. Compared to treatment, prevention has as a "cost" the consequently greater numbers of untreatable illnesses. After that cost has been included, we then go on to our central issue of whether treatment should have priority over equally or somewhat more cost-efficient prevention.

so-called "high-risk circumstances" is a reaction to the fact that the *situation* in which we are getting the reduction in risk is one in which our lives are at higher risk. But part of it is also due to a somewhat different factor: What we are willing to spend to reduce risk rises more than proportionately with the amount of the *reduction* in risk we are paying for. In that respect a circumstance is viewed as "high-risk" when the care we are deciding whether or not to purchase accomplishes a greater reduction in the risk than care does in other circumstances. Deciding not to provide a particular item of treatment to an already ill person will be "low-risk" if the amount of *reduction* in an admittedly high risk that is passed up is very small. It might be considerably smaller than the amount of reduction in a lower risk that is forgone by failing to give preventive care.

Because of this, *prior consent and willingness-to-pay may not generate any priority at all for treatment which accomplishes a smaller reduction in a higher risk than prevention does.* Whether they do depends on whether a smaller reduction in risk accomplished by treatment more powerfully inclines toward prevention than the higher-risk situation itself inclines toward treatment. In any case, we should not think that ill people warrant some greater investment in treatment just because their life or health is in greater jeopardy. We need to consider the comparative reductions in jeopardy accomplished by treatment and prevention.

Out of all these considerations emerges some priority for most treatment, but *how* much emerges? That simply depends on two factors: How much greater the treatment's reduction in risk is, and how much higher is the actual jeopardy to the health and life of the treatment's recipient. These determine how much greater is the willingness to pay for treatment than for prevention, and therefore how powerfully the prior consent argument inclines toward treatment. How great this difference in willingness to pay will be is an empirical matter to be determined by the variation in people's actual preferences in different risk situations. The ball will be thrown to empirical observers, and ultimately to patients.

Nonrational Preferences
Undoubtedly some critics will argue that these actual preference differences are irrational, but this characterization of the preference for present over future benefits is incorrect. Admittedly, these preference variations are probably ultimately *non*rational. But as was articulated earlier (2.3), why should that bother us one bit? What *ultimate* prefer-

ences are *not* nonrational? We can hardly eliminate nonrational preferences from moral relevance without wreaking havoc with our attempts to put value on anything.

The greater preference for present as opposed to future benefits has also been characterized as a simple lack of emotional response to the distant and the unknown. As mentioned earlier (2.3), there are of course the disturbing experiments by Milgram: The amount of known harm a person is willing to inflict varies directly with how immediately and vividly the person sees or hears the victim suffer.[52] These variations are admittedly irrational and cannot be grounds for giving any priority to treatment. But why are they irrational? Because the *victim* does not share them. Milgram's subjects who inflicted the harm were not also the victims—they did not have their actions imposed back upon themselves. If they had had, they would not have evidenced the distancing effect which Milgram notices. The effect is therefore irrational.

Precisely in this respect, however, the preferences which constitute the low-risk distancing effect that lies behind priority for treatment are not *ir*rational. They are accepted by people for themselves. Though they may be *non*rational, they are surely not irrational in the sense that the Milgram reactions are. Admittedly, *part* of the preference of people for their own treatment over their own prevention probably stems from their failure to imagine the more distant sufferings which prevention avoids. That part is ignorant or irrational. But clear that out, and clear it out completely, and undoubtedly there is still a residuum of willingness to spend more per life saved on more immediate and highly threatened lives.

Preferring How to Die

This entire prior-consent argument for a qualified priority for treatment should not be confused with a different point. Glover relates an interesting example.[53] At a certain point in the Allied effort in World War II, a pilot's chances of dying in his thirty bombing missions were three in four. If the fuel load were reduced and the bomb load thereby increased, it was suggested, the resulting one-way but almost certainly fatal missions would need only half as many pilots to accomplish the same military objectives. Selection for the one-way missions could be by lot, and when the lots were drawn half the original group of pilots

52. Milgram 1973.
53. Glover 1977, pp. 212–13.

would escape altogether and half would go to certain death. Yet despite the one-in-two rather than three-in-four chances of death for the initial group of pilots, the one-way missions were rejected. Probably the pilots themselves would not have voted for them. Glover comments that we seem to have an "extreme horror ... at the thought of being in a position where we can see certain death ahead." We are prepared "to accept *some* additional risk of death in preference to risking a condemned-cell situation ... during which certain death could be anticipated."

As Glover makes clear, however, as strikingly as the example shows that we prefer some kinds of death over others, it provides no basis for a moral preference for identifiable over statistical lives. It suggests only that "we ought to give some additional weight to avoiding slow (and certain) rather than sudden and unexpected (or uncertain) death." The point can be applied to prevention and treatment. The bombing example tends to show that we should try to prevent slow, certain death before we try to prevent sudden or uncertain dyings, and that we should spend more to do so, for the example apparently reveals a qualified preference for dying less certain deaths.[54] Yet none of that transfers easily to the question for this chapter. Not offering preventive care usually exposes its recipient to a death which is less certain *at that time* than not treating an already ill person is at its time. Yet prevention itself might be the prevention of what would later on be a very slow and certain death. Whether the bombing mission generates any weight for the priority of treatment over prevention will depend on the kinds of death prevented. If they are deaths that are later, slow, and at that time relatively certain, then Glover's consideration generates no less weight for prevention than for treatment.[55]

Variations in our willingness to spend money to reduce the risk of death typically do generate some moral priority for treatment over prevention. Preferences about how to die—or how we most want not

54. I do not mean to say that the example shows we would *always* prefer relatively unexpected deaths. See the next paragraph of the text for further clarification.

55. The bombing example also does not show that *in general* we prefer an unexpected death over a slow one which we know to be certain. In some cases we may prefer precisely the opposite. Perhaps the bombing mission example shows only that dying a slow, certain, *premature* death from "unnatural" causes is not preferred to dying an unexpected premature death. In any case, it does not show that knowledge of an assured, imminent death is a more radical torture than other suffering. It only shows that alleviating suffering, not just saving lives, is important. This general point, though not in relation to the bombing mission example which I use here, is made by Fried 1970, pp. 228–29.

to die—are less indicative of any moral priority which treatment might have.

6. FAIRNESS TO THE ALREADY ILL

Suppose that sometime when we are well, all of us have the opportunity to choose between a policy of priority and one of equivalence. If we all choose to maximize our chances of survival at that time by opting for equivalence, none of us will have any complaint later when we become ill and find ourselves without treatment because almost all health-care resources are devoted to prevention.

Suppose that later some of the people, who are then ill, try to raise an objection of justice: "Here we have in fact become ill, presumably through no fault of our own. You who are well have not (yet) been burdened with such misfortunes, and still you get the bulk of the care. Of course when we were in your shoes, we, too, opted for prevention. But now we stand in a relation of injustice to you: Your individual lifetime net welfare is greater than ours. Thus, despite our previous vote against giving priority to treatment, now justice as equality of net benefits demands that we get some extra care as compensation for our misfortunes."

Our reply comes easily. This objection ignores the injustices prevented by preventive care. By hypothesis the situation we are considering is one in which a greater amount of future misfortune can be avoided by prevention than by treatment of the present illness. If we were to claim that the lesser number and degree of present injustices create a weightier claim for treatment than the greater number and degree of future injustices do for prevention, we would surely be begging the very issue at hand. Justice is as much a result-oriented moral principle as welfare or utility are, only justice is concerned about a different result—equalities, not aggregate utility.[56]

The objection also fails to give full respect to the autonomy of the ill who complain. After all, earlier they found it in their interest to vote for a policy of equivalence. To be sure, it may be unjust that they have become ill, and it is unjust that we not give them all the care that might help to make their net lifetime benefits more equal to ours. But they freely chose to trade away later rectification of the injustice of becoming ill in order to get the benefit of maximizing their chance of

56. This is at least one of our principles of justice. There are other very basic complications in our concept of justice which I am overlooking for the moment. See 8.2 and 8.3 for their development.

not *getting* ill. That *chance* was a real benefit that then they actually got, *whether or not they end being free from illness*.[57] Only if society does not give in to later demands for the priority of treatment can the benefit which the original chance constitutes be preserved. As a matter of policy, it wouldn't be consistent for those presently ill to have earlier had their cake and now to be eating it, too. Honoring their original, knowledgeable, autonomous choice requires that we reject their demand for any treatment that is less cost-effective than prevention. Insofar as *actual* people consent to a policy of equivalence, there is nothing whatsoever unfair about later denying them treatment.[58]

But now note that there remains one huge, seemingly intransigent problem: *Some people do not stand to benefit from a policy of equivalence adopted from now on*. These people fall into two groups: (1) those in current generations who are already seriously ill, and who are not likely to benefit enough from the ensuing prevention to offset the treatment that they would lose in a policy of equivalence, and (2) those in future generations who are congenitally ill, whose path toward later tragic demise cannot likely be prevented once they are born. Since these people have not consented to a policy of equivalence (or never would have, and never will), isn't it unfair to deny them treatment merely because it is less cost-effective than prevention? They wouldn't consent to equivalence even if they were perfectly rational. It is not so much that they are ill before they have the opportunity to *vote* on this issue; it is that *at no point in time can they be said to stand a chance, as real individuals, of benefiting* from a policy of equivalence which might now be adopted. Even in future generations, some congenitally ill people, once they are born, will not have a chance of benefiting from a policy of equivalence.[59] And in the present

57. Some will not view a chance from which one does not actually later benefit to have ever been a *real benefit*. To the contrary, I think it is. We must say it is a real benefit, for example, to explain our conviction that it is unjust for people to vote in an attempt to influence the outcome and then shirk all obligation to obey the resultant policies when the opposition wins. They had a chance to win, and it would be unjust for them to get that equal benefit from voting without also sharing equally the burden of obedience necessary to make winning a benefit worth trying to obtain. See Singer 1974, p. 55. See also n. 59 below.

58. I choose the term "unfair" here rather than "unjust." If I freely choose to accept an admittedly unjust inequality when I am on its short end because I will likely be even worse off in a society without it, the accepted inequality is fair. Fairness is justice modified by autonomous consent. See chap. 1, n. 49.

59. To be sure, from the present vantage point it can be said of these future, possible, not-yet-real persons that "they stand a chance of benefiting" from a program of preventing their diseases. If we can talk about such future possible persons as having now benefited from a program of prevention that still leaves them later as unlucky in-

generation, while sometime in the past many adults did have a chance of benefiting from a policy of equivalence, that policy was not then adopted. Now it is too late.

Prevention's Defense

Defenders of prevention may acknowledge this point: Some people will never be in a position to vote for prevention as in their self-interest. Weale then argues, however, that to make prevention morally equivalent to treatment, one need not claim "that there is an actual (universal) consent, even of the tacit variety." Instead, the maximize-benefits strategy of a policy of equivalence should be understood as an "hypothesis about the sort of argument to which it would be *rational* for people to consent at any given level of expenditure on health services."[60]

Weale's argument has to go further, however. Suppose, like Weale, we disregard actual consent and focus on hypothetically rational consent instead. We still cannot say it would be rational for *all real* people to consent to a policy of equivalence. It would not be rational, for example, for the already ill, when they would not themselves gain sufficient benefit from prevention. The only way then to save equivalence is to focus on the rational consent of *hypothetical persons*. But it is *actual* disadvantaged persons whom it is necessary to hear, if we are to take claims of justice seriously (see Appendix).

Defenders of prevention may then press another, and equally problematic, strategy. Just separate off from others, they will say, the already seriously ill who do not themselves have a chance of benefiting sufficiently from subsequent prevention. Treat them as if their treatment had priority over others' equally beneficial prevention, but apply to all the others a policy of equivalence. Only if this separation

---

dividuals with the disease, we will think of them as having contracted to implement a later policy of equivalence for their actual lives. But that surely stretches too far the notion of that having a *chance* to benefit actually is a benefit (see n. 57). As the real persons that they are, *they* never had even a chance of benefiting. If we insist on saying that in some morally relevant sense they did have a chance of benefiting, we will also have to say such odd things as that everyone has had an equal chance of coming out well in the natural lottery, and thus that equality of opportunity does not demand any help for the ill by the well. Real persons, not merely possible persons, need to be heard.

This is not itself a criticism of the ability of Rawlsian hypothetical contract reasoning by theoretical (and in that sense "possible") persons to generate principles which obligate actual individuals. It may lead in that direction, but that is another matter (see Appendix). Here I only deny that every real person's "possible person" analogue before birth can obligate the actual person with its contracts. Whether appropriately restricted, veil-of-ignorance, hypothetical persons can do that is another issue.

60. Weale 1979, emphasis added.

cannot be made should we adopt a general policy of priority for treatment of all people in order to avoid treating the already seriously ill unfairly.

In most areas of health care it is doubtful that we could implement such a separation. Even if we could, of course, the argument is only a partial one for equivalence. With people who cannot now be helped by prevention, particularly the chronically ill, we should put more resources into less cost-effective treatment of *their* illnesses than into the more cost-effective prevention of *other* problems. In relation to people with these other problems the case for equivalence is stronger. We need to note, however, that even here it does not generate a final equality of prevention with treatment. We need to go back to the argument of the previous section. These other people—individuals who would seemingly benefit from voting for equivalence—still know they are willing to spend less to preserve life in the typically low-risk perspective of prevention. According to that prior-consent argument for treatment, even they will not prefer a policy of strict equivalence.

In general, then, the argument for priority for treatment that is based on fairness to people who are already ill is persuasive.

A Qualification

The fairness argument for some priority for treatment, however, must not be overstated. We are justified in giving priority to treatment of the already ill, who never find it rational to vote for a policy of equivalence. Note that *this never allows us to downgrade prevention of their own types of illnesses.* Suppose that their treatment does take priority over more cost-effective prevention of *others'* different but equally severe diseases—those which arise, for example, simply at a later time in life. Isn't it still morally just as important to prevent as to treat *their* type of illness—the very type that precludes its victims from the opportunity of ever voting rationally for equivalence? Ironically, *the very unfairness argument which creates some priority for these people's treatment makes prevention of their own kinds of illnesses equally morally urgent.* It is not only more important to treat their kinds of illnesses than to prevent other equally severe ones; it is also more important to prevent their kinds of illnesses than to prevent others.

This point is vital in assessing the importance of preventing congenital, chronically disabling diseases for future persons. Here the claim for prevention is as weighty as the claim for treatment of those in the present generation whom these diseases afflict, and in any case, it is weightier than the claim to prevent other, equally cost-effective, preventable diseases which do not preclude their victims from sometime having a rational self-interest in a policy of equivalence. The practical implications are immensely important. For example, *treatment of defective newborns may properly take priority over many types of prevention, but it should not take priority over prevention of future, similar, neonatal defects.* An appeal to a local health-planning council to expand a neonatal intensive-care unit, for example, should not be granted until equal-marginal-benefit-producing funds are devoted to educational programs to prevent future birth defects.

Thus, the fairness argument generates these priorities: (1) The first priority is the treatment *and* the prevention of those illnesses which from now on make it never rational for their victims to vote for equivalence. (2) A lower priority is prevention of other illnesses.[61]

7. SUMMARY

While there are many very weak arguments for the priority of treatment, two arguments, highly qualified, are persuasive. (1) People consent to spending proportionately less per life saved in low-risk contexts (often prevention) than they do in high-risk ones (often treatment). Where the reduction in risk attributable to a given treatment is less than the reduction in risk accomplished by prevention, however, no

61. Where does *treatment* of these "other" illnesses—those in my second category—fall? Is treatment of them as important as the treatment and prevention of the different illnesses in the first category, no more important than the prevention of those in the second category, or intermediate? If practically we cannot separate their care from the care of illnesses in category one, shouldn't we make their treatment an equally high priority? But that would probably amount to saying that their prevention cannot be separated out into second priority either, and then we would have no distinguishable groups to rank at all. Suppose that in some cases they are separable, however. The earlier prior-consent argument will generate priority for many cases of treatment of these illnesses over their prevention. We are still left in doubt, though, about whether their treatment is as important as the treatment and prevention in category one, or intermediate between categories one and two. Intermediate, most of us will probably think, but why is not very clear.

It is also natural to ask how *much* priority the treatment and prevention of illnesses in category one has over the prevention of the illnesses in category two. The fairness argument itself contains no elements which help us determine this. If there were some way to determine where treatment of the illnesses in the second category falls in relation to the first, then we could determine the amount of priority of the first over the second, for the prior-consent argument already provides us with a way of determining the rough degree of priority which treatment of these illnesses has over their prevention. We simply do not know how to do that.

priority for treatment may be created at all.[62] (2) It is unfair to presume that those who are already too ill to stand a chance of benefiting much from prevention would ever consent to a policy of equivalence. They will veto it. Others who stand to benefit from equivalence, of course, may veto the opposite policy of priority for treatment, yet the two vetoes are morally different. The already ill person's veto is a complaint of injustice and unfairness, not just a claim of self-interest; by contrast, the claim of those who vote for equivalence is largely a claim of self-interest—they are not yet seriously disadvantaged. However, the prevention of those illnesses which preclude their victims from ever having the opportunity to consent self-interestedly to equivalence is morally equal to the treatment of those same illnesses, and at least equal to other illnesses' treatment.

These highly qualified arguments mean that the distinction between preventive and rescue medicine has variable moral weight. Overall, "because the person needs help now" is never *by itself* a sufficient reason for giving even prima facie priority to a particular instance of treatment. Similarly, merely to say that some particular care is preventive and its benefits more distinct is not enough reason for giving it second priority.

These persuasive reasons for a qualified priority for treatment must not be inflated by reasons that have not a strand of moral fiber. Some of these were mentioned in the first section of this chapter, for example, the self-interested collusion of the medical profession, or capitalist interests about the workplace. While we should guard against the underemphasis on prevention which these factors may generate, there is no reason to retract the qualified defense of treatment's priority simply because that defense comes down for a moment on their side of the fence. Not only politics but morality makes for strange but perfectly admissible bedfellows. We only want morality not to be raped or seduced in the process.

When all this is said and done, we also need to keep in perspective the precise issue discussed in this chapter. We should not exaggerate its role in the prevention/treatment debate. Some critics of our current emphasis on expenditures for treatment may not be contesting the greater moral claim to be rescued of those already in trouble.

62. I say it *may* be the case that no priority is created. It is possible that some priority will be created, however, even when treatment's *reduction* in risk is less than prevention's. The *situation* in which the treatment is set might constitute a risk that is enough higher than that in the situation of prevention to lead people still to prefer less cost-effective treatment.

Their attack on the emphasis on treatment may be more exclusively an economic one: We can simply save money that would later be spent on treatment if we spend a lot more now on prevention. Our monetary ceiling on costworthy treatment is not too high, they might admit, and morally we should spend more per life saved on treatment than on prevention. Still, we are foolish not to spend more on prevention. If we spend more, although the per patient cost of treatment will not go down, fewer persons will need treatment. If the savings will more than make up for the cost of the additional earlier prevention, additional prevention will cost nothing at all. To forgo that saving is simply to waste our resources. *Don't shrink our commitment to treatment; just spend more on prevention, since we are committed to spend very large sums to rescue a person who does get in trouble. Despite— nay, because of—treatment's moral priority, we should bring spending on prevention up to the same cost-benefit level.*[63]

8. PRIORITIES IN RESEARCH

That concludes the main discussion of the chapter. Two ancillary considerations remain. One is determining what the relative emphasis on prevention and treatment should be in research.

Defenders of equivalence should consistently oppose priority of actual treatment over research as much as they oppose any priority of treatment over prevention. Since research is itself a kind of prevention, it, too, takes no back seat to treatment. Isn't it shameful, for example, that Western countries use very costly existing treatments while passing up what is probably much more cost-effective research on tropical diseases that afflict huge numbers of people in the third world?[64] Equally cost-effective research on the one hand, and developed prevention and treatment on the other, will be seen as morally equivalent.

None of this is surprising. Something else, however, is: Even if we are of another persuasion and think that treatment has moral priority over prevention, research to develop treatments may have no priority over research to develop preventive care. Freedman argues that in de-

63. Susan Predmore has privately suggested to me this more exclusively economic argument for a policy of near equivalence.

64. Some of the statistics are stunning. Walsh and Warren (1979) suggest that the most cost-effective way of dealing with developing countries' diseases may be research on cheaper and more effective treatments and preventions. In 1978, for example, the total spent worldwide on research on all tropical diseases was $60 million per year. One disease, schistosomiasis, afflicts 175 million people, but in 1978 only $7 million ($.04 per *afflicted* person) was spent on its research. Compare these figures with the roughly $380 per *citizen* (not patient) and $85 billion total spent on hospital care in the U.S. in 1979.

ciding how to allocate funds among competing research projects, for example, we are not visibly engaged in trading off lives.[65] Unlike treatment itself, research for treatment is usually not aimed at benefiting known individual subjects. Research on treatment usually has as small a chance of benefiting those who might presently need it as research on prevention has of benefiting its recipients.

Yet look how suspicious this view is. To be sure, if we thought that prevention and treatment were morally equivalent, of course we would think that research for treatment and research for prevention were equivalent. But, according to Freedman's view, even if treatment does have moral priority over prevention, in research we should give no priority to treatment over prevention. Can it really be that we should give no priority to *developing* that to which we should give priority *if and when* it *is* developed? Knowing that treatment will have priority if it is developed, isn't it irrational to act as if developing treatment and developing prevention are now both the same?

Suppose, however, that we thought it was irrational. Ironically, we would be assuming precisely the maximize-the-results posture which the original case for the priority of treatment over prevention rejects. *Maximizing* the available treatments to which we can then choose to give priority is analogous to maximizing the amount of life saved or suffering avoided in the original choice about prevention and treatment. If the strategy of maximizing a good result is precisely what we disavow in that original choice, how can we be logically compelled to adopt it in a subsequent choice about research? Thus Freedman's odd-sounding posture starts to sound consistent. Research on prevention may be morally equivalent to research on treatment, even if we deny the equivalence of prevention and treatment themselves.

Still, all that this shows is that the two kinds of research *may* be morally equivalent. *Are* they? At this point the same prior-consent and fairness arguments that argued for a qualified priority of treatment come into play. Prior-consent considerations argue against Freedman's view. As we have seen, prior to the use of treatment that competes with prevention, knowledgeable people consent to some priority for treatment; they know that their pricing of life is higher the more threatening the situation is and the larger the reduction of that threat which health care provides. How will these same people look at research for prevention, as compared with research for treatment? If the research will develop treatments and preventions available to *them*, their different pricings of life which generated priority for treatment

65. Freedman 1977.

will also generate priority for research on treatment. Even if the research will likely succeed too late (that is, only for others), the same
priority will still be generated. If the initial variation in the pricing of
life is large enough to generate priority for treatment over prevention,
wouldn't it be presumptuous not to carry that over to future generations? Freedman's open door to equivalence in research priorities
starts to close.

Fairness considerations, however, do not lean toward priority for
treatment in research. Some people, to be sure, will object to a policy
of equivalence in research; they are already too ill to gain enough of
the possible benefit from successful research on prevention, so they
need research for treatment. Just as with the priority of actual treatment over prevention, however, the implications of this point seem
limited. It is important to try to alleviate the unfairness that stems
from people never having the opportunity to consent self-interestedly
to equivalence by developing treatments for the diseases which destroy that opportunity. But isn't it just as incumbent on us to avert
that unfairness in the first place by developing methods of preventing
these same illnesses? Research for treatment of *these* diseases has
priority over research on the prevention of other diseases, but research for their prevention has the same priority.

The matter is thus, finally, very complex. While Freedman has
raised the important possibility of exempting research from his own
argument for treatment's priority, the same prior-consent argument
which generates a highly qualified priority for actual treatment over
prevention apparently applies also to research.

9. COVERING AND ENCOURAGING PREVENTION

There is a second, ancillary issue: To what extent, if any, should government stimulate the use of preventive care by encouraging insurance coverage for it? Or should the forces of demand for prevention
instead be left to the market?

Doctors, hospitals, and insurers typically seem to underempha-
size prevention. That is understandable. As long as providers make
their incomes and fame largely by delivering rescue medicine, they
will have less economic interest in prevention. Additional moral and
cultural factors come in to create an even greater emphasis on treatment. Insurance companies have an incentive to cover and encourage
preventive services only when subscribers demand them or prevention averts later expensive treatment quickly enough to benefit the in-

surance company in the short term. But subscribers tend to demand less preventive care than treatment; for one thing, once covered for treatment, their demand for prevention to avoid expense diminishes. Insurers thus tend to downgrade prevention in comparison with other care.[66]

Doesn't government need to correct this by mandating or encouraging coverage of preventive care? Former senator Richard Schweiker (present secretary of DHHS), for example, sponsored legislation that would remove the exclusion/deduction from taxable income for premiums for any plan that does not cover comprehensive maternal care, well-baby clinic services, childhood immunizations, regular hypertension screening and pap smears, and periodic physical exams.[67] The same concern has led some people to support a national health service arrangement along British lines.[68]

The implications of the previous conclusion about treatment's qualified priority over prevention should be relatively obvious. The government must not become an across-the-board proponent of equivalence. While it is not inherently objectionable to correct the existing incentives in the marketplace, there are proper limits to that correction. How great should the correction be? That depends on the extent to which low consumer demand for preventive care stems from an irrational or ignorant failure to imagine the full dimensions of more distinct sufferings that would be avoided by prevention. We must not assume any across-the-board moral equivalence of equally beneficial treatment and prevention. A general governmental commitment to equivalence would fly in the face of the arguments for treatment's moral priority that have been defended here. A paternalistic justification could emphasize cost-effective prevention for citizens' own good, but it would also miss the point: It is ultimately these individual citizens' nonrational preferences which define their own "good," even if these preferences generate apparently inefficient policies.

66. Phelps 1978.
67. Senate Bill 1590 (1979); Butler 1980.
68. Endorsing an NHS in order to give greater encouragement to preventive care than a competitive, private market system does may be foolhardy. Prevention has not improved in Britain with the NHS, or not as much as it was hoped. There the capitation method for paying physicians (by patient, not by service) has led to offices that are overcrowded with sick people. It has quickly had to be supplemented with special fees for preventive inoculations and special preventive exams, a development which in turn has almost undermined the capitation system. See Glaser 1970, p. 271.

CHAPTER EIGHT

Competing Groups: Age, Severity, and Numbers

If we simply want to maximize the total benefits from our health-care dollars, we will invest more in preventing and treating a fatal disease of the young than a similar disease of the old. We will invest more in curing and preventing common, high-incidence diseases than rarer ones. And we will not devote additional care to a person with a highly burdensome disease when the same money devoted to someone who is less severely ill will produce greater improvement. Thus, we will spend less per older and fatally ill person than we spend per equally ill, younger one; we will direct care or research to rare diseases only after we have attended to more common ones of the same severity; and sometimes we will leave those who are most ill in less than the best state we could put them in, so that we can move on to make greater improvements in those who are not so badly off.

Should we make these decisions that way? Shouldn't we think in terms other than *years* of life and suffering, so we do not effectively disadvantage the old? Shouldn't we work valiantly on the most severe afflictions before we shift to the less severe? Shouldn't we give all individual victims of a disease an equal chance of benefiting from health care and research regardless of the incidence of their disease? How, after all, can we treat people justly if we count so heavily what is a mere accident, the "popularity" of their disease? Our practices and common assumptions gloss over most of these questions.

A different trade-off has received more attention: improving the quality of life, as opposed to extending it.[1] Ideally, we would like to die

---

1. For interesting statistics on the relative emphasis on quality of life versus extension of life in the research of the various National Institutes of Health, see Mushkin 1979, pp. 191–204. On this whole issue see Veatch 1979c.

'young as late as possible,' like the one-horse shay in Oliver Wendell Holmes's "Deacon's Masterpiece." The hundred-year-old vehicle was perfect, and then

> It went to pieces all at once
> All at once, and nothing first
> Just as bubbles do when they burst.[2]

But we can't often do that; quality of life competes with life itself. We can consider this trade-off through the concept of a "quality-adjusted life year," determined by the chance of death a person would risk in order to avoid a particular kind of suffering: The greater the chance of death a person is willing to take to alleviate suffering, the more severe the suffering is, and the more it therefore lowers the quality of life.[3]

This, however, is *not* the central trade-off at stake in the issues of age, severity, and numbers that are the focus of this chapter. Assume that an illness of the young and one of the old are equally disliked— that is, that in either case the years of life at stake get similar quality adjustments. Still, should we count *years* of life saved (or suffering avoided) in deciding whether the young or the old get medical attention? In the case of severity differences where there are trade-offs between degrees of suffering to be alleviated, but not between suffering and life itself, we will still have to ask whether we should continue to invest resources in treating the worst-off when their benefit per marginal dollar is less than it is for the less severely ill. And the quandary between rare and common diseases arises when for individuals they involve equal life extension, or relief of the same degree of suffering.

Some will say that in a market economy for health care none of these allocation decisions among care for the aged, the worst-off, and those with rare diseases ever need to be made: "Allocations" just emerge from the multitude of consumer decisions about insurance plans. Nevertheless, there are points at which our three dilemmas still insistently appear. Allocations of publicly funded research money still have to be made; all the dilemmas of this chapter crop up there. In a voucher arrangement, government still has to decide whether to prohibit an insurance plan's exclusion of very expensive care, and it might be that expensive because the disease it is for is very rare. In a market medical economy, common diseases have a more "economically rewarding," profit-making character. A disease of relatively high incidence about which enough is known to generate medium-term return on investment will attract research monies in private drug indus-

2. I first saw this delightful selection in Keller 1975, p. 65.
3. Zeckhauser and Shepard 1976; see chap. 2, n. 15.

try. Consequently, drugs such as multiple antibiotics, tranquilizers, antispasmodics, and painkillers have been developed, many of them similar in effect. Other drugs that would be of greater benefit to single individuals but would be used by fewer people are not economically profitable.[4] The same situation often results when drugs are developed with public funding; maximizing aggregate benefits with a given number of dollars can be the dominant rationale in public funding, too.

While there will always be "have" and "have-not" diseases in the battle for research monies, most commentators lament selection for political rather than scientific reasons.[5] Maximizing benefits is then often claimed to be a scientific reason. But is it? "Readiness" and the prospect of breakthroughs are clearly scientific considerations, but the competing issues which are the subject of this chapter reach beyond "scientific." Is maximizing aggregate benefits a "scientific" allocation principle? Hardly. Whether incidence is a good or a bad reason for allocation of research monies is an open and a moral, not a scientific, question. We still have to deal directly with these dilemmas.

1. AGE: YOUNG LIVES BEFORE OLD?

In 1975 60 percent of the $500 spent per person in the U.S. on health care was spent on people who died within one year. Most of these were the relatively elderly. To be sure, more than one-third of the total deaths in the country were of people under 65. But that just leads to doubt in the same direction: Shouldn't we be spending a lot more per life to prevent these many early deaths than to prevent older ones? The incidence of death in the 15–24 year age group rose 13 percent from 1960 to 1978, more than for all the other categories, and much more than for most. In 1971 sudden infant death syndrome received 1/2,000 of the federal research support that cancer got, but had 1/33 of its deaths. One critique of the present emphasis on crisis care for the elderly is entitled "Early Death: An American Tragedy." Considering both the enhanced quality of the younger years of life and the number of years of life that could be saved, its author argues, we are certainly spending too little on the young, and maybe also too much on the old.[6]

4. Garratini 1977.

5. Ingelfinger 1972; Strickland 1972 and 1978.

6. Vaupel 1976. The statistics earlier in the paragraph come from Bloom 1976; Lally 1977; Vaupel 1976; and *Washington Post*, 9 November 1979. For a philosophical discussion I do not take explicit account of in this entire section, see Daniels 1982.

The conflict harbors several different questions. (1) "Life-span" extension: Should we raise the typical age of death from the 65–80 range to, say, 75–90, or should we improve instead the health and quality of life of those under 75?[7] (2) "Life years": Should we count *years* of life saved—not lives saved—in determining what health-care programs are most cost-beneficial? And if we do, should a year of life at an old age be assigned the same value as a year of life at a younger age, presuming that each is the life of a normally healthy person? (3) Young life against the quality of older life: Should we improve the functioning health and *quality* of life for the elderly, or instead prevent the *deaths* of those much younger?

The life-span question will be only briefly addressed, as the quality-adjusted-life-years solution to it has already been mentioned. Most of this section will then focus on questions about life years. Finally, I will briefly discuss the young-life/quality-of-older-life issue.

Life-Span Extension
On this matter Callahan's position is unequivocal:

> The main problem for medicine now is to find ways to deal with those remaining diseases and conditions that stand in the way of living a full life. A by-product of that effort will be a longer life for most people. . . . But until some good reasons have been presented why a longer life *per se* is good, as distinguished from a long life where the evils of life have been . . . minimized, there is no public policy case to be made for the investment of so much as one cent in efforts to extend life for its own sake.[8]

This is a very attractive view. Our expectations, visions, and life plans are highly colored by the fact that most people die in their seventies. We do not expect that we will be seriously ill before that, though we know that such illness is not rare and we have usually taken precautions against it. If the typical life span were to be extended, these expectations would be reshaped. For an individual then to step back to the present average life span would be a disruption as serious as a younger person's illness presently is. Still, at age 70 as well as at 30, don't most of us presently care more about avoiding de-

---

7. I borrow the "life span" terminology from Veatch 1979a.

8. Callahan 1977, p. 37. It is interesting to note that the policy-influencing director of the National Institutes of Health, Donald S. Frederickson, at least partially concurs in philosopher Callahan's view: While the aging process should be studied to increase the quality of life, he says, high priority should not be given to lengthening normal life span. See Frederickson 1977, p. 167.

bilitating illness than about extending life from 75 to 85? That fact undergirds Callahan's view.

But doesn't extending the life span have *some* value? Is it ever clear that this value is *always* smaller than the value of a higher quality of life in earlier years? Surely Callahan is getting dogmatic when he says that extending life in the upper years without improving its quality is not worth the investment of so much as one cent. We all have preferences for a real trade-off here—we will give up only *some* chance of extending longevity a certain amount in old age in order to avoid a particular kind of suffering or limitation now. Nevertheless, the direction in which Callahan leans is undoubtedly correct: Life-span extension is low priority.

Equality is another, and more generally persuasive, reason for preferring higher quality of life to life-span extension. Devoting resources to life-span increases for those who are not suffering, or who are not threatened with early death, would divert resources from care for the least well-off group.[9] Some who had already lived a "normal" life would benefit at the expense of those who have not yet had the same fortune.

Life Years

If all this about life-span extension is correct, isn't it morally dubious to allocate resources on the basis of how many lives will be extended? Why should putting off a 70-year-old's death to 75 count as much as postponing a 25-year-old's death to a likely age of 75? The alternate, clean, and simple proposal is to count only the *years* of life saved.

Yet this way of proceeding doesn't seem to be correct, either, for two reasons. They are complicated, they pull in opposite directions, and they need to be developed at length.

(1) *The per-year monetary value of life varies with the length of the segment of life that we are pricing.* The longer the segment, the lower the *per-year* value of life. Thus the proposal simply to count years of life saved tilts too much toward the young.

To see this, we can take willingness-to-pay readings for different ages and different length extensions of life. Suppose a person of 25 is willing to spend $250,000 to reduce a 50 percent risk of dying very soon instead of living to a likely 75; that computes out to $500,000 for fifty years, or $10,000 per year.[10] But to get the same $10,000-per-year

9. Veatch 1979a.
10. The figure will be higher if we consider discounting. The $10,000 we pay now for a year of future life is paid for the discounted value of that future life. That is, since

value, she would have to be willing to pay only $5,000 to reduce a 50 percent risk of dying very soon and not living one more good year.[11] Wouldn't that same person more than likely be willing to pay considerably more than that? Suppose it is on the order of $50,000.

Now look at a 70-year-old with roughly the same assets, income, and cultural outlook facing a similar 50 percent risk of dying very soon instead of living one more good year. Wouldn't this person be willing to pay somewhat less than the $50,000 of the 25-year-old? The expectations of living are probably simply not as great, and perhaps he would think the overall quality of life at 70 to be a bit lower than at 25.[12] Suppose, therefore, that this 70-year-old would pay $40,000. Now take this same person with *five* years of additional life at stake: Wouldn't he be willing to pay more than the $25,000 that generates the $10,000-*per-year* value for the 25-year-old facing the threat to fifty years? After all, he was willing to pay $40,000 when only one year was at stake. Suppose a plausible figure here is $75,000. Probably the 25-year-old would pay somewhat more than this—say $100,000—to assure five more years of life.

The following chart summarizes all this:

Age	$ Paid to Reduce 1:2 Risk to 0	Total Value of Life Saved	Years at Stake	$/Year of Life Saved
(a) 25	$250,000	$500,000	50	$ 10,000/yr.
(b) 25	$100,000	$200,000	5	$ 40,000/yr.
(c) 25	$ 50,000	$100,000	1	$100,000/yr.
(d) 70	$ 75,000	$150,000	5	$ 30,000/yr.
(e) 70	$ 40,000	$ 80,000	1	$ 80,000/yr.

we are paying for it now while not getting the value of it as future life until later, its monetary value now should be discounted back from what it would be then. We can put the same point in reverse order: $10,000 paid now has a higher monetary value later, even disregarding inflation. There are two reasons why I do not account for this in the figures used here. First, it is very debatable what discount rate we should use. Second and more importantly, it is not clear that the non-inflation-adjustment part of discounting as clearly applies to life and the money spent to save life as it does to more usual uses of money. If now I have the option to buy future enjoyments, won't I be willing to spend more to enjoy the same experiences now? In the case of life, however, this difference is missing. I cannot postpone a present year of life until later; I cannot live more or fewer years now, nor more or fewer later.

11. A "good" year I will loosely construe as simply a functioning and relatively painless one.

12. The latter is very debatable. Things could very well even be the reverse—the quality of life could improve with age. This "older-tends-to-be-better" view is mentioned by Veatch 1979a, p. 216. One of its variants is the belief that "what is really valuable in life is its memories."

The point here has little to do with the particular members. Only the *order* of variation among the life-year monetary values is important.[13]

What these variations seem to reveal is this: If years of life rather than lives saved are what should be counted to determine the value of life-saving programs, the different monetary values of those years has to be taken into account. The varying values do not necessarily reflect a quality-of-life judgment about the different years; there is no reason to think that each one of the fifty years saved in example a is lower in quality than each year in b or d, or the one year in c and e. What these valuations do reflect is a kind of *diminishing marginal utility of life years*: Life years' value diminishes not so much with age itself as with the length of the segment of life which is threatened, and which we are paying to secure.

Is there any way to avoid drawing this conclusion from these responses? Perhaps, some will say, the real value of the segments of five years or fifty years should be computed sequentially: Add the values of each year of life in them as if each year is singly threatened at its respective time. Consider each year as it comes, so to speak. That would give us a per-year average of something between $40,000 and $50,000 for the 25–75 age segment of the 25-year-old's life. The practical consequence would be very close to considering just the number of years of life saved.

But why make the computation that way? In fact we are not looking at reducing each of one person's series of fifty sequential threats to one remaining year of life, starting at age 25. We are looking only at the threat at 25 to the whole rest of a life—likely fifty years. If reducing that threat to fifty years is what a health program accomplishes, why should we not measure directly the value of *that* reduction? To be sure, we can imagine what the alternately conceived sequence and sum of one-year valuations is, but how would we argue that we should use it in computing the value of reducing a threat to fifty years of life? That remains completely unclear. Our conclusion sticks.

(2) *People have a prima facie right to a minimal number of years.* Suppose that the straight counting of life years is correct in effectively giving more weight to saving a younger person's life than a much older one's. But does it lean strongly *enough* in that direction? Isn't it still objectionable simply to aggregate the units of value (years of life

13. I am not saying that in fact people will pay any of these amounts. I know of no empirical studies on these age and years-at-stake comparisons. I claim only that the chart reflects commonsensically plausible relationships between the values expressed at different ages for different lengths of life at risk.

saved) among a large group of people, regardless of how they are distributed? Should an additional five years for each of twenty 70-year-
olds morally outweigh an additional fifty years for one 25-year-old?
Other things being equal, use of the straight numerical life-years
method says they should. Yet just as the principle of equality leans
against letting one person go seriously malnourished in order that
millions get steak (even if some rationally and accurately calculated
aggregate value were thereby maximized), so also the principle of
equality does not let us bypass the one 25-year-old to save the twenty
elderly. Why in the world should *life* be any different than other values which there is a prima facie case for distributing equally?[14]
Doesn't equality generate a right to live a minimal number of years before others are *helped* to live longer?[15]

In part the issue comes down to whether the principle of justice
as equality applies only to people's individual average *per-year* net
benefits, or to their *lifetime* net benefits. Probably the latter. We aggregate different units of welfare and utility over time, for example, when
we talk about a person's general well-being—we do not take several
moments of time for one person as indicating several separate moral
entities. The identity of persons over time, as problematic a notion as
it is, powerfully shapes our thinking here.[16] Admittedly a person's
well-being over time may not be the only value we consider. But we
generally consider the units of utilitarian moral reference to be well-
being over lifetimes, not separate person-moments or person-years.
Don't we then have to view the *equality* principle as also applying to
whole lives? The *lifetime* net benefit, period, is the relevant focus of
the principle.

The principle of equality thus leans strongly toward a right to a
minimal number of years. That is, it leans toward saving the life of one
25-year-old before saving *any* number of 70-year-olds. If at some point
we reject or equivocate about this as a final conclusion, it is not because *equality* does not pull us that way. It is either because despite
the strong pull of equality toward saving the 25-year-old, we are un-

14. I reiterate something that I have repeatedly mentioned but is often overlooked:
The relevant moral equality is not equality of a particular benefit but equality of overall
net benefits between people. See chap. 1, n. 46.

15. This right is highlighted by the report of the Hastings Center Research Group
(1979). The report also emphasizes the goal of vitality and productivity, so the right is to
some minimal number of years of "vital and productive life." Veatch (1979a) also defends
the right to a minimal number of years and grounds it in his egalitarian notion of justice.

16. For a fascinating discussion of this relationship between our notions of personal identity and our basic moral viewpoint, see Parfit 1973.

sure what the "minimal" number of years is toward which this alleged right is directed. (Would we feel pulled toward saving one 50-year-old before saving any number of 75-year-olds?) Or it is because equality is not the only basic principle in our moral life. Equality might be neutralized—either outweighed by the principle of maximizing welfare, or canceled by autonomous consent.

Take consent. Unthreatened individuals at age 20 are not likely to choose to implement a lifelong policy of always saving one 25-year-old instead of very large numbers of 70-year-olds. Aren't their chances of benefiting more from modifying such a policy high enough that they will gladly commit themselves to a society-wide policy of sometimes saving the elderly who compete with the young?[17]

To be sure, some real individuals never find themselves at a point where such a modified policy will be in their own interest. From very young ages on, they run a high risk of dying in youth or mid-life. Some of them may die before expectations, visions, and plans develop very far, diminishing the moral pull of any right to a minimal number of years. For others, however, it will never appear to be a good bargain to modify that right; to them early death remains a particularly flagrant stunting of expectations.

Nevertheless, for *most* young people consent does seem to cancel out any right to a minimal number of years. It is simply in their interest to modify any policy of trying to guarantee people a minimal number of years before helping anyone older live longer. It is not clear just *what* agreement of that sort young people in our society are prepared to make, but it will hardly be simply the opposite extreme—the maximum life-years method. Very likely, some compromise will emerge.

Finally, therefore, we find ourselves with the following conclusions: The prima facie right to a minimal number of years of life is plausibly grounded in the principle of equality. Some, but not all, young people will bargain away at least part of that right to maximize their self-interest. That right might also be outweighed by the maximization of welfare which would result from saving a larger number of older persons' individually fewer years of life.

What do we do now with the larger issue? Should we use life years saved or lives saved to make our moral computations? Implicit in the previous points is a conclusion. Simply counting lives saved effectively overvalues the lives of the elderly, but the straight counting of life years undervalues them—the fifty years of a younger person's life

17. The same bargaining means that Vaupel (1976) should not so hastily claim that we would forgo all improvement in the standard of living so that in thirty years we would have almost no "early" deaths (those under 65).

that we might save have a lower *per-year* monetary value than the smaller number of remaining years of an older person's life. In a different respect, however, even the straight counting of life years overvalues the lives of the elderly: One young person has a qualified prima facie right to a minimal number of years of life, which should be saved before *any* number of aggregated life years of the elderly are saved. Perhaps these two competing points balance each other out: The straight counting of life years and its consequent tilt toward the young is probably roughly correct after all.

Young Lives Versus Quality of Older Lives
About life-span extension there is no universally correct trade-off. Everyone will prefer to forgo some extension of later life in order to enhance the quality of life before old age, but how much later additional life will be sacrificed for how much increased quality before then will vary from person to person and culture to culture. And younger life itself takes limited precedence over older life itself. Can anything be said about the somewhat different choice between improving the quality of older life and saving younger life itself?

Somewhat surprisingly, our previous conclusions do not imply that younger life prevails here. If saving young lives takes limited precedence over saving old ones, it may seem that saving young lives even more clearly takes precedence over merely improving the quality of older life. But it doesn't. While the elderly have little claim to having their lives extended before younger lives are saved, they may have a much stronger claim to improvement of the health and quality of the life which in any case they would live. Here again there is a sliding trade-off. What probability of dying are 25-year-olds willing to risk, in order to enhance the quality of their vividly imagined likely years from 65 to 75? More, surely, than they are willing to risk in order merely to extend their lives in old age. But how much more will undoubtedly vary.

Thus, when competing with the saving of younger lives, the claim of the elderly to improve the quality of their lives is stronger than their claim to extend them.[18]

Summary
(1) While the extension of life span does not automatically defer to the reduction of suffering and disability within the usual life span, both our preferences and considerations of equality relegate the extension

18. A similar position is defended by Yondorf (1975) in a revealingly titled article, "The Declining and the Wretched."

of life span to second priority. (2) When the very lives of young people compete with those of the old, counting only lives saved is unacceptable. The better method is counting the years of life saved. It represents a rough balance between two factors. One pulls for the elderly: the lower *per-year* monetary value of the longer segment saved in a younger person's life. Another pulls for the young: the prima facie right of an individual to a minimal number of years of life before any older lives, even great numbers of them, are prolonged. (3) In competing with the saving of younger lives, the claim of older people to improve the quality of their years is stronger than their claim to extend them.

2. SEVERITY: THE MORE AND THE LESS ILL

Veatch articulates the essential dilemma: "One disease that ranks high as an assault to the normal health of ... citizens may be within our capacity to treat, but only at a cost that could consume the health resources capable of treating a group hundreds of times as large, but less sick."[19]

There is little if any ethical quandary here when the "illnesses" of the "less sick" are as trivial, say, as baldness, unsightly but nonlethal skin diseases, ailments which prevent jogging, or the common cold. In competition with the claims of the more seriously ill, we tend to ignore the claims of persons with these ailments no matter how great the aggregate benefits of attending to them may be. While people should be able to purchase care for such minor afflictions, there is little moral pull on the well to help them. The real moral dilemma emerges when the less sick are still seriously ill. If it is significantly less cost-effective to give increased attention to the most ill than to attend to the not-so-ill, attending to the less ill will maximize benefits.[20] The direction in which justice pulls, however, remains unclear.

The quandary lies *within* justice; it is not just a conflict between justice and aggregate welfare. Serious illness seems unjust; its victims do not deserve it, and it is a major, sometimes definitive, barrier to enjoying the same opportunities which we have constructed an elaborate system of rights to protect. These characteristics, however, apply

19. Veatch 1976.
20. Through the notion of a quality-adjusted life year, we estimate, for example, whether freeing a hundred people from arthritis for ten years has greater benefits than freeing one person from the pain and death of bone cancer; see this chapter, p. 185. Death is ranked relative to suffering, and sufferings relative to each other. Then the degree of relative harm is multiplied by number of persons respectively afflicted.

to the less but still seriously ill as well as to the most ill. Why not *aggregate* the injustices that can be removed and then attend to the not-so-ill to minimize injustice as well as to maximize benefits? At this point, however, some will side with the worst-off: Justice in health care generally requires sufficient care to provide "an opportunity for a level of health equal, as far as possible, to the health of others.... The medically worst off have a complete claim of justice on health care resources in order to bring them, as far as possible, up to the level of the health of others."[21]

Does this reflect a realistic problem for our present-day health-care system? Perhaps we already do provide all the "available," presently developed care to the worst-off. Even if we are already doing that, however, there will always remain the question of what care we should develop. The worst diseases which both kill and cause great suffering—such as Huntington's chorea, spina bifida, and many forms of cancer—may compete for research funds with usually less assaultive ones—such as arthritis, asthma, ulcerative colitis, Crohn's disease of the intestine. Or emphysema, for which there is a very high incidence of "bothers all the time" or "bothers a great deal" responses in surveys of its victims, may compete with hernias or hip impairments.[22]

We could say we should distribute health care on the basis of "need," but that would resolve nothing. Suppose that we want to guarantee each person in actual society a right to equal access to health services. In turn that will require some further principle of distribution within the health-care system, and the usual candidate is need.[23] But the less ill have needs, too. When shifting attention to the needs of the less ill would be more cost-effective, it is unclear whether the needs of the worst-off should be attended to first.

The Distinction between Misfortune and Injustice

Consider the following argument. Misfortune and tragedy are different from injustice. That the worst-off are severely disabled or suffering is tragic, and commiseration and benevolence ought to be our response; they also ought to be part of the response of those who are seriously but less ill to the most ill. Still, moral outrage or resentment on the part of the worst-off that they are the worst-off is out of place.[24] They have no *claim* on others, especially not on the less ill. In relation to

21. Veatch 1976.
22. Mushkin 1979, p. 207.
23. Green 1976.
24. Stell 1978.

our current problem, then, the way is cleared for maximizing benefits by attending to the less ill.

But *is* moral outrage at natural misfortune out of place? To be sure, outrage at one's initial ill health should not be directed *toward people*; it is, after all, natural misfortune. Yet why cannot an appropriate kind of outrage be directed at the natural misfortune itself? Why is it *not* "cosmically unjust" that some people carry much greater natural burdens in life without compensating benefits and rewards? If it is "bad" that some person dies a death that is torturous as well as premature, though no one is responsible—that is, if it would be a "better" universe should no one have to undergo that—then why can't the same situation be called cosmically "unjust"? People morally react to the *inequalities* of burdens in the universe as much as they morally react to the pain and suffering that constitute those burdens.

Furthermore, we can reduce some of the burdens of the worst-off. Also, in using a distinction between misfortune and injustice to try to solve this problem, we are in danger of pulling the moral rug out from under the whole of medicine. Justice in health care is driven by a conviction that the well should help those who are ill through no fault of their own. This conviction is grounded not just in benevolence but also in justice. To be sure, those in need of aid may have no right to be helped. Still, it may be wrong not to help them, and it may be wrong not merely because of the bad we do not alleviate, but also because of the injustice we do not reduce.[25] The point is this: If, since it is wrong for people not to reduce reducible injustice, the well have an obligation to help the ill, don't the seriously but less ill have a prima facie obligation to help the worst-off?

Rawls's Rejection of a Policy of Redress

Perhaps we can seize on a point made by Rawls in his theory of justice. As Rawls sees it, even if justice requires institutions to have general structures and policies that maximize the well-being of represent-

25. Nozick's famous "kidney problem" surfaces here. See Nozick 1974, p. 206. A strict egalitarian sense of injustice would seem to require that we *take* a kidney or an eye from some of those with two good ones in order to save those with none (no good ones). We would and should not do that, and therefore Nozick asserts that any sense of injustice that requires us to do so must be mistaken. His conclusion, however, does not follow from the example. The principle of justice as equality does not say that finally we should take away natural assets that people already have, and somehow distribute them to those who are less fortunate. It may first of all admit a difference between redistributing natural assets and redistributing other assets to correct inequalities. Secondly, it only says there *is* an unjust inequality between one person with two eyes or kidneys and another with none. Whether it should finally be *corrected* will depend on other considerations as well, in particular, on autonomy and welfare.

ative worst-off persons, we need not try to level out natural talents and handicaps. Rational, original-position, veil-of-ignorance contractors will not adopt a policy of "redress"—giving enough additional attention to those with fewer native assets and social advantages to effectively equalize all these contingencies. Neither will actual worst-off people demand such redress. They will demand only that they gain from leaving the inequalities unredressed—that is, that the contributions of "unleveled," naturally advantaged persons spill back to give some benefit to the worst-off. While no one deserves initial advantages, we shouldn't eliminate them. Rawls's second principle of justice goes far enough; it ensures us that no one loses because of his or her initial disadvantages without also receiving compensating, long-run advantages.[26]

Does this show that Rawls can avoid the problem we are trying to resolve? Of course, when the benefits of not devoting more and more resources to heal the stubborn illnesses of the worst-off *do* trickle down to leave them better off than they would have been had they attracted those resources themselves, even the most ill will agree to use the resources elsewhere. But sometimes, surely, continuing to reduce the unequal disadvantages of the worst-off will still somewhat benefit them even though it is decreasingly cost-effective. Arrow then suggests that Rawls's second principle of justice leads to devoting so many resources toward the worst-off that the rest of society will be virtually impoverished.[27] A strict policy of maximin would seem to imply that we should do exactly that. One careful critic, Daniels, sees no way for Rawls to avoid this implication without castrating the second principle of justice and ensuring that it no longer provides any theory of health-care distribution at all.[28] Thus, Rawls's help in resolving our

26. Rawls 1971, pp. 100–02. In order to avoid the principle of redress perhaps Rawls has to de-emphasize his condition of the *equality of opportunity* of worst-off persons to compete for the more than equally advantaged positions that are justified because they raise the welfare of the worst-off. Equality of opportunity is an important part of his second principle of justice. But if he emphasizes *real* equality of opportunity to compete, won't he be driven back to the principle of redress? Perhaps he needs to put primary emphasis on the other part of his second principle—that the justified inequalities improve the well-being of the worst-off.

27. Arrow 1973. "Maximin": maximizing the minimum level of well-being.

28. Daniels 1979. I have not remotely done justice to Daniels's detailed and concise summary of the reasons why Rawls's possible moves in this connection fail. In a more recent article Daniels constructively revises Rawls to get a theory of justice for health care after all. See Daniels 1981. But even here, Daniels shows explicit indecision on the current problem: "We are not required to pour all our resources into the worst cases, for that would undermine our ability to protect the opportunity of many others. But I am not sure what ... [my] approach requires here, if it delivers an answer at all." For a complementary criticism of Rawls, see Ackerman 1980, pp. 261–70. On Daniels, see Buchanan 1982, pp. 27–44.

dilemma is doubtful. Either his theory straightforwardly reinforces the questionable conception of need that would direct almost all resources toward raising the level of the worst-off, no matter how little, or, in order to avoid the seeming unacceptability of that position, it can reject the policy of redress. But in the latter case the theory becomes effectively useless for health-care policy.

We can move on to more helpful suggestions for resolving the problem. All of them at some point defend *not* devoting more and more resources to the worst-off.

Aggregating Injustices
Thomas Nagel writes:

> It is more reasonable to accord greater urgency to large improvements somewhat higher in the scale than to very small improvements lower down.... [And] if the choice is between preventing less severe but still substantial hardship for those who are better off but still struggling for subsistence, then it is very difficult for me to believe that the numbers do not count.[29]

This constitutes a criticism of egalitarianism, if, as in Rawls, egalitarianism "establishes an order of priority among needs and gives preference to the most urgent *regardless* of numbers."[30]

But why shouldn't egalitarian notions of justice themselves take into account the numbers of people? Take the following example. One person most ill is at a welfare level -5. Five people, not quite so ill, struggle at welfare level -4. Fifty healthy people live at "normal" level 0. Suppose we have the ability either to raise the welfare of the one most ill to -4, the five already at -4 to -2, or the fifty normal people to $+0.5$. We have four options: (1) to preserve the status quo, (2) to raise the welfare of the worst-off person, (3) to raise that of the five who are the next worst-off, or (4) to raise that of the fifty who are healthy. For each of these options we can calculate not only utility but also aggregate inequality—by the multiplying the degree of inequality times the number of persons the inequality disadvantages.[31]

29. Nagel 1979, p. 125.
30. Nagel 1979, p. 117, emphasis added.
31. This is calculated by taking each unjustly related person, multiplying the amount of the welfare difference between him or her and the "normal," well, not unjustly situated person, and then adding up all these separate products. There are other ways of determining the degree and number of injustices, too, but they strike me as odd. In one, each person-to-person relationship is conceived to constitute a separate potential injustice, so that the status quo in the above example involves one worst-off person at -5 relating to five next-worst-off persons at -4 ($1 \times 5 \times -1 = -5$), that same

	Options			
	1 (status quo)	2	3	4
Worst-off person(s)	1 @ −5	6 @ −4	1 @ −5	1 @ −5
Next worst-off persons	5 @ −4	——	5 @ −2	5 @ −4
Healthy persons	50 @ 0	50 @ 0	50 @ 0	50 @ +0.5
Aggregate utility	−25	−24	−15	0
Aggregate inequality	$(1 \times -5) +$ $(5 \times -4) = -25$	$6 \times -4 = -24$	$(1 \times -5) +$ $(5 \times -2) = -15$	$(1 \times -5\frac{1}{2}) +$ $(5 \times -4\frac{1}{2}) = -28$

Probably no justification can be found for preserving the status quo. Option four maximizes aggregate utility. Option two has the advantage of minimizing the most extreme case of individual inequality. Option three minimizes aggregate inequality. Unlike the third option, the second represents a nonaggregating principle. Just as in some views of rights, one does not aggregate rights violations and try to minimize them,[32] so also a conception of justice as equality does not aggregate the injustices we are trying to minimize.

We should look more carefully at this comparison with the notion of rights to see if it helps us resolve our dilemma. Talking in terms of rights is most distinctive amidst our wider moral discourse when we do not permit, much less mandate, violating one person's rights in order to minimize violations of a larger number of other persons' similar rights. For example, the rights of other people not to be murdered restrain me from murdering an innocent person, even when that one murder is necessary to prevent a larger number of murders. These are "agent-centered" restrictions. Yet, as Nagel says in calling them that, the label does not go very far toward explaining them.

> A serious account would have to consider ... the relation between the agent and the person he is constrained not to treat in certain ways, even to achieve very desirable ends. The concern with what one is doing to

worst-off person relating to fifty healthy persons $(1 \times 50 \times -5 = -250)$, plus the five next-worst-off persons relating to fifty healthy persons $(5 \times 50 \times -4 = -1000)$, for a total injustice of -1255. This method effectively means that one society with twice as many healthy persons as a second society, but the same number of worst-off and next-worst-off persons at the same level of misfortune, would be nearly twice as unjust. While conceivable, that conclusion does seem dubious.

32. Nozick's conception of "side constraints" is such a view: It is not justifiable to violate one person's rights in order to minimize the equally grave violations of the rights of many others. See Nozick 1974, pp. 28–35.

whom, as opposed to what happens, is an important source of ethics that is poorly understood.[33]

Because it is so terribly difficult, however, to articulate this relation between an agent and the person to whom the agent is allegedly obligated not to do certain things, the arguments for one's right not to be murdered even to minimize the total number of murders seldom seem compelling. The numbers begin to gain their hold on us again. But just because it is difficult to argue against counting the numbers when the issue is the enforcement of rights, that is no reason to count the numbers when the issue is not rights, but whether to devote our decreasingly productive resources to the worst-off. In this latter issue, *all* proposed options aim at producing some *result*. Defenders of the worst-off, just as much as defenders of the less ill, emphasize not just an agent-centered act, but a result that will be someone's actual improvement. As Nagel himself notes, *egalitarianism as much as utilitarianism is an assessment of outcomes, not actions themselves.*[34]

Furthermore, from the standpoint of egalitarianism, equally good cases can be made for both sides of our current dilemma. Nagel calls the worst-off-absolutely-first policy "radically egalitarian."[35] But is there anything more "radically" egalitarian about reducing the inequality of one person from -5 to -4 than about reducing the serious inequalities of five people from -4 to -2, leaving the one person at -5? The two options just reduce *different* inequalities. There is, of course, a level of slight illness which we would not count as significant. But in the current example, even the less ill are still seriously ill—clearly ill enough to stand in an unjustly unequal relationship to healthy people.

Thus, neither the comparison with rights nor the meaning of "egalitarian" provide any help in resolving our dilemma. It is only clarified, not resolved, by noticing that injustices might be aggregated. Before we will make any substantive progress toward resolving the issue, we need to go further than just noting that option three minimizes aggregate inequality.

Prior Consent

Perhaps we can get some help from considering prior consent. What policy would people choose if they had to make their choice *before* they knew whether they were going to be among the worst-off, the

33. Nagel 1979, p. 115.
34. Nagel 1979, p. 117.
35. Nagel 1979, p. 123.

next worst off, or the healthy? Would they choose to reduce aggregate inequality?

Here Rawls's crucial conditions for concluding that rational contractors under a veil of ignorance would choose a strict "maximin" policy are missing.[36] First, Rawls's contractors do not know their odds; our people do. They know they are more likely to be among the next-worst-off than among the worst-off. The very policy they are deciding on—to aggregate inequalities—makes a difference when the next-worst-off are the greater number.[37] Second, Rawls contends that if even hypothetical contractors had to choose between raising themselves a small distance should they turn out to be among the worst-off, or raising themselves a great distance should they be among the less ill, they would choose the former. We would disagree. The "better off" are still seriously burdened. The question is not whether rational people are likely to gamble more than a strict maximin policy contends that they do. If I vote for strict maximin as our policy, I will be gambling in the face of very bad outcomes for myself as potentially the next-worst-off. In fact I will be gambling in the face of bad outcomes at least as much as I would as a worst-off person voting to minimize aggregate injustice. Won't both actual people and hypothetical contractors be inclined toward minimizing aggregate injustice?

Thus the case for aggregating inequalities based on prior consent begins to sound persuasive. But we now run into what for us is becoming an old problem. Fortunately it is not so vexing here.

Unfairness to the Congenitally Ill

There are actual persons for whom the model of prior self-interested consent does not so nicely resolve our dilemma. The worst-off who are already ill may never have—or never have had—a chance of benefiting from any policy other than strict maximin. These most clearly include those who are severely and congenitally ill. In chapter 7 we saw that fairness considerations lead to important restrictions on any policy of equivalence between rescue medicine and preventive care. It might appear that any sacrifice of strict maximin for the sake of aggregate justice would also face restrictions when we get to the congenitally worst-off.

36. Rawls 1971, pp. 154–57. See n. 27.

37. Rawls, of course, does not allow his original-position contractors to know even any of the odds of coming out here, there, or any particular place in the natural or social lotteries. See Rawls 1971, p. 154. His reasons have seemed questionable to some. In any case, in making this immediate point, I am not working within his framework of purely hypothetical contractors.

But the matter is not that simple. Some of the somewhat less ill are already burdened, too. Unlike rescue medicine's competitors, that is, the recipients of preventive care, they are now already situated in a known, distinctly unjust relationship to the well. The principle of justice as equality would thus seem to undergird their claim to aid as well as it undergirds the claim of the most ill. It would not do that, of course, if before the less ill had become ill, they had self-interestedly traded away their claim to priority over the most ill. A similar agreement not to claim further rescue medicine is precisely what the non-congenitally ill (who at the time were *not* ill) can be presumed to have given in the prior discussion of treatment and prevention.

In our present dilemma, too, the noncongenitally most ill can be said to have given tacit, rational consent to a policy of minimizing aggregate injustice and not always attending to the worst-off first. The *congenitally* worst-off, however, have given no such consent and probably would continue not to do so. In their probable, enduring refusal to agree to minimizing aggregate inequality, they stand at loggerheads with the congenitally next-worst-off who have refused to accept any policy of strict maximin. The arguments are neutralized. Consideration of the congenitally ill ends up generating no discernible conclusions for our present dilemma.

The Benevolence of the Worst-Off

Might the benevolence and sympathy of the worst-off for any much greater number of the next-worst-off lead them to accept a policy of minimizing aggregate inequality? Aren't the worst-off apt to sympathize with the less but still seriously ill who would gain greater benefit from equivalent resources? It is not that they see the less ill as having a claim of *justice* against their own decreasingly efficient use of resources; in the current dilemma the meaning of justice is precisely what is unclear. Their sympathy and benevolence stem from realizing the sheer magnitude of the reduction in suffering which could be accomplished by not claiming the resources less efficiently for themselves. Might not the most ill themselves pronounce, "That's enough, don't spend more on us, there are better things to do with the dollars"?

Perhaps it is precisely the focus on atomized self-interest, the sharp division into "we" and "they," the most ill and the less ill, which keeps us in our corner here. The most ill will not benevolently pronounce "That's enough" for the benefit of the less ill if they feel separated off from others. If, on the other hand, they are fully accepted by others into the life of the community, will they want for even one minute to have the lion's share of health-care resources poured into decreasingly efficient attempts to improve their own health? They themselves may see community integration as their deepest reward. That integration does not come without the well (or even the less ill) listening to their needs. Above all, it does not come without the most ill sharing in the joys and improvements of the less ill, though that sharing is admittedly terribly delicate. If and when this integration does come, it transcends claims to justice as equality. All along justice as equality has been a potentially terribly grudging moral ideal.

The proper conclusion to this section is both complex and tenuous. Realizing that inequalities can be aggregated only sharpens the dilemma between the most ill and the less. The case for minimizing aggregate injustices and not adopting a policy of strict maximin seems to be advanced by considering people's prior consent. Considerations of fairness to the congenitally ill neither confirm nor reject an aggregating principle. Furthermore, to the extent to which the most ill are benevolent and sympathetic toward the less, the tenuous case which prior consent establishes against any strict priority for the most ill is strengthened. The proper motto for health care is not just "the worst-off first."

3. NUMBERS: RARE AND COMMON DISEASES

In the United States the costs of developing and testing a drug for marketing may run as high as $10 million. In these circumstances it is much less likely that drugs for relatively rare diseases such as muscular dystrophy, multiple sclerosis, and amyloidosis will get much attention. Not only will costs per unit of the drug be much higher since the total costs have to be recouped from a smaller number of users, but total costs, too, may well be higher; there are smaller numbers of experimental subjects, they are harder to procure, and they are less likely to be in one place. The treatment of such "economically unrewarding," rare diseases, says Garratini, requires a political will to divert intellectual and economic resources to help their otherwise "stranded" victims.[38] These victims deserve an equal chance to regain their health. Their smaller numbers should not disadvantage them.

38. Garratini 1976. An interesting example of this very issue of drug development for rare diseases is the so-called "drug-orphan" legislation that the U.S. Congress passed in December 1982. It gives drug companies much larger tax write-offs for the expensive process of testing drugs for rare diseases than for testing drugs for more common ones. President Reagan finally signed the legislation into law, after his alleged opposition. See Wehr 1983.

In our general public life there is some precedent for not always saving the larger number. Glover cites another marvelous World War II example.[39] Britain thought of having one of its double agents send back false reports to the Germans that their rockets were falling north of London, when in fact they were right on target. If consequently redirected to the south, the rockets would kill fewer people. This option was finally rejected. An influential adviser argued that the government should not, in order to save more people, choose which citizens should be sacrificed. It should just let people be exposed to the rockets falling where they may.[40]

The competition for research funds harbors other examples. Some diseases have attained strong positions in that competition despite their relatively low incidence in the population. Witness sickle-cell disease, multiple sclerosis, Cooley's anemia, meophilia, cystic fibrosis, and sudden infant death syndrome. Their present status is due to pressure groups, not prevalence. From one point of view this is fortunate: To consider prevalence would be to leave the victims of rare disease stranded by virtue of the mere accident of their small numbers, denying each *individual* victim of a disease an equal chance of being saved. To others, however, heeding pressure groups and not the numbers is wasting our resources. It may even seem unfair—why spend more marginal resources *per life saved* on the victims of rare diseases than on the victims of more common, prevalent afflictions? For some it is a "demoralizing" selection for research money on the basis of "political rather than scientific reasons."[41] Lobbies both ignore scientific readiness for productive research and thumb their noses at the prevalence of the diseases on which they want our dollars to be spent.

This conflict comprises the pure numbers-counting issue. In an impure form the numbers-counting issue was involved in the previous section. There, however, the questions of whether the numbers should

39. Glover 1977, p. 102.
40. The example is admittedly not perfect for my present purposes. For one thing, if the British authorities had been genuinely interested in giving all Britain's citizens a more equal chance of surviving regardless of whether they were in the smaller or the larger group of potential victims, they would have flipped a coin to see whether the double agent plan would be adopted or whether the rockets would be left falling on London. For another thing, as Glover relates it, the reasoning which led them to leave the rockets falling on London seems dominated by the desire that wherever the bombs did fall, they would not seem to be in any way falling there because of a decision of the British government.
41. Ingelfinger 1972.

count and whether we should minimize aggregate inequality got mixed with differences in either the level to which the different groups would be raised or the amount of improvement that individuals would gain from the care. To focus on the numbers-counting issue per se, we need to eliminate those factors. We need to focus, first, on cases where a smaller number and a larger number of people at *equal levels of illness* compete for resources, and second, on cases where individual persons will each gain equally if they get care, regardless of which group they are in. Even then, can a smaller number of individuals persuasively argue that the resources *not automatically* go to the larger group?

For convenience we can label the two contrary views on this issue. *The Numbers Count:* we ought to spend the lowest number of marginal dollars per person and per unit of benefit. *Equal Chance:* we ought to give each individual victim of a disease an equal chance of benefiting from medical resources, even if in doing so we end up spending many more dollars to save the life of a person in the smaller than in the larger group.

Equal Chance has some considerable attractiveness at the level of microallocation, where particular health-care professionals and institutions determine which particular individuals shall receive an available resource. Should we really count out Mr. Smith as a candidate for kidney dialysis just because he requires more time on the machine than Ms. Jones? At the level of macroallocation, however, where no particular persons are literally knocking at our door, we more commonly count the numbers.[42] Yet even here, as the example of investment in drugs for rare diseases illustrates, it can be argued that the numbers should not count, or should not count so much. I will explicitly focus on the macroallocation context and not discuss the considerable literature on this issue at the microallocation level, particularly kidney dialysis.[43] It will be more interesting to see whether a relatively intractable moral dilemma remains even in cases where it seems more acceptable to count the numbers.

One version of the claim that the numbers don't count is extreme: They don't count even in determining what the outcome with the greatest aggregate *value* would be. To Taurek, for example, it is not only that it is not right to save five lives in preference to one because

42. One of the clearest examples would be citing the high prevalence of a disease in a developing country as a reason for concentrating on it first.

43. See Rescher 1969; Childress 1970; Westervelt 1976; and Basson 1979.

there are five; five lives are not even more *valuable* than one, or a hundred persons handicapped a *worse* state of affairs than two.[44] I will ignore this radical strategy for discounting the numbers and assume, first, that more people who are equally in pain constitute *more pain*; second, that this pain to each of five people is a *worse* total state of affairs than the same pain to one; and third, that the former is *five times as bad* as the latter. The central question, now pruned, remains: Under all these assumptions, is counting the numbers and maximizing welfare the right thing to do?

Equal Burdens

Consent may at first appear to provide a happy resolution. Won't people give their prior consent to counting the numbers? Rawls's hypothetical contractors will—in the situation there is no risk of one individual ending up at a lower level of well-being than any other individual. Thus there is no risk to which they could possibly be averse, since individuals in both the smaller and the larger numbers are threatened by equally serious outcomes. Actual persons who do not know they are in either group will also consent—by voting to count the numbers, they will maximize their chance of gain, without incurring any risk of greater loss.

Yet this brings us to the crux of the problem. Not all people can be presumed to consent, at some point in their lives, to a numbers-count policy for their futures. Some are born into, or very quickly become, an afflicted smaller number. Admittedly, they will have no grounds to claim that the resources should be directly devoted to themselves and not to the greater number.[45] (How could being in the

44. Taurek 1977. His reason is not that there is no way to measure the pains of one person relative to the pains of another. His is a more complex argument. With considerable help from Parfit (1978), I would piece it together as follows. (1) If we prefer the worse of two outcomes we are morally deficient. (2) People would not be morally deficient if they preferred to save themselves rather than to save a greater number of others. (3) Obligations are not "agent-relative" (that is, if it would not be wrong for you to save yourself rather than five others, it would not be wrong for me to save you rather than the five). Therefore, Taurek argues, (4) it would not be wrong for people to save a smaller rather than a larger number of others, and (5) the deaths, say, of five cannot collectively be a worse outcome than the death of one. As Parfit notes, it would seem more plausible just to retract either (1), (2), or (3) than to carry the argument through to (5).

45. As individuals they have no more claim directly to the resources than any individual in the larger number has. That no individual in the larger number has such a claim is the foundation for Anscombe's argument that the larger number do not have any claim to the resources: "No *one* of the larger number has any ground for accusing me of having wronged himself" if I save the smaller number. "What is *his* claim, except the claim that what was needed go to him rather than be wasted? But it was not

smaller number give them any such claim?) At most they will have only an argument for doing what may unpredictably generate their being saved—flipping coins, or random selection in one of its forms. That will give them an equal chance, something which *all individuals* in the smaller and larger groups alike can then be said to have. When the smaller number hold out for equal chance, they are not merely holding out for their interests; they can plausibly cite some moral principle of equality.

Does this whole line of thought, however, distort that principle? If no person in the smaller number is left worse off by counting the numbers than any person in the larger number would be if we flipped a coin and the larger number lost, how can equality be read to favor flipping coins? The smaller number have a very sound reply at this point. They can say: "Through the random, natural lottery we are afflicted with two curses. One is the same as that suffered by the equally ill of the larger number. But there is a second, additional curse—being in the smaller number! Before the numbers are counted, it looks as if we and the larger number have equal burdens. But in a society with a numbers-count policy, *our additional burden of having naturally fallen into the smaller number is a misfortune as great as having the disease to begin with.* It may mean that we die, and they live. The burdens are not equal after all."

Yes, they are not. Still, is this a relevant inequality? Being in the smaller number constitutes no greater natural burden in itself; it becomes a burden if and only if we make a decision to count the numbers. Other inequalities about which we have been worrying—inequalities between the more and less ill, for example—constitute burdens before anyone makes a policy decision. In deciding to count the numbers, we are treating people with equal concern and seeing them as having equal burdens *when* we make the decision.

But does any of that make any difference? Why should *presently* unequal burdens for actual persons be the only ones relevant to the question of whether counting the numbers is compatible with equal-

wasted"—it saved the smaller number. See Anscombe 1967, emphasis added. Ezorsky notes that Anscombe never asks "what kind of reason there might be for choosing to save fewer persons." By contrast, Ezorsky claims, there is a reason for saving the greater number—because otherwise more people will die. See Ezorsky 1972, p. 160. Yet as good as Ezorsky's reason may be against a person who wants to save directly the smaller number, her reason fails to take account of the turn in the discussion I am presently introducing: Critics of counting the numbers do not recommend choosing the smaller number, but only flipping coins. They are willing to save the smaller number only if that is what the toss dictates.

ity? Don't we need to take account of the *results* of our decisions? Results are relevant whether maximizing the value of consequences is all there is to our ethics or not. The persons for whom we make any of these decisions are immediately going to have unequal burdens if we adopt a moral policy of counting the numbers and not flipping coins. While there is no way to account for unequal burdens that fall on as yet unknown victims, other persons know already that they will lose by a numbers-count policy. Policy-makers, too, already know that these people will lose. Why isn't it as important to consider knowable inequalities that are contingent on a particular policy decision as to consider inequalities that are already present?

Bad Luck

In defense of counting the numbers, Parfit claims it is as fair to let one person die because we count the numbers as to let anyone—the five or the one—die because we flip coins.[46] It is simply the smaller number's misfortune that if we count the numbers their claims are outweighed. In a sense, of course, this is unfair, a kind of natural injustice as previously noted. But "such injustice cannot be removed by flipping coins. It could only be transferred. Natural injustice is bad luck. Making more depend on luck will not abolish bad luck." Others echo Parfit's sentiment: Why is a human lottery "any more moral than the natural lottery which made some on the life boat weaker and others stronger?"[47]

Yet the argument doesn't work. To be sure, flipping coins will not abolish what is still, in the last analysis, bad luck. But there are huge differences here. Bad luck may be more or less unjust, depending on the process out of which it has emerged. Fried poses an instructive case to show that sometimes the process of the natural lottery is fair. Would "a person who, after a shipwreck, had the good luck to find a spar big enough to support only one ..., have to submit to a lottery" if another survivor swam up? Fried summarizes that he would not:

> To be sure a lottery between the two survivors as they confront each other over the plank does give each an equal chance at that moment, but what is missing is any argument for making that moment determinative. Why, it can be argued, is not the finding of a plank a sufficiently random circumstance to allow the conclusion that the two survivors in question had equal opportunities in respect to it? And if that is a plausible point,

46. Parfit 1978, pp. 300–01.
47. Leiman 1978, p. 9.

then to make the fortunate survivor undergo a second lottery would be unfair to him. . . .

I do not wish to argue that there might not in the shipwreck example be devised explicit schemes which would randomize and equalize the benefits and burdens in that sort of situation better than letting the burdens fall where they may. . . . My argument is, rather, that in many situations in the absence of some explicit arrangements to which all involved parties have consented to be bound, there may be no better approximation to equality than the rough and ready randomization entailed by the principle of letting the loss lie where it falls.[48]

The point is persuasive for the shipwreck case: Reliance on the natural lottery of who finds the spar first was a good—even a very good—method of randomizing the burdens and benefits at the time the ship got wrecked. For the real individuals who thus found themselves in danger, this method does preserve the equal chance of all *at that time* to survive. *It is only because the natural lottery in this case reflects the equal chances of real individuals at the time they decide on a policy that the later bad luck for some is perfectly acceptable.*

Now contrast this case with another, say a very rare, *congenital* disease. Here the only sense in which the natural lottery can be said to have given its victims an equal chance is if we speak of the victims as individuals before they are born, nay, even conceived. Admittedly we are not very clear about why this is an inappropriate perspective from which to view the natural lottery. But *that* it is inappropriate we can be reasonably sure. Its implications are wholly unacceptable: From this perspective, no disease or natural misfortune of *any* sort could be regarded as morally unacceptable bad luck. As a purely hypothetical person before conception, *anyone* has had an equal chance of coming up lucky in the natural lottery. *If that should lead us to regard that lottery as fair, there would be no moral pull of justice to any claim of any of the ill to any assistance from the well.* It is because there are inequality-generating natural lotteries to which real individuals have *not* given some kind of prior consent that the well have some initial, basic obligation of justice to help the ill.

Human lotteries clearly are fairer than natural lotteries to which real persons cannot be presumed to consent. They give real, existing persons an equal chance. The bad luck of being in the smaller number is less acceptable, morally, than the bad luck of losing the toss of a coin.

48. Fried 1970, pp. 200–03.

Aggregate Injustice, and Benevolence

There is, however, another more persuasive argument to be made for counting the numbers. Can't the moral principle of equality itself be compromised more by flipping a coin than by counting the numbers? As we saw in the last section, if any initial, intuitively basic principle of equality focuses on differences in people's total net lifetime benefits, it would seem that inequalities of different people can be aggregated. As individuals, people are left disadvantaged—and just as disadvantaged—if we flip coins and chance saving the smaller number as if we straightforwardly count the numbers. Doesn't that total up to a greater inequality?

This is exactly the aggregation issue tackled in the last section. There the discussion was distinctly inconclusive. Here it should probably be also. There may be fundamentally good reasons why we cannot definitively affirm either a principle of equal chance for every actual individual, or the principle that here competes with it, that of minimizing aggregate inequality of results. Perhaps there just are two different, and competing, principles of equality at the base of our morality. One concerns results; it aggregates. Another concerns process; it emphasizes equal chance and opportunity.[49] Since we cannot rule out the aggregate principle of equality, we end up in a paradigmatically unstable position: While attracted for very good reason to an equal-chance policy, we are also pulled toward counting the numbers by a different but equally fundamental aspect of moral equality.

There is another argument which we tried in the previous section: The dilemma between the more and the less ill is tempered if the fewer, more gravely ill persons freely and benevolently pass up small improvements in their own condition so that others who are somewhat less ill can gain more. The final conflict between equal chance and counting the numbers might be tempered in the same way. Individuals in the smaller group may benevolently decide that aggregate welfare or aggregate equality of results takes priority over the equal chance for all actual individuals. Equal chance to benefit can remain the policy which initially expresses equal concern for each person. If all in the smaller number then benevolently lower their demand for an equal chance to benefit, all of them can still feel that the need for their consent already reflects equal enough concern for them as individuals.

49. The second seems to be what Ronald Dworkin emphasizes as the value of equal concern and respect for all real persons. He claims that Rawls's whole hypothetical-contract model does not generate this value but *depends on* it. See Dworkin 1974.

To be sure, the general weaknesses of presumptions of benevolence remain. In contrast to the previous section, here in addition there is no greater *individual* benefit for those who gain from counting the numbers that can pull the minority into benevolent consent. Nor, in any case, are those in the smaller number likely to give the necessary *unanimous* consent to counting the numbers. Unless either their actual sentiment for aggregate welfare and inequality can be increased, or the equal-chance side of equality can be shown to be bogus, we end up stuck with a significant dilemma that is generated at the most fundamental level of normative ethics.

Averaging Gains and Losses
In the realistic context of current health care, some of this resulting quandary, fortunately, may be softened. One of the initial ways the numbers-count issue surfaces is in asking whether the victims of a rare disease should have to pay more for their unique drugs. With insurance, this moral quandary about the numbers gets largely avoided. The issue might remain in reduced form, the higher cost of insurance to victims of rare diseases. We may properly not be much bothered by this inequity, if it is an inequity at all; only relatively manageable cost differences are at stake, not the care itself, much less life. The more bothersome issue, however, has still not disappeared. In some cases, the cost of a more expensive treatment of a rare disease can be ascertained in advance, and somebody, probably government, an insurer, or a prepaid plan, has to make a policy decision—whether to develop, distribute, or cover this service. Should we use the same dollar-per-benefit ceiling here that we use to make other decisions? If we do, those in the smaller number lose out. The original question still confronts us.

I have talked as if life or something of that order is at stake. Fortunately, often it may not be. We may be dealing with care that holds only a very marginal and statistical benefit for its patients. Even though with this disease they are in the smaller number, they may gain from a general policy of counting the numbers because they will benefit in many other respects. This is most likely to occur when their original, rare affliction is not that severe. Take people genetically predisposed toward migraine headaches, and suppose that a hundred times as many people suffer from much less severe, ordinary headaches. While the migraine sufferers were born into the smaller number and may never have had an equal chance of benefiting from a policy of counting the numbers in allocating resources between migraines and ordinary headaches, they can still be presumed to consent to a more general numbers-count policy. Because there are many other maladies in respect to which they stand to gain by such a policy, the gains and losses from *generally* counting the numbers *for care with less than huge stakes for given individuals* will even out over time. Counting the numbers in allocating resources for the wide variety of pains and sufferings that all people share will redound to *everyone's* benefit.

Admittedly, it is difficult to draw this line between the smaller stakes, where gains and losses do average out for everyone over time, and the larger ones, where they do not. But that it is the proper line, I am quite sure. On the side of the line where the stakes are smaller, there is no moral case that can be made against counting the numbers. Where the stakes are larger, we seem to be stuck with a serious and irresolvable quandary: Aggregate equality and welfare argue for counting the numbers, but principles of autonomous consent and more individualistic equal concern keep the equal-chance policy morally very much alive.

The last two sections of this chapter have brought to light a plurality of competing, morally fundamental principles and relatively intractable dilemmas. Perhaps Calabresi's and Bobbitt's observation of a pattern of serial emphasis on one value and then on another is fitting here. Societies have made noble use of different allocation principles by accepting all of them across time:

> A society which wishes to reject none of them can, by moving, with desperate grace, from one approach to another, reaffirm the most threatened basic value and thereby seek to assure that its function as an underpinning of the society is not permanently lost.... The alternative ... would be the final rejection of some fundamental values.[50]

This may not be just an historically astute observation about American society; it may offer us a philosophically attractive option. I end on this note of irresolution. Dilemmas like those of the last two sections are very difficult indeed. Our worst mistake may be to think that we have clearly resolved them. They may have only disappeared from our view.

---

50. Calabresi and Bobbitt 1979, p. 198.

CHAPTER NINE

Physicians' Incomes

1. THE ISSUE

Doctors have the highest average annual earnings of any occupational group in the United States—$81,000 in 1980. Some, like cardiac surgeons, average over $350,000.[1] The power over societal resources which health-care institutions have as a whole is directly reflected in the economic status and power of physicians.

Two very different things might be said about this. On the one hand, we could quote contemporary physician Eugene Diamond:

> If the return to health is the principal concern of the patient who is ill ..., the fee becomes his principal concern after he is well.... Our critics will acknowledge our long hours, sympathize with the tension of life and death decision-making and yet, scorn our affluence.[2]

Or, on the other hand, Adam Smith:

> We trust our health to the physician; our fortune and sometimes our life and reputation to the lawer.... Such confidence could not safely be reposed in people of a very mean or low condition. Their reward must be such, therefore, as may give them rank in the society which so important a trust requires.[3]

1. Glandon and Werner 1980 and Roe 1981.
2. Diamond 1977, p. 106.
3. Adam Smith, *The Wealth of Nations*, quoted in Glaser 1970, p. 1.

Some current facts appear to bear Smith out. For instance, for all their other variations in health-care delivery, Canada, France, Germany, the United Kingdom, and the United States all have virtually the same ratio of physician's income to average income of full-time employee. Among these five countries that ratio ranges only from 4.72 in the United States to 6.52 in Germany.[4] It looks as if, somehow, people need to know that their physicians are paid roughly five times what they are. Reputation, for example, seems to be considered important enough to warrant paying the attorneys who protect it more than twice the national average income. But, then, if health is more important than reputation, it is hardly surprising that doctors earn again twice that.[5]

In our current situation, however, we can hardly be so sanguine as to let the matter rest here and leave doctors' incomes as they are. To be sure, if life, and the saving of life which doctors often undertake to do, has no finite monetary value—no "price"—or if it does have a price, it is very, very high, even the marginally effective services of doctors will be worth every penny we now pay them. But nowadays we are often sceptical about how effective this or that medical procedure really is. And, in any case, even if a medical procedure is judged to be effective, its effectiveness is usually only a matter of statistics. The distinctly finite prices of life which emerge from willingness to pay for reductions of risk prevent doctors from convincing us that they are worth just anything they charge. If life, lifesaving, and health have a finite price, doctors' earnings are less likely to be worth our money. *Who gets paid what* is just as crucial an allocation question as how many of our resources are used on health care, and for whom.[6] Asking the most difficult and basic questions about the cost of health care will inevitably lead us to a discussion of physicians' incomes.

It is surprising how this has been ignored. At a time when talk of cost containment is common, little serious and comprehensive literature has been produced on the normative *justification* of physicians' incomes, as opposed to the mere description of what they are or the explanation of what causes them to be that way. One reason this question has been ignored is undoubtedly a misperception of some statis-

4. Newhouse 1976a.

5. U.S. Department of Labor, Bureau of Labor Statistics, *Occupational Outlook Handbook* (1980–81 edition) (Washington, D.C.: Government Printing Office, 1980), p. 378.

6. Newhouse 1976a.

tics. It is often noted that reducing doctors' net incomes 20 percent would decrease health-care expenditures only 3–4 percent. While physicians influence the allocation of the bulk of health-care dollars (e.g., the 44 percent that goes to hospitals), they themselves receive less than 20 percent of health-care dollars.[7] But that does not mean that the matter of reducing doctors' incomes is trivial. First of all, why should a *20* percent reduction be the parameter of the discussion, when $81,000 is the base income we start the discussion from? More importantly, even if the reduction of health-care expenses is only 3–4 percent, that $7–10 billion is far more than the cost of most of the procedures the cost-benefit analysis of which currently fills the health policy journals. While people should realize the modest financial proportions, $7–10 billion is nothing to sneeze at.

So we should persist. Even assuming that doctors are medically effective, are they worth what we pay them? And, if they are, do their earnings compare justly and fairly with other people's? In pursuing these questions, I want to focus primarily not on the very high earnings typical of a few specialties, but rather on the prevalent income level of physicians in general.

2. MORE FACTS

Doctors' incomes have risen from roughly $4,000 in 1940 to $12,000 in 1950, $42,000 in 1970, and $81,000 in 1980. In relative terms, too, they have risen. In 1940, physicians' incomes were less than twice those of a broad cross-section of professional and technical workers; by 1975 they were four times as great. Between 1940 and 1975 the percentage rise in physicians' incomes was twice as great as the average rise for workers. Furthermore, except in the 1970s, when other people, too, were seeing their increases eaten away by inflation, physicians have been gaining in real income. From 1970 to 1975 real income decreased 0.5 percent per year; from 1975 to 1979 it rose at the same rate, for a 0.1 percent per year drop for the entire decade.[8]

The following table compares incomes in various professions in 1978:[9]

7. Kridel and Winston 1978, p. 7; Moloney and Rogers 1979; Nagurney, Braham, and Reader 1979.
8. Dyckman 1978; Glandon and Werner 1980; Rayack 1977.
9. Compiled from U.S. Department of Labor 1980, pp. 125–397.

Profession	1978 Income	Proportion of Average Worker's Income ($15,000)
Physicians	$71,000	4.7
Airline pilots	$57,000	3.8
Dentists	$50,000	3.3
Lawyers[10]	$31,000	2.1
Veterinarians[11]	$30,000	2.0
Air traffic controllers	$25,400	1.7
Architects	$25,000	1.7
College or university professors	$22,400[12]	1.5
Nurses	$16,800	1.1
Firefighters	$15,000	1.0

The hours that physicians work partly explain their higher incomes: They worked an average of 51.4 hours per week in 1970, and 49.5 in 1980.[13] If we count the 9.5 hours above 40 per week as time-and-a-half and discount the $81,000 accordingly, we get $52,400 as an average doctor's income in 1980, over three times the average for all full-time workers.

Physicians in some specialties have much higher averages than physicians in general. As a group, orthopedists have often been highest; in 1977 two of every five exceeded $100,000 per year. Hospital-based pathologists and radiologists with percentage-of-department-revenue contracts had even higher earnings, roughly $160,000 and $145,000 respectively, more than double the earnings of the average physician. That is surprising to most of us; for one thing, pathologists and radiologists are not publically perceived as the most heroic or burdened of physicians. We are probably least surprised to hear that in 1981 the average annual earnings of cardiac surgeons were at least $350,000.[14]

Some attribute much of the rise in physicians' incomes in the last forty years to an increased use of medical specialties. Specialists, of

10. Business corporations, nonsupervisory.

11. An averaging of the $33,000 for private veterinarians and the $25,300 for government-employed ones.

12. The academic year average was $18,700. I have raised this by 20 percent for an annual figure.

13. These hour figures are from Glandon and Werner 1980. They are lower than the 62 hours per week used by Lindsay, based on *Medical Economics* questionnaires; see Lindsay 1973. Others regard the 62-hour figure as high; for one thing, doctors were asked to report their work for the "last full week." See Sloan 1976.

14. Dyckman 1978, p. 79; Roe 1981.

course, are paid more, for one thing because of their long residencies. The facts, however, do not support this explanation. While the proportion of specialists has increased markedly, the median income of general practitioners has increased at the same rate as the average income of all physicians.[15] The dramatic rise in the incomes of physicians in the last forty years has occurred almost across the entire profession.

Within the health-care sector as a whole, mean earnings are on a par with other industries, but the standard deviation is almost double. That is, the percentage of health-care workers at the very low end is much higher, as is the percentage earning twice the mean, and almost none have earnings that fall between the mean and twice the mean. Prepaid plans, which were expected to make greater use of middle-level "physician substitutes," are surprisingly no different. Though in legal services the overall pattern is much the same, in health care the extremes are much greater.[16] Physicians have great economic power and prestige in relation to other health workers as well as to workers in general.

3. SOME EXPLANATIONS

A considerable body of literature attempts to explain why doctors' earnings are as high as they are today. We need to review some of that literature's main suggestions before tackling the problem of justification itself. Four theories stand out: (1) "human capital" and investment in schooling, (2) monopoly control through the restriction of entry into the profession, (3) demand creation and the "target-income" phenomenon, and (4) the third-party reimbursement formula of "usual, customary, and reasonable" fees.[17]

Human Capital

According to this theory, variations in income generally reflect different investments in training—human capital.[18] Physicians' incomes

15. Rayack 1977.

16. Fuchs, Rand, and Garrett 1972.

17. For an exhaustive review of the literature on explanations of the distribution of income in general, see Sahoto 1978. I have found no similarly comprehensive review of the literature about the generation of physicians' incomes in particular. I have organized this section keeping in mind both Sahoto's more general review and the scattered literature on doctors' earnings in particular.

18. Two of the most seminal presentations of the theory are by Becker (1964 and 1967) and Mincer (1974 and 1976). Atkinson quotes Cannan in rejecting the entire theory

compensate for long years of schooling and residency as well as the pressure, deferred satisfaction, and debts which those years involve.[19] One author, Lindsay, claims that if we note the cost of medical education, consider the earnings forgone in the long years of schooling, account for the hours which physicians later work per week, and use a discount rate of 10 percent, then the costs of physicians' training give no more than the normal return on an educational investment.[20] Another critic, Leffler, calculates that doctors began receiving "rents" above and beyond a normal return on their investments only after Medicare legislation ballooned the demand for health-care services in the late 1960s.[21]

When applied to doctors, however, the human-capital theory of income distribution runs into problems. It would probably be more accurate to revise Lindsay's 62-hour physician work-week downward to a 50-hour figure, and that makes a significant difference in the calculations.[22] For that and other reasons, many critics have concluded returns to medical education are generous. Doctors' earnings would have to be reduced 23–30 percent to equal the return that university and college teachers receive for their training, 29–39 percent to compare with pharmacists, and 1–7 percent to compare with lawyers.[23]

This conclusion seems to be more realistic than that of Leffler and Lindsay. Still, their use of human-capital theory has made an important point about physicians' incomes: If we account for longer hours and investment in training, the ratio of a physician's to an average worker's earnings is not nearly as high as the apparent 4.7:1. A conservative hour adjustment brings 4.7 down to 3.5. If we also account for the cost and forgone earnings of medical education, and if we discount for interest, we move closer to 2.0. That is not much higher than the similarly adjusted earnings of lawyers, and about twice the adjusted earnings of university teachers. So now our question is not whether physicians' labor is worth five times the average worker's, but whether it is worth a little more than twice as much.

as implausible: If generally there actually were equality of net advantages, "we should find well-to-do parents in doubt whether to make their sons civil engineers or naval stokers, doctors or roadsweepers." See Atkinson 1975, p. 86, quoting Cannan 1914, p. 207.

19. Forty-six percent of residents' medical school debts exceeded $20,000 in 1980. That is expected to rise to $50,000 shortly; see French 1981. Tuitions of $12,000 are not at all unusual. Interns' and residents' incomes are relatively low, often below $1,000 a month, so that little of the debt can be paid back until after residency.

20. Lindsay 1973.
21. Leffler 1978.
22. Glandon and Werner 1980.
23. Sloan 1976 and Mennemeyer 1978.

And it is not whether doctors' time is worth twice as much as lawyers', but whether it is worth only a bit more.

Monopoly Control: Restricting Supply

The lack of competition in the health-care economy has many dimensions.[24] The control which physicians have over medical services leans toward monopoly. The uneasiness that health-care consumers feel about relying on their own medical understanding and their relative lack of information about fees sets the stage. Physicians expand this into fully monopolistic control, it is claimed, by their ability to limit the entry into the profession of others who may be willing to do the same work for less. The output of medical schools is kept artificially low, and licensing requirements are strict. Physicians are then able more or less to target their incomes.

Have medical schools thus conspired with organized medicine? Many economists and antitrust scholars argue that they have.[25] Of course conspiracy charges are always notoriously difficult to defend. The actual debate on medical schools' conspiracy with organized medicine has largely focused on a preliminary point: Has there indeed been any shortage of physicians? One definition of "shortage" emerges directly from our discussion of human capital: The number of physicians is optimal if the rate of return on occupational investment for marginal entrants to medical schools is normal.[26] If the properly adjusted, real returns to medical education have been no greater than for college education in general, one will think there has been no shortage, or at least that there has been no shortage severe enough to give medicine monopolistic control over its earnings. Whatever shortage defined in other ways may still exist can then be attributed to a combination of the high standards for admission which the nature of the profession may demand, and medical education's strained financing (the bulk of support for medical schools comes not from entrants investing in their future earning power, but from outside donors).[27]

These last points are well taken. But if, as is likely, real returns to medical education are considerably higher than the returns to most other college education, we should nevertheless conclude that there has been some shortage. The huge investment that medical schools

24. See, for example, Enthoven 1980.
25. Fein and Weber 1971; Friedman and Kuznets 1954; Kessel 1958; and Rayack 1977.
26. Hall and Lindsay 1980.
27. Lindsay 1976; Hall and Lindsay 1980.

put into screening applicants may be necessary for quality, but the very sharp competition and the disputes about the necessity of certain admission standards leave us thinking that restricted supply is still a likely part of the story. The mere fact that there seem to be more applicants who are qualified than the number who are admitted to medical school, or that there certainly would be if the process were not known to be so competitive, indicates that the balance of expected rewards and costs is more favorable for a career in medicine than for other occupations.[28]

There is, however, other much more definitive evidence for a shortage. The number of positions for interns and residents rose from 21,500 in 1950 to 56,300 in 1973, while the percentage of these positions filled by foreign medical-school graduates rose from 9.6 to 32.7.[29] In 1967, in fact, about 46 percent of all newly licensed physicians in the U.S. were foreign graduates. There is other evidence, too. Pressure has increased to find lower-cost substitutes to do much of the same work that physicians do.[30] Why should we pay a physician $81,000 to do much of what a nurse practitioner is capable of doing and willing to do for $30,000? Through control over licensing, of course, physicians retain largely monopoly power. The recent decades have been replete with these continuing jurisdictional battles—with nurse practitioners and midwives, for example. A plausible recommendation is to take away organized medicine's *control* over licensing. Of course, doctors should be advisers to the licensing body, but why should they set policy?[31] Then, too, if the AMA's goal were only to ensure quality, not also to restrict supply, it would advocate requirements for *re*licensure that were as high as those for original licensure or medical-school admission.[32]

In conclusion, while the picture is mixed, physicians have undoubtedly gained some monopolistic leverage by tough medical-school admissions policies and licensure requirements.[33]

28. Newhouse 1978, p. 100.
29. Rayack 1977.
30. Rayack 1967.
31. Rayack 1977.
32. Kessel 1970. Others writing on this general issue are Friedson, who generally backs Rayack's views, and Leffler and Lindsay, who generally oppose them. See Friedson 1976 and Lindsay and Leffler 1976.
33. A sidelight of this whole discussion is whether physicians' "price discrimination"—charging more to the wealthy and less to the poor—reflects their charity or their monopoly power. If physicians had no monopoly power, they would seemingly lose to other physicians any wealthy patients whom they charged more; in the long run that would remove any physician's capacity to give price reductions to the poor. See primar-

Demand Creation

Such talk of shortages, however, may only apply to a bygone era. An oversupply of 70,000 doctors has been forecast for 1986 by the Graduate Medical Education Advisory Committee.[34] Yet if anyone thinks that this will lower physicians' incomes, they may be wrong. Even physicians in excess supply seem to be able to create demand for their services, either by prescribing more services or by charging higher prices. They target their incomes and hit that target no matter how large the supply of doctors grows.

The clearest (though admittedly limited) example of this occurs in highly specialized fields like neurosurgery. If one neurosurgeon for every 200,000–500,000 people is adequate but in a city of a half a million five have taken up residence, what happens? The number of operations per surgeon may drop as low, say, as three a month.[35] The "usual, customary, and reasonable" fee for the procedure floats up to the level necessary to maintain these doctors' original or expected incomes. Patients have little incentive or information on the basis of which to look for a surgeon in another area; for one thing, most patients are insured. The several neurosurgeons in the area all know each other; without ever conspiring on the matter, none of them will reduce their prices in order to force others to leave, nor will they lower their charges.

To a lesser extent this also happens with primary-care physicians. When supply increases relative to population, more physicians in the area then prescribe more or better services, probably to more people. None of this need be deliberate provision of "unnecessary" care, though much of it may be care only marginally or questionably worth its cost. Some reduction in work load will probably also occur, but at least some of the attendant drop in an individual doctor's income can be made up by gradually increased fees. Insurance makes that possible.[36]

Some will dispute this picture, attributing income levels to heavy hours and investment in training, not to demand creation and targeting of income.[37] But we have already seen the limits of that human-capital explanation, and even if it were correct, one would still wonder

---

ily Kessel 1958. See also Rayack 1977, Somers and Somers 1961, and Masson and Wu 1974. For an opposite view see Ruffin and Leigh 1973.

34. Emery 1981.

35. Blackstone 1978.

36. Evans 1974; L. Jensen 1979; and Schroeder and Showstack 1979.

37. Leffler 1979.

why incomes do not drop when a particular area becomes saturated. We can conclude that the thesis of demand creation and resultant target income contains considerable truth.[38]

The "Usual, Customary, and Reasonable" Fee (UCR)

In a fee-for-service system, an insurer can reimburse either the patient by category of medical problem (not by services used), the patient for the actual expenses, or the doctor for the patient's expenses. The last two methods can either be by standard fee schedule or by a more flexible formula like UCR, which is adaptable to the needs of a particular patient. The first method of reimbursement, "indemnity" insurance, assures neither patient nor doctor that what actually has been done will be paid for. A standard fee schedule may not do that either; more importantly, it leaves the physician no incentive to perform particularly fine work in more intricate cases. For all these reasons, Medicaid, Medicare, Blue Shield, and most private companies have gravitated increasingly toward the more flexible UCR formula. Within the formula, "usual" denotes the typical fee of the particular individual physician, "customary" any fee below the 90th percentile of doctors' fees for that procedure in the area, and "reasonable" any exceptions in special medical circumstances. This formula was not merely concocted by and for the medical profession. Insurance company competition for subscribers was for the most part what stimulated the adoption of UCR. UCR guaranteed patients the maximum coverage of the cost of their care.[39] We asked for it; we got it.

But obviously, in doing this, third-party payers also played into the hands of physicians. UCR preserves neither the independence of third-party payers nor competition among physicians. Fees all gravitate up to the "customary" level in the area; though technically secret,

38. In its reply to Dyckman's 1978 Council on Wage and Price Stability Report, the AMA notes that while fees are higher where physician density is greater, net incomes are lower. See American Medical Association 1978, pp. 18, 22. The AMA cites Sloan as well as Benham, Maurizei, and Reder, but also notes that the findings of Redisch et al. show the opposite. See Sloan 1968; Benham, Maurizei, and Reder 1968; and Redisch et al. 1977.

This part of the reply is in any case weak. Unless physicians had something more than their usual leverage from a free-market situation, they would be unable to raise fees at all when supply increased. Though net incomes may actually have dropped somewhat when supply increased, a good deal of the target-income effect may still be present. To be sure, however, this is a complex and disputed matter. Steinwald and Sloan (1974) report studies not generally consistent with the demand-creation/target-income hypothesis. Newhouse (1970) and Redisch et al. (1977) report studies supporting the hypothesis, and Newhouse and Phelps' results (1976) are consistent with it.

39. Korcok 1979.

it is easy for a physician to find out this level by charging a higher fee and noting what happens. More importantly, while "customary" keeps reimbursement below the 90th percentile of fees in the area, many specialties are small enough in number on the local level that a very few (or even one) of them can actually raise the UCR fee level simply by charging more themselves. UCR also gives physicians an incentive to raise their fees tacitly in concert with each other over time.[40] Thus UCR seems to augment whatever monopolistic power physicians already have.

To some critics, of course, this is a small point; the entire fee-for-service method of paying for medicine is their target. George Bernard Shaw is often quoted: "That any sane nation, having observed that one could provide for the supply of bread by giving bakers a pecuniary interest in baking for you, should go on to give a surgeon a pecuniary interest in cutting off your leg, is enough to make one despair of political humanity."[41] In particular, fee-for-service favors discrete, technology-intensive, non-time-intensive services, and some estimates are that a physician can triple net earnings by emphasizing tests.[42] This may explain the high average incomes of radiologists and pathologists.

It would be rash, however, to pin too much on the fee-for-service method of payment per se and then be too quick to favor alternate methods like capitation or salary instead. Comparative evidence between countries gives no indication whatsoever that fee-for-service generates higher doctors' earnings. Witness Britain, for example, with its emphasis on capitation in the NHS and its still-high 5:1 ratio of physician's income to average worker's. Furthermore, capitation tends to encourage underdoctoring and the recruitment of only the healthiest patients, and the salary method offers doctors little incentive to be either productive or oriented toward patients rather than toward the party that pays the salary.[43] Glaser's classic, internationally comparative study of payment methods should remind us that no single method is either culprit or panacea.[44] No single method so far devised discourages both overdoctoring *and* underdoctoring, while at the same time encouraging quality care for "unprofitable" patients, proper referral, and good specialty and geographic distribution.

40. Butler 1980; Delbanco, Meyers, and Segal 1979; and Roe 1981. Roe's attack on the UCR "boondoggle" is particularly clear and pointed.
41. *The Doctor's Dilemma*, preface, p. 226 in Shaw, *Collected Plays with Their Prefaces* (1911, 1971).
42. Shroeder and Showstack 1979.
43. Abel-Smith 1976, pp. 70–71.
44. Glaser 1970. See also Roemer 1962.

4. JUSTIFICATION

What finally does all this mean? Are physicians' earnings too high?

We can infer several things from the previous section reasonably safely. Physicians' incomes are currently higher than they would be if they were determined by a free market of informed, autonomous consumers bidding for the services of suppliers who do not prevent competing qualified suppliers from entering the profession. Thus, even if we assume that the incomes resulting from free-market decisions are justified, we cannot conclude that current physicians' incomes are. Doctors' incomes cannot be counted on to reflect either the value of their contributions to people's welfare or the value of their labor and training in comparison with that of other potential suppliers.

In the larger discussion of justification, two different strategies can subsequently be pursued: We can try to ascertain what income levels would in fact be generated in a free market of doctors' services, or we can go directly to some independent criterion for the justness of an income. In what follows I will use some of both approaches; I will connect them, looking briefly at the relationship between a just income and one that is generated by a free market.

Justice and the Market

There is one particularly strong connection between justice and incomes generated by a truly free market. The fact that there are certain rewards and burdens in every occupation brings directly into play the principle of justice as distributive equality: All persons' individual overall net welfare in life should ideally be equal—if their burdens increase, so should their benefits.[45] Thus, if the total rewards of an occupation, monetary and non-monetary, stand in the same relationship to its compensating burdens as they do in other occupations, that occupation is justly paid.

Non-monetary rewards and burdens, of course, are absolutely crucial to include. But how can we possibly judge how great the non-monetary rewards or burdens are in a career in medicine? This is an extremely vexing problem, and yet it must be solved if we are to get anywhere in determining a just level of earnings. We could theorize forever, arguing ad nauseum about how much of a reward or a burden this or that aspect of a particular job really is. Right at this crucial point, however, the market provides a ready test: If only so many people are willing to take on these burdens in order to get these rewards,

45. Ake 1975.

and if that supply generates, say, $50,000 incomes, we have the best indication we ever could have for saying that a $50,000 income is necessary to make the overall benefit/burden ratio of this job equal to that of competing occupations. Thus, to obtain a justified earnings-level figure, we need to simulate the market. Then we should discount present levels of doctors' earnings by the amount of skewing we judge to be caused by restriction of entry and creation of demand. That will put us as close to a just monetary reward as we know how to get, either practically or theoretically.

This is the *market-based* solution to the question. It is distinctly superior to merely regarding the actual income which physicians earn in the existing market as just, but it must still confront serious problems. It may just happen that many, many buyers are bidding each other up for the use of one person's natural talent, while very few buyers are bidding each other up for another's. Furthermore, some suppliers may get low incomes simply because many people happen to like a particular kind of reward and therefore want to join in that occupation, or because many have the required natural talents for that occupation. Others may get very high incomes because there happen to be few such people. Suppose you are one of the former and I one of the latter. You might earn $10,000 and I $100,000. How can that be just? The difference, after all, is a function of something that is morally purely arbitrary, the frequency of certain dispositions or talents in the population. It is no more just for individuals to luck into fortune this way when others do not than it is for one person to be left to suffer with one disease while another with a different disease fortuitously gets cured.[46] (Here we are not concerned with some proverbial gold nugget we luck into on a Sunday stroll, but with people's whole work and livelihood. People will likely consent ahead of time to an unrestricted, finders-keepers policy on lucky treasure; they won't likely do that when it comes to livelihoods.)

Is there any reason to think that something akin to this arbitrary fortuitousness is happening in the market for medicine? Probably not, or at least not much. It is apparent that the non-monetary rewards of a medical career are appreciated by more than a few people. And while the natural talents required to become a heart surgeon may be

46. These are the problems with Nozick's conclusion to his celebrated Wilt Chamberlain case. To be sure, each basketball ticket buyer freely contributes to Wilt's $250,000 salary only because each is really getting his or her money's worth out of the transaction. Still, what is just about a universe in which there are many of those buyers, so few people with the natural talent to be basketball stars, and so few buyers for many other natural talents? See Nozick 1974, pp. 161–64.

rare and the talents needed to become any sort of physician very great, the latter at least are hardly esoteric or rare enough to create a natural shortage of suppliers. On the other hand, there probably is a naturally stronger demand for a physician's services than for most of the other jobs people do. Doctors thus have some natural advantage in any free-market generation of income. Since it is very hard to estimate the extent of this advantage, we might be inclined to leave the advantage undisturbed. We should hardly allow it, however, to be augmented by monopolistic factors like restriction of entry or creation of demand. Restricting entry in order to get physicians of the very highest quality might not be objectionable in itself, if doctors had no power to create demand for their services, and demand creation in itself might be acceptable if there were free entry to drive down any high earnings and equalize doctors' and others' overall net benefits. To allow restriction of entry when demand can be created, however, surely invites unjustly high earnings.

Should Doctors Be More than Equal?

The previous analysis inclines us to conclude that physicians are currently paid too much. It is driven by the principle of justice as distributional equality, applied to occupational income in particular: Everyone's net total occupational benefits, monetary and non-monetary, should be equal. But shouldn't some people, perhaps, like doctors, get *greater* than equal net benefits?

Most claims that they should would appear to warrant the label "elitist." What, for example, would justify the view that doctors *deserve* greater than equal *net* benefits? After all, we have already built compensation for greater burdens or deferred earnings into "net" benefits. To say, subsequently, that doctors deserve greater than equal benefits because of *who* they are is surely elitist, and objectionably so. It is of no avail to argue that since society gets enough people into medicine and there is open competition for positions, net total benefits must be as great for the last entrant into medicine as for the marginal entrant into other occupations—there is no truly open competition in medicine. Nor can we cite some particular compatibility between high earnings and the tasks performed by doctors. With business executives, for example, we might argue that the people who get attracted by high earnings are also precisely the people likely to have the monetary ambition necessary for efficient, profit-making activity. Where is there any similar qualitative link between high earnings and the goals and nature of medicine? Are *monetarily* ambitious people likely to be better doctors than monetarily nonambitious people? One could even argue that in medicine the relationship is the reverse.

We are left to consider one further argument. Doctors are saving life and restoring health, it will be said. There simply is no way we can doubt that that is worth two or three times what other services are, regardless of what the net benefits are to physicians. Despite the unusual control over their incomes and the attendant greater net benefits which physicians enjoy, their *product* is still *worth* every dollar we pay. Wouldn't only an ungrateful, grudging patient keep harping on the issue of whether doctors' net benefits are greater than others'? We have an honorific desire to pay our physicians very highly, *regardless* of calculations of human capital and comparative net benefits. That is partly gratitude and partly a trust-creating act on our part—we want doctors to be very special persons, and what we pay them reflects that.

This argument, however, is woefully misconceived. At best it thumbs its nose at considerations of justice and equity. At worst, it also reflects an arrogance about some allegedly priceless value of medical services rooted in the mistaken belief that life and health have no price. Every profession, of course, claims to warrant higher pay—it thinks "the problems it specializes in solving are particularly threatening to society, that society *must* be eager for salvation at any cost."[47] But if, as I have argued, risk-reducing care does have a finite dollar value, and if the blank check that has been given to medicine on society's resources should be withdrawn (that's partly what cost containment is all about), why should we continue to give individual physicians blank checks? To be sure, we do want physicians to gain a healthy income. That is very different, however, from giving them monopolistic control or greater-than-equal net benefits.

Furthermore, to say that physicians must be the highest-paid professionals in society, or, even more dubiously, that pathologists and radiologists have to earn more than $200,000 a year, is a strange kind of vicarious materialism *even if life has no price*. We do want greater material well-being ourselves, and we know doctors do, too. But why should giving sheer opulence to our physicians give us any reason to trust, honor, or respect them more for the allegedly invaluable services they provide? Our confidence in another's *professional* prestige is misplaced if we focus so much on material well-being. That we do that may be an understandable side effect of American ambition and materialism. It is nonetheless perverse. For physicians to en-

47. Glaser 1970, p. 290.

courage this mentality in us in order to keep their economic power is a lamentable straying from their allegedly primary loyalty to patient welfare.[48]

High doctors' incomes have other unfortunate side effects. A considerable number of patients in fact lose some of their trust. When doctors become directors of banks, real estate speculators, owners of shopping centers, and so on, are we sure that they can be objective in prescribing services, that they are not at all motivated unconsciously by the exigencies of an economic career?[49] More importantly, as they grow more distant from the poor, doctors become less and less willing to make services accessible to them, and they certainly become less willing to deliver in good conscience the kind of care which represents the poor's lower ceiling of costworthiness. Doctors may also be inclined to believe that the level of their occupational liberties should be as high as their economic well-being. For example, they may believe that government development of strong incentives to practice in underserved areas and disincentives to practice in oversupplied ones is a violation of their right to live and work where they please. But as it has been pointed out, if a particular college professor's liberties are not violated by not being able to teach in Berkeley Heights, why should a doctor's be by not being able to practice there? "The appearance that there is an enshrined liberty under attack is a legacy of an historical accident . . . , namely that physicians have been more independent of institutional settings for the delivery of their skills than many other workers. . . ."[50]

Conclusion

When adjusted for hours and training, the income of the average physician is not as much greater than incomes of other professions as the initial statistics would lead us to think. Nonetheless, doctors have unusual control over their incomes. A significant number of them use that power to make much greater incomes than even the average physician. To determine a just monetary reward for their labors, we may take their actual income level as the starting point, then discount for their monopolistic power over entry and demand and peculiar prac-

48. Alford goes further: Rather than "a societal consensus giving doctors their power, it is the doctors' power which generates the societal consensus. Or . . . the existence of a network . . . of institutions which guarantees . . . that their dominant interests will be served comes to be taken for granted as legitimate, as the only possible way in which these health services can be provided." See Alford 1975, p. 17.

49. Diamond 1977, p. 109.

50. Daniels 1981.

tices like "usual, customary, and reasonable" reimbursement, and finally account for the additional leverage which they get from the naturally pervasive demand for health care. Neither the peculiar value of
their services nor the need of patients to go to respected, prestigious
members of their communities requires they be given additional economic power. The argument should not so much focus on the particular question of whether two, three, or five times the average worker's
earnings is the proper income level for doctors; instead it should account for these disparities of power. It is utterly hypocritical for doctors, health-care administrators, academic analysts, and policy makers
to close their eyes to the level of doctors' incomes amidst an otherwise
vigorous concern for making health care worth the increasing money
we pay for it.

Hypothetical Contract Reasoning in Ethics

There are a number of ethical frameworks that might have been used in developing the arguments in this book. As explained in the last section of the Introduction, I have chosen a pluralistic framework in which aggregate human welfare, justice as distributive equality of net benefits, and consent (individual autonomy) are separate, irreducible, basic moral principles. This admittedly detracts from a fuller coherence and unification which one might have hoped my arguments to have. A more unitary viewpoint has not been chosen; in the last analysis I simply doubt if any such viewpoint is more correct. A utilitarian position, for example, seems woefully inadequate in explaining our stubborn and fundamental convictions about equality. Even if egalitarian distributions are actually utility-maximizing, the *reason* they are *just* is still not merely their contribution to the pie of aggregate utility. Why must *distributions* of goods among individuals be at bottom supported by what the distributions contribute to aggregate utility? The same sort of point could be made about an exclusively libertarian position which considered the moral attractiveness of welfare and equality to emerge from free choices. We need not—and should not—permit the thirst for reductionism to sweep slighted principles under the rug.

A defense of pluralism seems relatively easy to make against reductionist utilitarianism, libertarianism, or egalitarianism. It is undoubtedly more difficult to make against a hypothetical-contract framework for moral reasoning such as the one proposed by John Rawls.[1] Allegedly a more sophisticated viewpoint, it claims to honor our most fundamental, different values, give short shrift to none, and efficiently provide a method of rationally adjudicating and balancing them when they conflict. Why should I not appropriate that model? My final reason is essentially the same as for rejecting other, simpler,

1. Rawls 1971.

reductionist positions: Admittedly, hypothetical-contract reasoning is more effective than a pluralistic model in resolving many of the conflicts between fundamental values, but it finally fails to adjudicate conflicts between different fundamental principles; at important points it begs questions for or against some of them. Given the importance of Rawls's work in the past decade, my view needs explaining.

The attractiveness of hypothetical-contract reasoning is that we need somehow to escape the partiality that our particular circumstances create in any of our attempts to adopt a set of basic moral principles. Actual circumstances, the argument goes, are not the appropriate setting for adopting those principles. For one thing, it would be unfair to allow biologically or socially inherited advantages, which a person in no way deserves, to influence one's initial, basic, moral tilt. Furthermore, some greater agreement about basic moral principles is needed than can be obtained from actual persons. These attractions of hypothetical contract cannot be denied.

Yet the hypothetical contract model does not really avoid presupposing that some other particular moral values are fundamental. Obviously not just any hypothetical contracting will do. We have to impose the *right* hypothetical limitations. What are they? What veil of ignorance is appropriate within the model? Rawls's first suggestion comes right out of our intuitions about fairness and desert: We should not know our biological talents or handicaps or our social inheritances, since we do not deserve them. While perhaps it cannot be said that we deserve *not* to have them, Rawls can still claim that we do not deserve *to* have them, and that makes taking them into account unfair. Most of us quickly agree. But *why* do we? Our agreement is not likely some isolated intuition. I suspect that a fundamental principle about equality drives Rawls's thinking and our reactions right here.

At a crucial later point in Rawls' clarification of the veil of ignorance, he also expunges any knowledge of probabilities—for example, the probability that we will turn out economically advantaged, or destitute, or ill. Again, it is hard to see that there is any final argument for doing this which is not itself the statement of a moral conviction. If in fact we do buy Rawls's move here, isn't it finally because we think it unfair for real persons in a small, disadvantaged minority to have had moral principles decreed for them by hypothetical contractors who found it easy to slight potential but real disadvantages since they knew how improbable it was that they themselves would be afflicted by them in actual life? That intuition reflects the seriousness with which we take *each actual individual* in morality, regardless of how many people are similar.

It is considerations like this which lead to the sort of critical observation expressed by Ronald Dworkin: Some moral principle of the equality of actual individuals *undergirds* Rawls's whole model.[2] It is not just rationally generated by it. Rawls's hypothetical contract then cannot be read as a more fundamental level of reasoning which adjudicates conflicts between subordinate princi-

2. Dworkin 1974.

ples of welfare, equality, and consent. A principle about the equality of all actual persons as individual persons is favored in shaping the very environment
for the contract. Rawls "adjudicates" between equality and aggregate welfare
only by begging the question in favor of equality. (I am less sure he begs any
question in favor of equality when it conflicts with consent. Rawls does give
priority to his first principle of justice—equal liberty—over the relatively egalitarian distribution of goods demanded by his second principle. That priority
probably does not beg the question in favor of consent, however, since he derives the priority of liberty from an original position which is fashioned by
considerations that already reflect a principle of equality. Also, the liberty that
has priority is equal liberty.)

Rawls's dependence on considerations of equality can be read into his
model in yet another way. As mentioned, a very important reason for initially
embarking on any path of hypothetical contract is to gain leverage for impar-
tiality over the self-interested perspectives of actual persons who might otherwise reject any moral principle that looked as though it would not work in
their favor. In one respect most of us would agree: Our fundamental moral
principles should not be subject to veto by the *advantaged* persons of this
world. Thus, properly, Rawls is not terribly bothered by Nozick's puzzlement:
What will Rawls say to the rich who complain when his yardstick of justice
demands that they transfer some of their holdings to the poor?[3] The advantaged rich are simply not in an appropriate position to lodge a moral complaint of *injustice*. That is due, I think, to something like the principle of justice as distributional equality. Rawls can so easily dismiss any rejection of his
principles by the advantaged only because he already has available, at the
ground floor of his own theory, the relevant principle of equality for shoring
up his defenses against Nozick. Note that any actual *dis*advantaged person's
complaints against injustice in the results of Rawls's principles then get a
much firmer platform for moral pronouncement. To be sure, Rawls can often
end up quieting those complaints more directly; he can persuade the most
disadvantaged to accept his second principle of justice, which permits inequalities of primary goods (not liberty) that still leave the worst-off representative persons better off. However, this is a matter of their *consenting to what
is still real injustice*. The reasoning that such inequalities are just, then, derives in part from consent; it is not a matter of rock-bottom justice itself.[4]

This leads to my second fundamental dissatisfaction with hypothetical
contract reasoning: Rawls's position fails to represent adequately some of our
bottom-line convictions about justice. Take the consideration just raised. An
actual person, disadvantaged, is living under Rawls's second principle. A
greatly unequal distribution of goods is permitted because it benefits even this
worst-off person. To be sure, in one respect that person will not complain; he
or she would be even worse off if the inequality were not permitted. But he or

3. Nozick 1974, pp. 195–96.
4. Ake 1975.

she could surely lodge another plausible complaint. It would run something like this: "If the best-off have their advantages partly because of their not deserved natural talents, and if I am so much worse off partly because of my natural or socially inherited disadvantages, how can it be just that others have so much more than I? To be sure, given the realities of this world, I would not want to reduce their advantages. Still, the world into which they and I were born is unjust if they undeservedly end up with so much more than I." Ake, then, is precisely right: What we have here is a case of stubborn injustice which is accepted by its victims because they cannot realistically do any better.[5] Principles of consent and welfare override equality.

The problem is not limited to this case of happy, merely verbal disagreement about how to describe what the parties substantively agree on—in which what Rawls calls an instance of justice is what Ake and I call an injustice consented to by actual individuals for their own welfare. In other cases, disadvantaged actual individuals will not agree with Rawls's substantive conclusions, even if they think through their position in terms of hypothetical contract and speak out of genuinely considered intuitions. Rawls's second principle ensures only that *representative* worst-off persons will be as high in well-being as they can be in this real world. Some actual individuals will be worse off than that and could be better off under different distribution policies. Unless *they* contracted for some "representative person" version of the second principle over some "every actual person" version, wouldn't they as actual persons still have a legitimate complaint? After all, actual persons just aren't "representative persons."

There is another weakness in Rawls's reasoning. His reply to the worst-off person who complains is that he or she is still better off with the inequality. That is treacherously dependent on Rawls's ability to make good his arguments for maximin. If these arguments will not stick in a hypothetical-contract model, the model faces even more strenuous and persuasive objections from actual individuals. What will surely stick is the inequalities created by policies that would be knowingly consented to by actual persons, often before they are disadvantaged. The acceptability of these inequalities just reflects the dominance of actual over hypothetical contract.

Do these considered complaints of actual persons, even the very disadvantaged, miss the basic reason that any hypothetical-contract model is used at all in ethics? Shouldn't we excise our intuitions about anything which is permitted by the decisions of the ideal contractors, since it is the hypothetical contract, not our intuitions, that should tell us what we ought to do? But this is hardly a reply which Rawls himself would make. His methodology is "reflective equilibrium": The ideal contractors' environment is to be adjusted if the contract's results do not finally gain the consent of our open-minded, considered, finally stubborn intuitions.

The reflective-equilibrium methodology, however, may appear to save hy-

5. Ake 1975.

pothetical-contract reasoning from an earlier criticism. Earlier I argued that use of the model will beg questions in favor of one moral principle over another by the way any use of it will set up the original position. That is a misleading appearance, it might be claimed. Rawls's theory of ethical truth is a coherence theory: You use the contract model, consider its implications, and then adjust the original position and the veil of ignorance if these implications are unacceptable to your most stubborn and considered intuitions. You are in equilibrium only when everything finally coheres. But then there is no point of logical foundation that "starts" the system, and we cannot say that some implicit principles used in setting up the original position really beg important moral questions in these principles' favor.

Still, what is the difference between begging a question by letting certain initial assumptions reign—not a coherence theory—and begging it within a coherence framework, by letting certain considered intuitions stand stubbornly at the end in accord with conditions of the original position that those very same intuitions have helped to shape (or reshape)? We can at least make a very important observation at this point: If no questions are begged, hypothetical contract has no way to reconcile the conflicting views of persons with different stubborn intuitions. Those people adjust the conditions for the original position in different ways, then cling stubbornly their respective reflective equilibria. Pluralism seems to be the end result after all.[6]

We can conclude, then, that hypothetical contract reasoning fails to adjudicate between conflicting basic moral values without begging questions— that is, without presupposing rather than generating some fundamental principle of equality. It may also fail to represent adequately some fundamental starting points in ethics—for one, the existence of actual, disadvantaged, autonomous persons who stand in distributive relationships to others. A more frankly pluralistic theory is not as elegant in form or as complete in its conclusions, but it is not therefore less correct or finally less satisfactory.

6. Rawls himself may even admit this. See Rawls 1971, pp. 579–85, and Rawls 1980, especially pp. 565–72.

Bibliography

Abel-Smith, Brian. *Value for Money in Health Services*. New York: Saint Martin's, 1976.

Ackerman, Bruce A. *Social Justice and the Liberal State*. New Haven and London: Yale University Press, 1980.

Acton, Jan Paul. "Evaluating Public Programs to Save Lives: The Case of Heart Attacks." Santa Monica, Calif.: The Rand Corporation (R-950-RC). 1973.

————. "Nonmonetary Factors in the Demand for Medical Services: Some Empirical Evidence." *Journal of Political Economy* 83, no. 3 (June 1975): 595–614.

————. "Measuring the Monetary Value of Lifesaving Programs." *Law and Contemporary Problems* 40, no. 4 (Autumn 1976): 46–72.

Adams, J. G. U. "... And How Much for Your Grandmother?" In Rhoads, ed., 1980, pp. 135–46.

Ake, Christopher. "Justice and Equality." *Philosophy and Public Affairs* 5, no. 1 (Fall 1975): 69–89.

Albee, George W. "Does Including Psychotherapy in Health Insurance Represent a Subsidy to the Rich from the Poor?" *American Psychologist* 32, no. 9 (September 1977): 719–21.

Alford, Robert R. *Health Care Politics: Ideological and Interest Group Barriers to Reform*. Chicago: University of Chicago Press, 1975.

Allen, Jodie T. "The Concept of Vertical Equity and Its Application to Social Program Design," in P. Brown et al., eds., 1981, pp. 87–108.

Altman, Stuart H., and Blendon, Robert, eds. *Medical Technology: The Culprit behind Health Care Costs?* Washington, D.C.: Government Printing Office, 1979.

Altman, Stuart H., and Wallack, Stanley S. "Technology on Trial—Is It the Culprit behind Rising Health Costs? The Case For and Against." In Altman and Blendon, eds., 1979, pp. 24–38.

American Medical Association. *Critique and Comment on the Council on Wage and Price Stability's Staff Report*. Chicago: American Medical Association, 1978.

Anderson, Odin W. *Health Care: Can There Be Equity? The U.S., Sweden, and England*. New York: John Wiley & Sons, 1972.

————. "PSROs, the Medical Profession, and the Public Interest." *Milbank Memorial Fund Quarterly* 54, no. 3 (Summer 1976): 379–88.

Andersen, Ronald; Kravits, Joanna; and Anderson, Odin W., eds. *Equity in Health Services: Empirical Analyses in Social Policy*. Cambridge, Mass.: Ballinger, 1975.

Andrews, William D. "Personal Deductions in an Ideal Income Tax." *Harvard Law Review* 86, no. 2 (December 1972): 309–85.

Annas, George J. "Allocation of Artificial Hearts in the Year 2002: *Minerva v. National Health Agency*." *American Journal of Law and Medicine* 3, no. 1 (Spring 1977): 59–76.

————. "The Courts and Philip Becker." *Hastings Center Report* 9, no. 6 (December 1979): 18–20.

Anscombe, G. E. M. "Who Is Wronged?" *Oxford Review* 5 (1967): 16–17.

Arras, John D. "Health Care Vouchers for the Poor." *Hastings Center Report* 11, no. 4 (August 1981): 29–39.

Arrow, Kenneth J. "Uncertainty and the Welfare Economics of Medical Care." *The American Economic Review* 53, no. 5 (December 1963): 941–69.

————. "The Economics of Moral Hazard: Further Comment." *The American Economic Review* 58, no. 3 (June 1968): 537–39.

————. "Some Ordinalist-Utilitarian Notes on Rawls' Theory of Justice." *Journal of Philosophy* 70, no. 9 (1973): 245–63.

Arthur, John, and Shaw, William H., eds. *Justice and Economic Distribution*. Englewood Cliffs, N.J.: Prentice-Hall, 1978.

Atkinson, Anthony B. *The Economics of Inequality*. Oxford: Clarendon Press, 1975.

————, ed. *The Personal Distribution of Incomes*. London: Allen & Unwin, 1976.

Bailey, Martin J. *Reducing Risks to Life: Measurement of the Benefits*. Washington, D.C.: American Enterprise Institute, 1980.

Baker, C. Edwin. "The Ideology of the Economic Analysis of Law." *Philosophy and Public Affairs* 5, no. 1 (Fall 1975): 3–48.

Ball, Robert M. "Response" (to Schelling, 1976). In Perpich, ed., 1976, pp. 39–44.

————. "National Health Insurance: Comments on Selected Issues." *Science* 200, no. 4344 (26 May 1978): 864–70.

Barker, Karlyn. " 'I Was Just Infuriated.' " *Washington Post*, 16 May 1980, pp. A-1, A-37.

Basson, Marc D. "Choosing among Candidates for Scarce Medical Resources." *Journal of Medicine and Philosophy* 4, no. 3 (September 1979): 313–33.

Bayles, Michael D. "National Health Insurance and Noncovered Services." *Journal of Health Politics, Policy, and Law* 2, no. 3 (Fall 1977): 335–48.

————. "The Price of Life." *Ethics* 89, no. 1 (October 1978): 20–34.

Beauchamp, Dan E. "Public Health as Social Justice." *Inquiry* 13, no. 1 (March 1976): 3–14.

Beauchamp, Tom L. "The Regulation of Hazards and Hazardous Behaviors." *Health Education Monographs* 6, no. 2 (Summer 1978): 242–57.

Beauchamp, Tom L., and Childress, James F. *Principles of Biomedical Ethics* New York: Oxford University Press, 1979.

Beauchamp, Tom L., and Faden, Ruth R. "The Right to Health and the Right to Health Care." *Journal of Medicine and Philosophy* 4, no. 2 (June 1979): 118–31.

Beck, R. G. "The Effects of Co-payment on the Poor." *Journal of Human Resources* 9, no. 1 (Winter 1974): 129–42.

Becker, Gary S. *Human Capital.* New York: National Bureau of Economic Research, 1964.

————. *Human Capital and the Personal Distribution of Income: An Analytical Approach.* Ann Arbor: Institute of Public Administration, University of Michigan, 1967.

Bell, Nora K. "The Scarcity of Medical Resources: Are There Rights to Health Care?" *Journal of Medicine and Philosophy* 4, no. 2 (June 1979): 159–69.

Benham, L.; Maurizi, A.; and Reder, M. W. "Migration, Location, and Remuneration of Medical Personnel: Physicians and Dentists." *The Review of Economics and Statistics* 50, no. 3 (August 1968): 332–47.

Bishop, Jerry E. "Soaring Medical Costs and the Mayo 'Epidemic.' " *Wall Street Journal,* 26 February 1980.

Blackstone, Erwin A. "Market Power and Resource Misallocation in Medicine: The Case of Neurosurgery," *Journal of Health Politics, Policy, and Law* 3, no. 3 (Fall 1978): 345–63.

Bloom, Barry R. "Health Research and Developing Nations." *Hastings Center Report* 6, no. 6 (December 1976): 9–12.

Blumberg, Mark S. "Health Status and Health Care Use by Type of Private Health Coverage." *Milbank Memorial Fund Quarterly* 58, no. 4 (Fall 1980): 633–55.

Blumstein, James F. "Constitutional Perspectives on Governmental Decisions Affecting Human Life and Health." *Law and Contemporary Problems* 40, no. 4 (Autumn 1976): 230–305.

Blumstein, James F., and Zubkoff, Michael. "Perspectives on Government Policy in the Health Sector." *Milbank Memorial Fund Quarterly* 51, no. 3 (Summer 1973): 395–431.

Bok, Sissela. "The Ethics of Giving Placebos." *Scientific American* 231, no. 5 (November 1974): 17–23.

Brandt, Richard B. *A Theory of the Good and the Right.* New York: Oxford University Press, 1979.

Branson, Roy, et al. "The Quinlan Decision: Five Commentaries." *Hastings Center Report* 6, no. 1 (February 1976): 8–19.

Braybrooke, David. "Let Needs Diminish That Preferences May Prosper." *Stud-*

ies in Moral Philosophy American Philosophical Quarterly Monograph Series, no. 1. Oxford: Blackwells, 1968.

Brock, Daniel. "Distribution of Health Care and Individual Liberty." Prepared for the President's Commission for the Study of Ethical Problems in Medicine and Biomedical and Behavioral Research, Washington, D.C., 1982, photocopy.

Brody, Howard. "On Placebos." *Hastings Center Report* 5, no. 2 (April 1975): 17–18.

———. *Placebos and the Philosophy of Medicine.* Chicago: University of Chicago Press, 1977.

Bromberg, Robert S. "Financing Health Care and the Effect of the Tax Law." *Law and Contemporary Problems* 39, no. 4 (Autumn 1975): 156–82.

Broome, John. "Trying to Value a Life." *Journal of Public Economics* 9, no. 1 (February 1978): 91–100.

Brown, E. Richard. *Rockefeller Medicine Men: Medicine and Capitalism in America.* Berkeley and Los Angeles: University of California Press, 1979.

Brown, Leo E., and Ellis, Effie O., eds. *Quality of Life. Vol. 3: The Later Years.* Acton, Mass.: Publishing Sciences Group, Inc., 1975.

Brown, Peter G.; Johnson, Conrad; and Vernier, Paul, eds. *Income Support: Conceptual and Policy Issues.* Totowa, N.J.: Rowman & Littlefield, 1981.

Buchanan, Allen. "The Right to a 'Decent Minimum' of Health Care." Prepared for the President's Commission for the Study of Ethical Problems in Medicine and Biomedical and Behavioral Research, Washington, D.C., 1982, photocopy.

Bunker, John P.; Barnes, Benjamin A.; and Mosteller, Frederick, eds. *Costs, Risks, and Benefits of Surgery.* New York: Oxford University Press, 1977.

Butler, Stuart M. "The Competitive Prescription for Health Costs Inflation." *Backgrounder* (The Heritage Foundation) 111 (25 February 1980).

Cahill, George F., Jr.; Gurin, Joel; and Wechsler, Henry, eds. *The Horizons of Health.* Cambridge: Harvard University Press, 1977.

Calabresi, Guido. "The Decision for Accidents: An Approach to Nonfault Allocation of Costs." *Harvard Law Review* 78 (1965): 713ff.

Calabresi, Guido, and Bobbitt, Philip. *Tragic Choices.* New York: W. W. Norton, 1979.

Callahan, Daniel. "On Defining a 'Natural Death.'" *Hastings Center Report* 7, no. 3 (June 1977): 32–37.

Callahan, Daniel, and Engelhardt, H. Tristram, Jr., eds. *Knowing and Valuing: The Search for Common Roots.* Hastings-on-Hudson, N.Y.: The Hastings Center, 1980.

Cannan, E. *Wealth.* London: Staples, 1914.

Carlson, Rick J. *The End of Medicine.* New York: John Wiley, 1975.

Cazort, Ralph J. "Another View: We Need Quality and Equality." (A reply to Gerber, 1975.) *Prism,* October 1975, pp. 22–23.

Chase, Samuel B., Jr., ed. *Problems in Public Expenditure Analysis.* Washington, D.C.: The Brookings Institution, 1968.

Childress, James F. "Who Shall Live When Not All Can Live?" *Soundings* 43, no. 4 (Winter 1970): 339–62. Also in Veatch and Branson, 1976, pp. 199–212.

―――. "A Right to Health Care?" *Journal of Medicine and Philosophy* 4, no. 2 (June 1979): 132–47.

―――. "Priorities in the Allocation of Health Care Resources." In Mappes and Zembaty, eds., 1981, pp. 561–68. Or see the original and longer version in *Soundings* 62 (Fall 1979).

Christianson, Jon B., and McClure, Walter. "Competition in the Delivery of Medical Care." *New England Journal of Medicine* 301, no. 15 (11 October 1979): 812–18.

Coburn, Robert C. "Imposing Risks." *Pacific Philosophical Quarterly* (August 1981).

Cochrane, A. L. *Effectiveness and Efficiency: Random Reflections on Health Services.* London: Nuffield Provincial Hospitals Trust, 1972.

Cohen, Carl. "The Justification of Democracy." *The Monist* 55, no. 1 (January 1971): 1–28.

―――. "Medical Experimentation on Prisoners." *Perspectives in Biology and Medicine* 21 (Spring 1978): 357–72.

Cohen, William J., and Friedman, Milton. *Social Security: Universal or Selective?* Washington, D.C.: American Enterprise Institute, 1972.

Conley, Bryan C. "The Value of Human Life in the Demand for Safety." *The American Economic Review* 66, no. 2 (March 1976): 45–55.

Conley, Bryan C.; Cook, Philip J.; and Jones-Lee, M. W. "The Value of Human Life in the Demand for Safety: Comment, Extension, and Reply." *The American Economic Review* 68, no. 4 (September 1978): 710–20.

Cooper, Barbara S., and Gaus, Clifton R. "Controlling Health Technology." In Altman and Blendon, eds., 1979, pp. 242–52.

Cooper, Barbara S., and Rice, Dorothy P. "The Economic Value of Human Life." *American Journal of Public Health* 57, no. 11 (November 1967): 1954–56. Also in Rhoads, ed., 1980, pp. 19–36.

―――. "The Economic Cost of Illness Revisited." *Social Security Bulletin* 39, no. 2 (February 1976): 21–36.

Cullis, John G., and West, Peter A. *The Economics of Health: An Introduction.* Oxford: Martin Robertson, 1979.

Cummings, Nicholas A. "The Anatomy of Psychotherapy under National Health Insurance." *American Psychologist* 32, no. 9 (September 1977): 711–18.

Daniels, Norman. "Rights to Health Care and Distributive Justice: Programatic Worries." *Journal of Medicine and Philosophy* 4, no. 2 (June 1979): 174–91.

―――. "Health-Care Needs and Distributive Justice." *Philosophy and Public Affairs* 10, no. 2 (Spring 1981): 146–79.

―――. "Am I My Parents' Keeper?" *Midwest Studies in Philosophy*, vol. 7 (1982). Special issue on social and political philosophy.

―――. ed. *Reading Rawls: Critical Studies in "A Theory of Justice."* New York: Basic Books, 1974.

Delbanco, Thomas L.; Meyers, Katherine C.; and Segal, Elliot A. "Paying the Physician's Fee: Blue Shield and the Reasonable Charge." *New England Journal of Medicine* 301, no. 24 (13 December 1979): 1314–20.

Diamond, Eugene F. *This Curette for Hire.* Chicago: ACTA Foundation, 1977.

Dickerson, O. D. *Health Insurance.* Rev. ed. Homewood, Ill.: Irwin, 1963.

Donabedian, Avedis. "The Quality of Medical Care." *Science* 200, no. 4344 (26 May 1978): 856–64.

Dworkin, Ronald. "The Original Position." In Daniels, ed., 1974, pp. 16–53.

———. *Taking Rights Seriously.* Cambridge: Harvard University Press, 1977.

———. "Liberalism." In Hampshire et al., 1978, pp. 114–43.

Dyckman, Zachary Y., and U.S. Council on Wage and Price Stability. *A Study of Physicians' Fees: Staff Report.* Washington, D.C.: Government Printing Office, 1978.

Ehrlich, Isaac, and Becker, Gary S. "Market Insurance, Self-Insurance, and Self-Protection." *Journal of Political Economy* 80, no. 4 (July–August 1972): 623–48.

Eisenberg, John M., and Rosoff, Arnold J. "Physician Responsibility for the Cost of Unnecessary Medical Services." *New England Journal of Medicine* 299, no. 2 (13 July 1978): 76–80.

Eliot, George. *Middlemarch.* 1872. New York: New American Library, 1964.

Emery, Julie. "Oversupply Pressures Beginning to Affect U.S. Medical Schools." *Seattle Times*, 28 May 1981, p. B–2.

Engelhardt, H. Tristram, Jr. "Case Studies in Bioethics: A Demand to Die." *Hastings Center Report* 5, no. 3 (June 1975): 10–11.

———. "Autonomy: The Blessings and Banes of Living Freely." Washington, D.C.: The Kennedy Institute, 1980, photocopy (a).

———. "Doctoring the Disease, Treating the Complaint, Helping the Patient: Some of the Works of Hygeia and Panacea." In Callahan and Engelhardt, eds., 1980, pp. 225–49 (b).

Enthoven, Alain C. "Consumer Choice Health Plan." *New England Journal of Medicine* 298, 12 (March 23, 1978): 650–658 and 298:13 (March 30, 1978): 709–20 (a).

———. "Cutting Costs without Cutting the Quality of Care." *New England Journal of Medicine* 298, no. 22 (1 June 1978): 1229–38 (b).

———. "Health Care Costs." *National Journal*, 26 May 1979, pp. 885–89. Also in U.S. Senate, 1979b, pp. 285–89 (a).

———. "Incentives and Innovation in Health Services Organization." In U.S. Senate, 1979b, pp. 264–84 (b).

———. *Health Plan: The Only Practical Solution to the Soaring Cost of Medical Care.* Reading, Mass.: Addison-Wesley, 1980.

Enthoven, Alain, and Noll, Roger. "Regulatory and Nonregulatory Strategies for Controlling Health Care Costs." In Altman and Blendon, 1979, pp. 213–34.

Evans, Robert G. "Supplier-induced Demand: Some Empirical Evidence and Implications." In Perlman, ed., 1974, pp. 162–73.

Ezorsky, Gertrude. "How Many Lives Shall We Save?" *Metaphilosophy* 3, no. 2 (April 1972): 156–62.

Fain, Tyrus; Plant, Katherine C.; and Milloy, Ross, eds. *National Health Insurance: Public Documents Series*. New York: R. R. Bowker, 1977.

Fein, Rashi. "The Economics of Health Research." In Cahill et al., 1977, pp. 369–79.

Fein, Rashi, and Weber, G. I. *Financing Medical Education: An Analysis of Alternative Policies and Mechanisms*. New York: Carnegie Commission on Higher Education and the Commonwealth Fund, 1971.

Feldstein, Martin S. "The Rising Price of Physicians' Services." *Review of Economics and Statistics* 2 (May 1970): 121–33.

———. "A New Approach to National Health Insurance." *The Public Interest*, Spring 1971, pp. 93–104. Also in Lindsay, 1976, pp. 241–56.

———. "The Welfare Loss of Excess Health Insurance." *Journal of Political Economy* 81:2, pt. 1 (March–April 1973): 251–80.

———. "How Tax Laws Fuel Hospital Costs." *Prism*, January 1976, pp. 15–19.

Feldstein, Martin S., and Taylor, Amy. "The Rapid Rise of Hospital Costs." Harvard Institute of Economic Research, Discussion Paper no. 351, January 1977.

Fine, Max W. "The Case for National Health Insurance." *Current History* 73, no. 428 (July–August 1977): 13–16.

Fineberg, Harvey V. "Clinical Chemistries: The High Cost of Low-Cost Diagnostic Tests." In Altman and Blendon, 1979, pp. 144–65.

Fineberg, Harvey V., and Hiatt, Howard H. "Evaluation of Medical Practices: The Case for Technology Assessment." *New England Journal of Medicine* 301, no. 20 (15 November 1979): 1086–91.

Fitzpatrick, Garry; Neutra, Raymond; and Gilbert, John P. "Cost Effectiveness of Cholecystectomy for Silent Gallstones." In Bunker, Barnes, and Mosteller, 1977, pp. 246–61.

Fogarty International Center. *Priorities for the Use of Resources in Medicine*. Proceedings, no. 40. Washington, D.C.: Department of Health, Education, and Welfare (NIH-77-1288), 1977.

Frederickson, Donald S. "Health and the Search for New Knowledge." In Knowles, 1977, pp. 159–70.

Freedman, Benjamin. "The Case for Medical Care, Inefficient or Not." *Hastings Center Report* 7, no. 2 (April 1977): 31–39.

French, Francis D. "The Financial Indebtedness of Medical-School Graduates." *New England Journal of Medicine* 304, no. 10 (5 March 1981): 563–65.

Fried, Charles. "The Value of Life." *Harvard Law Review* 82, no. 7 (May 1969): 1415–37.

———. *An Anatomy of Values*. Cambridge: Harvard University Press, 1970.

———. "Rights and Health Care—Beyond Equity and Efficiency." *New England Journal of Medicine* 293, no. 5 (31 July 1975): 241–45.

———. "Equality and Rights in Medical Care." *Hastings Center Report* 6 (February 1976): 29–34.

————. *Right and Wrong.* Cambridge: Harvard University Press, 1978. Especially pp. 109–31.

Friedman, Milton. *Capitalism and Freedom.* Chicago: University of Chicago Press, 1962.

Friedman, Milton, and Kuznets, Simon. *Income from Independent Professional Practice.* New York: National Bureau of Economic Research (publication no. 45), 1954.

Friedson, Eliot. "Response" (to Petersdorf). In Perpich, ed., 1976, pp. 87–93.

Fromm, Gary. "Comment" (on Schelling, 1968). In Chase, ed., 1968, pp. 166–76.

Fuchs, Victor R. *Who Shall Live? Health, Economics and Social Choice.* New York: Basic Books, 1974.

————. "Economics, Health, and Post-industrial Society." *Milbank Memorial Fund Quarterly* 57, no. 2 (1979): 153–82.

————, ed. *Essays in the Economics of Health and Medical Care.* New York: National Bureau of Economic Research, 1972.

Fuchs, Victor R., and Newhouse, Joseph P. "The Conference and Unresolved Problems." *Journal of Human Resources* 13: Supplement (1978): 5–17.

Fuchs, Victor R.; Rand, Elizabeth; Garrett, Bonnie. "The Distribution of Earnings in Health and Other Industries." In Fuchs, ed., 1972, pp. 119–31.

Garratini, S. "Research for the Treatment of Economically 'Unrewarding' Diseases." *Biomedicine* 26 (1977): 162–63.

Gaus, C. R.; Cooper, B. S.; and Hirschman, C. G. "Contracts in HMO and Fee-for-Service Performance." *Social Security Bulletin* 29 (May 1975): 3–14.

Gauthier, David. "Unequal Need: A Problem of Equity in Access to Health Care." Prepared for the President's Commission for the Study of Ethical Problems in Medicine and Biomedical and Behavioral Research, Washington, D.C., 1982, photocopy.

Gerber, Alex. "Let's Forget about Equality of Care." *Prism,* October 1975, pp. 20–27.

Gibbard, Allan. "The Prospective Pareto Principle and Equity of Access to Health Care." *Milbank Memorial Fund Quarterly* 60 (1982): 399–428.

Gittelsohn, Alan M., and Wennberg, John E. "On the Incidence of Tonsillectomy and Other Common Surgical Procedures." In Bunker, Barnes, and Mosteller, 1977, pp. 91–106.

Glandon, Gerald L., and Werner, Jack L. "Physicians' Practice Experience during the Decade of the 1970's." *Journal of the American Medical Association.* 244, no. 22 (5 December 1980): 2514–18.

Glaser, William J. *Paying the Doctor: Systems of Remuneration and Their Effects.* Baltimore: Johns Hopkins University Press, 1970. Ann Arbor, Mich.: University Microfilms, 1978.

Glover, Jonathan. *Causing Death and Saving Lives.* New York: Penguin Books, 1977.

Godber, George. "Comment" (on address by Marc Lalonde). In Perpich, ed., 1976.

Goldberg, Lawrence G., and Greenberg, Warren. "The Effect of Physician-controlled Health Insurance: *U.S. v. Oregon State Medical Society.*" *Journal of Health Politics, Policy, and Law* 2, no. 1 (Spring 1977): 48–78.

Gori, Gio B., and Richter, Brian J. "Macroeconomics of Disease Prevention in the U.S." *Science* 200 (9 June 1978): 1124–30.

Gray, J. A. Muir. *Man against Disease: Preventive Medicine.* New York: Oxford University Press, 1979.

Green, Ronald M. "Health Care and Justice in Contract Theory Perspective." In Veatch and Branson, eds., 1976, pp. 111–26.

Greenberg, Daniel S. "Health Care Colossus." *Washington Post,* 18 December 1979, p. A-19.

———. "A Bonus for Empty Beds?" *Washington Post,* 15 January 1980, p. A-15 (a).

———. "Cost-Conscious Medicine." *Washington Post,* 25 March 1980, p. A-15 (b).

Greenwald, John. "Those Sky-High Health Costs." *Time,* 12 July 1982, pp. 54–55.

Griner, P. F. "Treatment of Acute Pulmonary Edema: Conventional or Intensive Care?" *Annals of Internal Medicine* 77 (1972): 501–06.

Grossman, Michael, and Colle, Ann D. "Determinants of Pediatric Care Utilization." *Journal of Human Resources* 13: Supplement (1978): 115–58.

Hall, Thomas D., and Lindsay, Cotton M. "Medical Schools: Producers of What? Sellers to Whom?" *Journal of Law and Economics.* 23:1 (April 1980): 55–80.

Hampshire, Stuart, ed. *Public and Private Morality.* Cambridge: Cambridge University Press, 1978.

Hapgood, Fred. "Risk-Benefit Analysis: Putting a Price on Life." In Rhoads, ed., 1980, pp. 313–24.

Hare, R. M. *The Language of Morals.* Oxford: Clarendon, 1952.

———. *Freedom and Reason.* Oxford: Clarendon, 1963.

Harris, John. "The Survival Lottery." *Philosophy* 50 (January 1975): 81–87.

The Hastings Center. "Values, Ethics, and CBA in Health Care." In Office of Technology Assessment, 1980, pp. 168–82.

Hastings Center Research Group. "Values and Life-extending Techniques." In Veatch, ed., 1979, pp. 29–79.

Havighurst, Clark C. "Regulation of Health Facilities and Services by 'Certificate of Need.'" *Virginia Law Review* 59 (1973): 1143–94.

———. "Separate Views on the Artificial Heart." In Veatch and Branson, eds., 1976, pp. 247–55.

———. "The Ethics of Cost Control in Medical Care." *Soundings* 60, no. 1 (Spring 1977): 22–39.

Havighurst, Clark C.; Blumstein, James F.; and Bovbjerg, Randall. "Strategies in Underwriting the Costs of Catastrophic Disease." *Law and Contemporary Problems* 40, no. 4 (Autumn 1976): 122–95.

Havighurst, Clark C., and Hackbarth, J. D. "Private Cost Containment." *New England Journal of Medicine* 300, no. 23 (7 June 1979): 1298–1305.

Hellegers, Andre E. "Reflections on Health Care and Its Possible Future." *The Kennedy Institute Quarterly Report* 5, no. 1 (Summer 1979): 1–6.

Helms, Jay; Newhouse, Joseph P.; and Phelps, Charles E. "Copayments and the Demand for Medical Care: The California Medicaid Experience." *Bell Journal of Economics* 9, no. 1 (Spring 1978).

Heysell, Robert M. "Controlling Health Technology: A Public Policy Dilemma." In Altman and Blendon, 1979, pp. 262–72.

Hoffman, Ronald, and Steuerle, Eugene. "Tax Expenditures for Health Care." *Office of Tax Analysis Papers*, no. 38, April 1979 (U.S. Department of the Treasury).

Hough, Douglas E., and Misek, Glen I., eds. *Socioeconomic Issues of Health, 1980.* Chicago: American Medical Association, 1980.

Illich, Ivan. *Medical Nemesis: The Expropriation of Health.* London: Calder & Boyars, 1975.

Ingelfinger, Franz J. "Haves and Have-Nots in the World of Disease." *New England Journal of Medicine* 287 (7 December 1972): 1198–99.

Jencks, Christopher. "Giving Parents Money for Schooling: Education Vouchers." *Phi Delta Kappan* 52, no. 1 (September 1970): 49–52.

Jensen, James E. "Rationale of the Medical Expense Deduction." *National Tax Journal* 7 (1954): 274–84.

Jensen, Lynn E. "The Social and Economic Milieu of Health Care Provision: Quality, Access, and Cost." A report of the AMA Center for Health Services Research and Development. *Journal of the American Medical Association* 241:13 (30 March 1979): 1345–47.

Jones-Lee, M. W. "The Value of Changes in the Probability of Death or Injury." *Journal of Political Economy* 82 (July–August 1974): 835–49.

———. *The Value of Life: An Economic Analysis.* Chicago: University of Chicago Press, 1976.

Jonsen, Albert R. "The Totally Implantable Artificial Heart." *Hastings Center Report* 3, no. 5 (November 1975): 1–4.

Joskow, Paul L., and Schwartz, William B. "Medical Efficiency Versus Economic Efficiency: A Conflict in Values." *New England Journal of Medicine* 299, no. 26 (28 December 1978): 1462–64.

Keller, Martin D. "Living with Pathology—The One-Horse Syndrome." In Brown and Ellis, 1975, pp. 65–70.

Kessel, Reuben A. "Price Discrimination in Medicine." *Journal of Law and Economics* 1 (1958): 20–53.

———. "The A.M.A. and the Supply of Physicians." *Law and Contemporary Problems* 35 (1970): 267ff.

Kingsdale, Jon M. "Marrying Regulatory and Competitive Approaches to Health Care Cost Containment." *Journal of Health Politics, Policy, and Law* 3, no. 1 (Spring 1978): 21–42.

Klarman, Herbert E. "Application of Cost-Benefit Analysis to the Health Services and the Special Case of Technologic Innovation." *International Journal of Health Services* 4, no. 2 (1974): 325–52.

———. "The Financing of Health Care." In Knowles, 1977, pp. 215–33.

———. "Observations on Health Care Technology: Measurement, Analysis, and Policy." In Altman and Blendon, 1979, pp. 273–91.

Knowles, John H., ed. *Doing Better and Feeling Worse: Health in the United States.* New York: W. W. Norton, 1977.

Korcok, Milan. "U.S. Physicians' Earnings." Part 1: "They Spend More but Still Keep More." Part 2: "Usual, Customary, and Reasonable." *Canadian Medical Association Journal* 120 (20 January and 3 February 1979): 187–89, 227, 378–82.

Kridel, Russell W. H., and Winston, Donald S., eds. *Cost-Effective Medical Care: A Guide on Cost Consciousness for Physicians in Training.* Chicago: American Medical Association, 1978.

Krizay, John, and Wilson, Andrew. *The Patient as Consumer: Health Care Financing in the U.S.* Lexington, Mass.: D. C. Heath, 1974.

LaFollette, Hugh. "Licensing Parents." *Philosophy and Public Affairs* 9, no. 2 (Winter 1980): 182–97.

Lally, John J. "Social Determinants of Differential Allocation of Resources to Disease Research: A Comparative Analysis of Crib Death and Cancer Research." *Journal of Health and Social Behavior* 18, no. 2 (June 1977): 125–38.

Lees, D. S. *Health through Choice.* Hobart Paper no. 14. London: Institute of Economic Affairs, 1961.

Leffler, Keith B. "Physician Licensure: Competition and Monopoly in American Medicine." *Journal of Law and Economics* 21, no. 1 (April 1978): 165–89.

———. "Doctors' Fees and Health Costs." *Rhode Island Medical Journal* 62, no. 7 (July 1979): 286–90.

Leiman, Sid Z. "The Ethics of Lottery." *The Kennedy Institute Quarterly Report* 4 (Summer 1978): 8–11.

Lembcke, P. A. "Measuring the Quality of Medical Care through Vital Statistics Based on Hospital Service Areas. Part I: Comparative Study of Appendectomy Rates." *American Journal of Public Health* 42 (1952): 276–86.

Lewis, Charles E.; Fein, Rashi; and Mechanic, David. *A Right to Health Care: The Problem of Access to Primary Medical Care.* New York: John Wiley, 1976.

Lindsay, Cotton M. "Real Returns to Medical Education." *Journal of Human Resources* 8, no. 3 (Summer 1973): 331–48.

———. "More Real Returns to Medical Education." *The Journal of Human Resources* 11, no. 1 (Winter 1976): 127–30.

———, ed. *New Directions in Public Health Care: An Evaluation of Proposals for National Health Insurance.* San Francisco: Institute for Contemporary Studies, 1976.

Lindsay, Cotton M., and Leffler, Keith B. "The Market for Medical Care." In Lindsay, ed., 1976, pp. 63–102.

Lomasky, Loren E. "Medical Progress and National Health Care." *Philosophy and Public Affairs* 10, no. 2 (Winter 1981): 65–88 (a).

———. "The Small but Crucial Role of Health Care Vouchers." *Hastings Center Report* 11, no. 4 (August 1981): 40–42 (b).

Luft, Harold S. *Poverty and Health: Economic Causes and Consequences of Health Problems.* Cambridge, Mass.: Ballinger, 1977.

———. "How Do Health Maintenance Organizations Achieve Their 'Savings'? Rhetoric and Evidence." *New England Journal of Medicine* 298, no. 24 (15 June 1978): 1336–43.

———. "Assessing the Evidence on HMO Performance." *Milbank Memorial Fund Quarterly* 58, no. 4 (Fall 1980): 501–36.

Luft, Harold S., and Frisvold, Gary A. "Decisionmaking in Regional Health Planning Agencies." *Journal of Health Politics, Policy, and Law* 4, no. 2 (Summer 1979): 250–72.

Macklin, Ruth. "Commentary" (on Smurl, 1980). *Man and Medicine* 5:2 (1980): 126–32.

McClure, Walter. "Choices for Medical Care." *Minnesota Medicine* 61, no. 4 (April 1978): 261–71.

McGinnis, J. Michael. "Trends in Disease Prevention: Assessing the Benefits of Prevention." *Bulletin of the New York Academy of Medicine* 56, no. 1 (January–February 1980): 38–44.

McKeown, Thomas. *Medicine in Modern Society.* London: Allen & Unwin, 1965.

———. *The Role of Medicine: Dream, Mirage, or Nemesis.* Princeton: Princeton University Press, 1980.

MacLeod, Gordon K. "The Hospital Bond Disaster." *Washington Post,* 8 January 1980.

Mappes, Thomas A., and Zembaty, Jane S., eds. *Biomedical Ethics.* New York: McGraw-Hill, 1981.

Marshall, John M. "Moral Hazard." *The American Economic Review* 66, no. 5 (December 1976): 880–90.

Masson, Robert T., and Wu, S. "Price Discrimination for Physicians' Services." *The Journal of Human Resources* 9, no. 1 (Winter 1974): 63–79.

Mather, H. G., et al. "Myocardial Infarction: A Comparison between Home and Hospital Care for Patients." *British Medical Journal* 1, no. 6015 (17 April 1976): 925–28.

Maynard, Alan. *Experiment with Choice in Education.* Hobart Paper no. 64. London: Institute of Economic Affairs, 1975.

Mennemeyer, Stephen T. "Really Great Returns to Medical Education?" *Journal of Human Resources* 13, no. 1 (Winter 1978): 75–89.

Menzel, Paul T. "Are Killing and Letting Die Morally Different in Medical Contexts?" *Journal of Medicine and Philosophy* 4, no. 3 (September 1979): 269–93.

Meyer, Jack A. *Health Care Cost Increases.* Washington, D.C.: American Enterprise Institute, 1979.

Milgram, Stanley. *Obedience to Authority.* New York: Harper & Row, 1973.

Mill, John Stuart. *On Liberty.* 1859. Reprint. New York: Appleton-Century-Crofts, 1947.

Mincer, Jacob. *Schooling, Experience, and Earnings.* New York: National Bureau of Economic Research, 1974.

————. "Progress in Human Capital Analyses of the Distribution of Earnings." In Atkinson, ed., 1976, pp. 136–92.

Mishan, E. J. "Evaluation of Life and Limb: A Theoretical Approach." *Journal of Political Economy* 79, no. 4 (1971): 687–706.

Mitchell, Bridger M., and Vogel, Ronald J. "Health and Taxes: An Assessment of the Medical Deduction." *Southern Economic Journal* 41, no. 4 (April 1975): 660–72.

Moloney, Thomas W., and Rogers, David E. "Medical Technology—A Different View of the Contentious Debate over Costs." *New England Journal of Medicine* 301, no. 26 (27 December 1979): 1413–19.

Montefiore, Alan, ed. *Philosophy and Personal Relations: An Anglo-French Study.* Montreal: McGill-Queens University Press, 1973.

Mooney, Gavin. *The Valuation of Human Life.* London: Macmillan, 1977.

Moore, Stephen. "Cost Containment through Risk Sharing by Primary-Care Physicians." *New England Journal of Medicine* 300, no. 24 (14 June 1979): 1359–62.

Morillo, Carolyn R. "As Sure as Shooting." *Philosophy* 51 (January 1976): 80–89.

Mosteller, Frederick. "Dilemmas in the Concept of Unnecessary Surgery." *Journal of Surgical Research* 25, no. 3 (September 1978): 185–92.

Mushkin, Selma J. *Biomedical Research: Costs and Benefits.* Cambridge, Mass.: Ballinger. 1979.

Mushkin, Selma J., ed. *Consumer Incentives for Health Care.* New York: Prodist, 1974.

Nagel, Thomas. "Equality." In Nagel, *Mortal Questions.* Cambridge: Cambridge University Press, 1979.

Nagin, Joshua G. F. "The Limits of Modern Medicine." *The Pharos,* October 1978, pp. 14–18.

Nagurney, John T.; Braham, Robert L.; and Reader, George G. "Physician Awareness of Economic Factors in Clinical Decision-making." *Medical Care* 17, no. 7 (July 1979): 727–36.

National Heart and Lung Institute. Artificial Heart Assessment Panel. "The Totally Implantable Artificial Heart: Economic, Ethical, Legal, Medical, Psychiatric, and Social Implications." In Veatch and Branson, eds., 1976, pp. 219–46.

Navarro, Vincente. *Medicine under Capitalism.* New York: Prodist, 1976.

Needleman, Lionel. "Valuing Other People's Lives." *The Manchester School of Economics and Social Studies* 44, no. 4 (December 1976): 309–42.

Neuhauser, Duncan, and Lewicki, Ann M. "What Do We Gain from the Sixth

Stool Guaiac?" *New England Journal of Medicine* 293, no. 5 (31 July 1975): 226–28.

———. "National Health Insurance and the Sixth Stool Guaiac." *Policy Analysis* 2, no. 2 (Spring 1976): 175–96.

Newhouse, Joseph P. "A Model of Physician Pricing." *Southern Economic Journal* 37, no. 2 (October 1970): 174–83.

———. "Allocation of Resources in Medical Care from an Economic Viewpoint." Santa Monica, Calif.: The Rand Corporation (P-5590), 1976 (a).

———. "Inflation and Health Insurance." In Zubkoff, ed., 1976, pp. 210–24 (b).

———. *The Economics of Medical Care: A Policy Perspective.* Reading, Mass.: Addison-Wesley, 1978.

Newhouse, Joseph P., and Phelps, Charles E. "New Estimates of Price and Income Elasticities of Medical Care Services." In Rosett, ed., 1976, pp. 261–320.

Newhouse, Joseph P.; Phelps, Charles E.; and Schwartz, William B. "Policy Options and the Impact of National Health Insurance." *New England Journal of Medicine* 290, no. 24 (13 June 1974): 1345–59.

Nozick, Robert. *Anarchy, State, and Utopia.* New York: Basic Books, 1974.

Office of Technology Assessment. U.S. Congress. *The Implications of Cost-Effectiveness Analysis of Medical Technology.* Washington, D.C.: Office of Technology Assessment, U.S. Congress, 1980.

Outka, Gene. "Social Justice and Equal Access to Health Care." *The Journal of Religious Ethics* 2 (Spring 1974): 11–32. Also in Veatch and Branson, eds., 1976, pp. 79–98.

Parfit, Derek. "Later Selves and Moral Principles." In Montefiore, ed., 1973, pp. 137–69.

———. "Innumerate Ethics." *Philosophy and Public Affairs* 7, no. 4 (Summer 1978): 285–301.

Pauker, Stephen G., and Kassirer, Jerome P. "Therapeutic Decision Making: A Cost-Benefit Analysis." *New England Journal of Medicine* 293, no. 5 (31 July 1975): 229–34.

Pauly, Mark V. "The Economics of Moral Hazard: Comment." *The American Economic Review* 58, no. 3 (June 1968): 531–37.

———. "Health Insurance and Hospital Behavior." In Lindsay, 1976, pp. 103–29.

Pellegrino, Edmund D. "Medical Morality and Medical Economics." *Hastings Center Report* 8, no. 4 (August 1978): 8–12.

Pellegrino, Edmund D., and Thomasma, David C. *A Philosophical Basis of Medical Practice: Toward a Philosophy and Ethic of the Healing Professions.* New York: Oxford University Press, 1981.

Perlman, Mark, ed. *The Economics of Health and Medical Care.* New York: John Wiley, 1974.

Perpich, Joseph G., ed. *Implications of Guaranteeing Medical Care.* Washington, D.C.: National Academy of Sciences, 1976.

Phelps, Charles F. "Demand for Health Insurance." Santa Monica, Calif.: The Rand Corporation, July 1973.

———. "Illness Prevention and Medical Insurance." *Journal of Human Resources* 13: Supplement (1978): 183–207.

Platt, Michael. "Commentary: On Asking to Die." *Hastings Center Report* 5, no. 6 (December 1975): 9–12.

Posner, Richard A. *Economic Analysis of Law.* 2d ed. Boston: Little, Brown & Company, 1972.

Randal, Judith. "Coronary Artery Bypass Surgery." *Hastings Center Report* 12, no. 1 (February 1982): 13–18.

Rawls, John. *A Theory of Justice.* Cambridge: Harvard University Press, 1971.

———. "Kantian Constructivism in Moral Theory." *The Journal of Philosophy* 78, no. 9 (September 1980): 515–72.

Rayack, Elton. *Professional Power and American Medicine: The Economics of the American Medical Association.* Cleveland: World Publishing Co., 1967.

———. "The Physicians' Service Industry." In Adams, ed., 1977, pp. 401–41.

Redisch, Michael A. "Physician Involvement in Hospital Decision Making." In Zubkoff, Raskin, and Hanft, eds., 1978, pp. 217–43.

Redisch, Michael A., et al. "Physician Pricing, Costs, and Income." Paper presented at Western Economic Association Meeting, Anaheim, Calif., 20 June 1977.

Rescher, Nicholas. "The Allocation of Exotic Medical Lifesaving Therapy." *Ethics* 79, no. 3 (April 1969): 173–86.

Rettig, Richard A. "The Policy Debate on Patient Care Financing for Victims of End-Stage Renal Disease." *Law and Contemporary Problems* 40, no. 4 (Autumn 1976): 196–230.

———. "End-Stage Renal Disease and the 'Cost' of Medical Technology." In Altman and Blendon, eds., 1979, pp. 88–115.

Rhoads, Steven E. "How Much Should We Spend to Save a Life?" *The Public Interest* 51 (Spring 1978): 74–92. Also in Rhoads, ed., 1980, pp. 285–312.

———, ed. *Valuing Life: Public Policy Dilemmas.* Boulder, Colo.: Westview Press, 1980.

Rice, Dorothy P. "Alternative Approaches to the Use of Medical Care Resources in the U.S." In Fogarty International Center, 1977, pp. 55–73.

———. Address presented at the annual meeting of the Institute of Medicine, Washington, D.C., October 1979.

Rice, Dorothy P., and Cooper, B. S. "The Economic Value of Human Life." *American Journal of Public Health* 57, no. 11 (November 1967): 1954–56. Also in Rhoads, ed., 1980, pp. 19–36.

Rich, Spencer. "Kidney Program Boon to Patients—and to Clinics." *Washington Post,* 26 May 1980, pp. A-1, A-2.

Roberts, Jennifer A. "Economic Evaluation of Health Care: A Survey." *British Journal of Preventive Social Medicine* 29 (1974): 210–16.

Roe, Benson B. "The UCR Boondoggle: A Death Knell for Private Practice." *New England Journal of Medicine* 305, no. 1 (2 July 1981): 41–45.

Roemer, Milton. "On Paying the Doctor and the Implications of Different Methods." *Journal of Health and Human Behavior* 3, no. 1 (Spring 1962): 6–7.

Rosett, Richard N., ed. *The Role of Health Insurance in the Health Services Sector.* New York: National Bureau of Economic Research, 1976.

Ruffin, Roy J., and Leigh, Duane E. "Charity, Competition, and the Pricing of Doctors' Services." *Journal of Human Resources* 8, no. 2 (Spring 1973): 212–22.

Rushefsky, Mark E. "A Critique of Market Reform in Health Care: The 'Consumer-Choice Health Plan.'" *Journal of Health Politics, Policy, and Law* 5, no. 4 (Winter 1981): 720–41.

Russell, Louise B. *Technology in Hospitals: Medical Advances and Their Diffusion.* Washington, D.C.: The Brookings Institution, 1979.

Rutstein, David. *Blueprint for Medical Care.* Cambridge: MIT Press, 1974.

Sagoff, Mark. "On Markets for Risk." Center for Philosophical and Public Policy, University of Maryland, December 1981, photocopy.

Sahoto, Gian Singh. "Theories of Personal Income Distribution: A Survey." *The Journal of Economic Literature* 16, no. 1 (March 1978): 1–55.

Salkever, David S., and Bice, Thomas W. "Certificate-of-Need Legislation and Hospital Costs." In Zubkoff, Raskin, and Hanft, eds., 1978, pp. 429–60.

Scanlon, Thomas M. "Preference and Urgency." *Journal of Philosophy* 72, no. 19 (6 November 1975): 655–69.

Schelling, Thomas C. "The Life You Save May Be Your Own." In Chase, ed., 1968, pp. 127–62.

———. "Medical Care Guarantees: Economics of Choice." In Perpich, ed., 1976, pp. 23–37.

———. "Standards for Adequate Minimum Personal Health Services." *Milbank Memorial Fund Quarterly* 57, no. 2 (Spring 1979): 212–33.

———. "Economic Reasoning and the Ethics of Policy." *The Public Interest* 63 (Spring 1981): 37–61.

Schroeder, Steven A., and Showstack, Jonathan A. "The Dynamics of Medical Technology Use: Analysis and Policy Options." In Altman and Blendon, eds., 1979, pp. 178–212.

Schwartz, Harry. "Conflicts of Interest in Fee-For-Service and in HMO's." *New England Journal of Medicine* 299, no. 19 (9 November 1978): 1071–73.

Schwartz, William B., et al. "Decision Analysis and Clinical Judgment." *American Journal of Medicine* 55, no. 4 (October 1973): 459–72.

Schweitzer, Stuart O. "Incentives and the Consumption of Health Care Services." In Mushkin, ed., 1974, pp. 34–60.

Scitovsky, Anne A., and Snyder, Nelda M. "Effect of Coinsurance on Use of Physician Services." *Social Security Bulletin* 35, no. 6 (June 1972): 3–19.

Seidman, Laurence S. "Hospital Inflation: A Diagnosis and Prescription." *Challenge,* July–August 1979, p. 18.

Self, Peter. *Econocrats and the Policy Process: The Politics and Philosophy of Cost-Benefit Analysis*. Boulder, Colo.: Westview Press, 1975.

Shaw, George Bernard. *The Doctor's Dilemma*. In *Collected Plays with Their Prefaces*. 1911. Reprint. London: The Bodley Head, 1971.

Sidel, Ruth, and Sidel, Victor W. *A Healthy State: An International Perspective on the Crisis in U.S. Medical Care*. New York: Pantheon, 1977.

Siegler, Mark. "A Right to Health Care: Ambiguity, Professional Responsibility, and Patient Liberty." *Journal of Medicine and Philosophy* 4, no. 2 (June 1979): 148–57.

Simmons, A. John. "The Principle of Fair Play." *Philosophy and Public Affairs* 8, no. 4 (Summer 1979): 307–37.

Simons, Henry. *Personal Income Taxation: The Definition of Income as a Problem of Fiscal Policy*. Chicago: University of Chicago Press, 1938.

Singer, Peter. *Democracy and Disobedience*. New York: Oxford University Press, 1974.

————. "Utility and the Survival Lottery." *Philosophy* 52 (1977): 218–22.

Skipper, J. K., et al. "Physicians' Knowledge of Costs: The Case of Diagnostic Tests." *Inquiry* 13 (June 1976): 194–98.

Sloan, Frank A. "Economic Models of Physician Supply." Ph.D. diss., Harvard University, 1968.

————. "Lifetime Earnings and Physicians' Choice of Specialty." *Industrial and Labor Relations Review* 24 (October 1970): 47–56.

————. "Real Returns to Medical Education: A Comment." *The Journal of Human Resources* 11, no. 1 (Winter 1976): 118–30.

Smurl, James F. "Distributing the Burden Fairly: Ethics and National Health Policy." *Man and Medicine* 5, no. 2 (1980): 97–125, 133–37.

Somers, Anne R., and Somers, Herman M. *Doctors, Patients, and Health Insurance*. Washington, D.C.: The Brookings Institution, 1961.

————. *Health and Health Care: Policies in Perspective*. Germantown, Md.: Aspen Systems Corporation, 1977.

Stason, William B., and Weinstein, Milton C. "Allocating Resources: The Case of Hypertension." *Hastings Center Report* 7, no. 5 (October 1977): 24–29.

————. *Hypertension: A Policy Perspective*. Cambridge: Harvard University Press, 1976.

Steinbock, Bonnie, ed. *Killing and Letting Die*. Englewood Cliffs, N.J.: Prentice-Hall, 1979.

Steiner, Hillel. "The Just Provision of Health Care: A Reply to Elizabeth Telfer." *Journal of Medical Ethics* 2, no. 4 (December 1976): 185–88. Response by Telfer, pp. 188–89.

Steinwald, Bruce, and Sloan, Frank A. "Determinations of Physicians' Fees." *The Journal of Business* 47, no. 4 (October 1974): 493–511.

Stell, Lance K. "Rawls on the Moral Importance of Natural Inequalities." *The Personalist* 59, no. 2 (April 1978): 206–15.

Stevens, William K. "Education Voucher Plan Making Slow Progress." *New York Times*, 2 July 1971.

Streeter, Deborah. "Ethical Issues in Human Reproduction Technologies: Analysis by Women." *The Bioethics Letter* 1, no. 2 (15 February 1980): 3–4.

Strickland, Stephen P. *Politics, Science, and Dread Disease: A Short History of U.S. Medical Research Policy.* Cambridge: Harvard University Press, 1972.

————. *Research and the Health of Americans: Improving the Policy Process.* Lexington, Mass.: D. C. Heath, 1978.

Sullivan, Ronald. "New York's Hospitals Will Gain by Filling Fewer Beds." *New York Times*, 31 December 1979, p. A-13.

Taurek, John M. "Should the Numbers Count?" *Philosophy and Public Affairs* 6, no. 4 (Summer 1977): 293–316.

Telfer, Elizabeth. "Justice, Welfare, and Health Care." *Journal of Medical Ethics* 2, no. 3 (September 1976): 107–11.

Terleckyj, Nestor E., ed. *Household Production and Consumption.* New York: National Bureau of Economic Research, 1976.

Thaler, Richard, and Rosen, Sherwin. "The Value of Saving a Life." In Terleckyj, ed., 1976.

Thomasma, David C. "An Apology for the Value of Human Lives." *Hospital Progress* 63, no. 3 (April 1982): 49ff. Reply by P. Menzel, May 1982.

Thurow, Lester C. "Government Expenditures: Cash or In-Kind Aid?" *Philosophy and Public Affairs* 5, no. 4 (Summer 1976): 361–81.

Trammell, Richard L. "Saving Life and Taking Life." *Journal of Philosophy* 72, no. 5 (13 March 1975), pp. 131–57.

Trammell, Richard L., and Wren, T. E. "Fairness, Utility and Survival." *Philosophy* 52 (1975): 331–37.

U.S. Department of Health, Education, and Welfare. *Health Research Principles, vol. 2: Documents Relating to the Development of Final Health Research Priorities for the DHEW.* Bethesda, Md.: National Institutes of Health (no. 80-2057), 1979.

U.S. Department of Labor. Bureau of Labor Statistics. *Occupational Outlook Handbook.* 1980–81 ed. Washington, D.C.: Government Printing Office, 1980.

U.S. Health Care Financing Administration. *Health Care Financing Trends* 3, no. 1 (June 1982).

U.S. Health Services Administration. Department of Health, Education, and Welfare. *Forward Plan for the Health Services Administration, F.Y. 1979–83.* Washington, D.C.: Government Printing Office, 1977.

U.S. House of Representatives. Committee on Interstate and Foreign Commerce. Subcommittee on Oversight and Investigations. *Reports on Cost and Quality of Health Care: Unnecessary Surgery.* 1976.

U.S. Public Health Service. Department of Health, Education, and Welfare. *Forward Plan for Health, 1977–81.* Washington, D.C.: Government Printing Office (DHEW Publication no. 05-76-50024), 1976.

U.S. Senate. Committee on Finance. "Summary of Senate Finance Committee Action on Health Legislation as of June 29, 1979." Washington, D.C.: Government Printing Office (CP 96-22), 1979 (a).

———. *Hearings: Presentation of Major Health Insurance Proposals.* 19 and 21 June 1979. Washington, D.C.: Government Printing Office, 1979 (b).

Vaupel, James W. "Early Death: An American Tragedy." *Law and Contemporary Problems* 40, no. 4 (Autumn 1976): 73–121.

Veatch, Robert M. "What Is a 'Just' Health Care Delivery?" In Veatch and Branson, 1976, pp. 127–53.

———. "Justice and Valuing Lives." In Veatch, ed., 1979c, pp. 197–224 (a).

———. "Just Social Institutions and the Right to Health Care." *Journal of Medicine and Philosophy* 4, no. 2 (June 1979): 170–73 (b).

———. "Voluntary Risks to Health: The Ethical Issues." *Journal of American Medical Association* 243, no. 1 (4 January 1980): 50–55.

———. *Theory of Medical Ethics.* New York: Basic Books, 1982.

———, ed. *Life Span: Values and Life-extending Technologies.* San Francisco: Harper & Row, 1979 (c).

Veatch, Robert M., and Branson, Roy, eds. *Ethics and Health Policy.* Cambridge, Mass.: Ballinger, 1976.

Viscusi, W. Kip. "Labor Market Valuations of Life and Limb: Empirical Evidence and Policy Implications." *Public Policy* 26, no. 3 (Summer 1978): 359–86.

Von Magnus, Eric. "Rights and Risks." Center for the Study of Values, University of Delaware, 1980, photocopy.

Walsh, Julia A., and Warren, Kenneth S. "Selective Primary Health Care: An Interim Strategy for Disease Control in Developing Countries." *New England Journal of Medicine* 301, no. 18 (1 November 1979): 967–74.

Walzer, Michael. "In Defense of Equality." *Dissent,* Fall 1973, pp. 399–408.

Ward, Richard A. *Economics of Health Resources.* Reading, Mass.: Addison-Wesley, 1975.

Warner, Kenneth E., and Luce, Bryan R. *Cost-Benefit and Cost-Effectiveness Analysis in Health Care: Principles, Practice, and Potential.* Ann Arbor: Health Administration Press, 1982.

Wasserstrom, Richard A., ed. *Morality and the Law.* Belmont, Calif.: Wadsworth, 1971.

Weale, Albert. *Equality and Social Policy.* London: Routledge & Kegan Paul, 1978.

———. "Statistical Lives and the Principle of Maximum Benefit." *Journal of Medical Ethics* 5, no. 4 (December 1979): 185–95.

Wehr, Elizabeth. "Victims of Rare Diseases Urging Approval of 'Orphan Drug' Bill." *Seattle Times,* 2 January 1983.

Weinstein, Milton; Shepard, Donald; and Pliskin, Joseph. "The Economic Value of Changing Mortality Probabilities: a Decision-Theoretic Approach." Discussion Paper no. 46D, Public Policy Program. Cambridge: Harvard University, November 1976.

Wennberg, John W. "Professional Uncertainty and National Priorities for the Use of Resources." In Fogarty International Center, 1977, pp. 301–18.

Westervelt, Frederic B. "The Selection Process as Viewed from Within: A Reply to Childress." In Veatch and Branson, 1976, pp. 213–18.

White, Robert B. "Case Studies in Bioethics: A Demand to Die." *Hastings Center Report* 5, no. 3 (June 1975): 9–10.

Wikler, Daniel I. "Coercive Measures in Health Promotion: Can They be Justified?" *Health Education Monographs* 6, no. 2 (Summer 1978): 223–41.

Wildavsky, Aaron. "Doing Better and Feeling Worse: The Political Pathology of Health Policy." In Knowles, 1977, pp. 105–23.

Will, George F. "The Case of Philip Becker." *Newsweek*, 14 April 1980, p. 112.

Willems, Jane S., et al. "The Computed Tomography (CT) Scanner." In Altman and Blendon, 1979, pp. 116–43.

Williams, Alan. "Measuring the Effectiveness of Health Care Systems." *British Journal of Preventive and Social Medicine* 28, no. 3 (August 1974), pp. 196–202.

Williams, A. P., et al. *Policy Analysis for Federal Biomedical Research.* Santa Monica, Calif.: The Rand Corporation (R-1945-PBRP/RC), 1976.

Wynder, E. L., and Hoffman, D. "Tobacco and Health: A Societal Challenge." *New England Journal of Medicine* 300, no. 16 (19 April 1979): 894–903.

Yondorf, Barbara. "The Declining and Wretched." *Public Policy* 23, no. 4 (Fall 1975): 465–82.

Zeckhauser, Richard. "Procedures for Valuing Lives." *Public Policy* 23, no. 4 (Fall 1975): 419–64.

Zeckhauser, Richard, and Shepard, Donald. "Where Now for Saving Lives?" *Law and Contemporary Problems* 40, no. 4 (Autumn 1976): 5–45.

Zimmerman, Roger. "Coercive Wage Offers." *Philosophy and Public Affairs* 10, no. 2 (Spring 1981): 121–45.

Zubkoff, Michael, ed. *Health: A Victim or Cause of Inflation?* New York: Prodist, 1976.

Zubkoff, Michael; Raskin, Ira E.; and Hanft, Ruth S., eds. *Hospital Cost Containment: Selected Notes for Future Policy.* New York: Prodist, 1978.

Index